Freeman Miller, MD
Co-Director, Cerebral Palsy Program
Alfred I. duPont Hospital for Children
Nemours Foundation
Wilmington, Delaware

Physical Therapy of Cerebral Palsy

With CD-ROM

Illustrations by Erin Browne, CMI

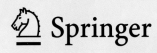
Springer

Freeman Miller, MD
Co-Director, Cerebral Palsy Program
Alfred I. duPont Hospital for Children
Nemours Foundation
Wilmington, DE 19899
USA

Library of Congress Control Number: 2006933715

ISBN-10: 0-387-38303-4   Printed on acid-free paper.
ISBN-13: 978-0-387-38303-3

9 8 7 6 5 4 3 2 1

springer.com

Physical Therapy of Cerebral Palsy

Preface

Cerebral palsy is a lifelong condition that affects the individual, family, and immediate community. Therefore, the goal of allowing the individual with cerebral palsy to live life with the least impact of the disability requires complex attention to the individual and the family. Furthermore, society needs to be sensitive and to accommodate individuals with disabilities by limiting architectural impediments and providing accessible public transportation and communication. The educational system provides the key means for helping the individual prepare to function in society to his or her maximum ability. In many ways, the medical care system probably has the least significant role in preparing the child with cerebral palsy to function optimally in society. However, the medical care system is the place where parents first learn that their child has developmental issues outside the expected norm. It is almost universally the place where parents also expect the child to be made normal in our modern society. In earlier times, the parents would expect healing to possibly come from the doctor, but also they would place hope for healing in religion. As this belief in spiritual or miraculous healing has decreased, a significant font of hope has decreased for parents of young children with disabilities.

The text aims to help the child with cerebral palsy to develop into an adult in whom the effects of the disability are managed so that they have the least impact possible on adult function. This intention is in the context of the fact that the magnitude of improvement in the disability that occurs with ideal management of the musculoskeletal system during growth may be only a small improvement. Probably the more significant aspect of good musculoskeletal management through childhood is helping the child and family to maintain realistic hope for the successful adult life of the growing child. This aim requires the medical practitioner to get to know the child and family and to communicate in a compassionate way realistic expectations of the child's function. For many reasons, the greatest difficulty in providing this kind of care is the limited time practitioners have to spend with the individual patient. There is also the sense, especially among orthopedic physicians, that cerebral palsy cannot be cured (cannot make the child function normally), and thus it is a frustrating condition with which to work. The physician must maintain a balance between communicating hopelessness to the patient and family; and feeling the need to do something, usually a heel cord lengthening, because the parents are frustrated that the child is not progressing. All medical decisions, including a surgical option, should always consider both the short- and long-term impact. With every decision the medical practitioner should ask, "What will be the impact of this recommendation by the time the child is a mature adult?" This is the most difficult perspective, especially for young practitioners with little experience. This text is intended to provide this insight as much as possible.

Another issue is the poor scientific documentation of natural history and treatment response in cerebral palsy, which has become clearer to me in the course of writing this book. With little scientifically based natural history and few long-term studies, much of what is written in this text is expert-based observation. The goal of writing this is not to say that it is absolute fact, but to provide the starting point of gathering information with the hope that others will be stimulated to ask questions and pursue research to prove or disprove the concepts.

The research, which is of help in treating children with cerebral palsy, needs to be planned and evaluated with consideration of its long-term impact on the child's growth and development. All treatment should also consider the negative impact on the child. As an example, a number of moderately good studies have analyzed the impact of wearing ankle orthotics on the young child. Although the orthotics may provide an immediate benefit by improving the child's gait, there is probably no long-term benefit. Thus, if the child develops a strong sense of opposition to wearing the brace at 10 years of age because of peer pressure, the brace wear cannot be justified on a cost–benefit analysis.

It is also important to consider the quality of the scientific evidence, ranging from double-blinded protocols to case reports, but it is equally important not to get hung up on this being the final answer. For example, excellent double-blinded studies show that botulinum toxin decreases spasticity and improves gait for a number of months. Therefore, these studies need to be considered in the context of our goal, which is to give the child the maximum possible function at full maturity. Because no evidence currently suggests that botulinum has either a negative or a positive effect on this long-term goal, the family and physician should decide together if botulinum injection has a positive cost–benefit ratio, as its effects will last only for approximately 6 months. In comparison, no double-blind studies show that Achilles tendon lengthenings improve gait three or six months after the surgery, and no such studies are needed because the goal of surgery is to make an improvement in gait several years later and to have improvement at maturity. Most important is that surgery create no disability at maturity. From this perspective, it would be much more useful to have a good controlled case series with a 15-year follow-up than a double-blinded study with six months follow-up.

This book should stimulate research that will improve the knowledge base which is focused on the long-term outcome of treatments. However, just because the scientific knowledge base is poor does not mean that we should not apply the best knowledge available to current patients. In addition to research, an individual professional can best extend his or her knowledge base through personal experience. This means that the child and family should be followed over time by the same practitioner with good documentation. By far, my best source of information has been the children whom I have followed for 10 to 20 years with videotapes every year or two. Practitioner experience is extremely important for augmenting the relatively poor scientific knowledge base for musculoskeletal treatment. Careful ongoing follow-up is also crucial to providing hope for the families and the individuals with cerebral palsy.

How to Use This CD

The CD included with this text is opened with a Web browser. Because the data on the CD is coded with XML and JAVA, only browsers released after

2002, such as Netscape 7.0, Explorer 6.0 or Safari, will be fully able to access this data. Some of the text in the book is organized in topics and is displayed in the section entitled "Main." All references on the CD have the abstract available on the CD by activating the link associated with the reference. Cases can also be activated from these references in the Main section. There is also a section called "Cases," which lists all the cases by name as listed in the text of the book. Following these cases are short quiz questions, which can be used to test understanding or study the material on line. There is also a section called "Quizzes," which lists the quizzes by name of the cases. These quizzes can be opened and answered referring to the full case descriptions. The answers from the quizzes will be tabulated to keep a running total of correct answers for each session. After a quiz is accessed, it will also change color to remind the reader that he has already reviewed that quiz. The section entitled "Decision Trees" is the treatment algorithms, which are present at the end of each chapter in the book. These decision trees are set up so that area of interest is linked to the text in "Main" for further reading. The section called "Search" is an electronic index to search for specific subjects with in the chapter of the section "Main." Because of space limitations, only individual chapters can be searched at one time. So if you want to search for "crutches," you first should activate the Durable Medical Goods chapter, and then search. The results of the search allow you to directly link to the area of interest. The section "History" keeps a running history of the areas that have been assessed, so if you want to return to an area you were reading earlier in the session you can open the history and it will allow you to return to that area. The section "About" includes information on the use of the CD and acknowledgments.

In summary, the CD includes videos, case study quizzes, and reference abstracts, which are not inclnded in the book. The book includes significant portions of text not included on the CD, sections on rehabilitation techniques, and a surgical atlas. The book and the CD are intended to complement each other but each can also be used alone.

Acknowledgments

The production of this book and CD was only possible because of an extensive network of support that was available to me. The support of the administration of the Nemours Foundation, especially the support of Roy Proujansky and J. Richard Bowen in giving me time to work on this project was crucial. It was only through the generous support in caring for my patients by my partners and staff, Kirk Dabney, Suken Shah, Peter Gabos, Linda Duffy, and Marilyn Boos, that I was able to dedicate time to writing. I am very grateful for the generous material provided by all the contributors and for the extensive and extremely important role of the feedback given to me by the consultants. In spite of having an extremely busy practice, Kirk Dabney still found time to read all of the Book. With his wide experience, Michael Alexander made an excellent contribution in the editorial support of the section on rehabilitation. The task of writing and editing would have been impossible without the dedicated work of Kim Eissmann, Linda Donahue, and Lois Miller. Production of the CD involved a significant amount of detailed editing and HTML coding, most of which was performed by Linda Donahue. To add a personal touch to the cases, a unique name was assigned by Lois Miller. The CD required a great effort of technical programming to make it work intuitively on all computer formats. Tim Niiler patiently persisted with this frustrating task until it all worked. Videos were masked and formatted by Robert DiLorio. Production of the graphics was a major effort in understanding the complex material in which Erin Browne excelled. This production would have been impossible without her dedication to understanding the concepts and bringing them to visual clarity. Thanks to Sarah West for modeling for the graphics. I would also like to thank the staff of Chernow Editorial Services, especially Barbara Chernow. Without the long support through out the evolution of this book by Robert Albano and his staff at Springer, this project would also have been much more difficult. And finally, I am most grateful for the many families and children who have allowed me to learn from them what it is like to live with the many different levels of motor impairments. It is to the families and children that I dedicate this work in the hope that it will lead to improved care and understanding by medical professionals.

Freeman Miller, MD

Contents

Contributors

Associate Editors

Kirk Dabney, MD
Michael Alexander, MD

Contributors

Mary Bolton, PT
Kristin Capone, PT, MEd
Diane Damiano, PhD
Jesse Hanlon, BS, COTA
Mozghan Hines, LPTA
Diana Hoopes, PT
Elizabeth Jeanson, PT
Marilyn Marnie King, OTR/L
Deborah Kiser, MS, PT
Liz Koczur, MPT
Maura McManus, MD, FAAPMR, FAAP
Betsy Mullan, PT, PCS

Denise Peischl, BSE
Beth Rolph, MPT
Adam J. Rush, MD
Carrie Strine, OTR/L
Stacey Travis, MPT

Consultants

Steven Bachrach, MD
John Henley, PhD
Douglas Heusengua, PT
Harry Lawall, CPO
Stephan T. Lawless, MD
Gary Michalowski, C-PED
Edward Moran, CPO
Susan Pressley, MSW
James Richards, PhD
Mary Thoreau, MD
Rhonda Walter, MD

SECTION I

Cerebral Palsy Management

1

The Child, the Parent, and the Goal

Cerebral palsy (CP) is a childhood condition in which there is a motor disability (palsy) caused by a static, nonprogressive lesion in the brain (cerebral). The causative event has to occur in early childhood, usually defined as less than 2 years of age. Children with CP have a condition that is stable and non-progressive; therefore, they are in most ways normal children with special needs. Understanding the medical and anatomic problems in individuals with CP is important; however, always keeping in mind the greater long-term goal, which is similar to that for all normal children, is important as well. The goal for these children, their families, medical care, education, and society at large is for them to grow and develop to their maximum capabilities so that they may succeed as contributing members of society. This goal is especially important to keep in perspective during the more anatomically detailed concerns discussed in the remainder of this text.

How Different Is the Child with CP?

When addressing each of the specific anatomic concerns, the significance of these anatomic problems relative to the whole child's success needs to be kept in the proper context. The problems of children with CP should be evaluated in the perspective of normal growth and development similar to any normal children with an illness, such as an ear infection, who need medical treatment. However, keeping the specific problems of children with CP in the proper context is not always easy. The significance of this proper context is somewhat similar to the significance of having a child do spelling homework on Wednesday evening to pass a spelling examination on Thursday. Likewise, practicing the piano is necessary to succeed in the piano recital. Even though each of these acts is important toward the final goal of having a confident, educated, and self-directed young adult who is making a contribution in society, the exact outcome of each event may not be all that important in the overall goal. Often, the success of a minor goal such as doing well on a specific test is less important than a major failure, but the measure of failure or success may be hard to recognize until years later. As with many childhood events, the long-term effect may be determined more by how the event was handled than by the specific outcome of the event.

For children with CP, in addition to all the typical childhood experiences is the experience of their CP treatment. Different children may experience events, such as surgery and ongoing treatment (including physical and occupational therapy), very differently. The long-term impact of these events from the children's perspectives is often either negative or positive, depending on their relationship with both therapists and physicians. These children have physical problems, which are the major focus of this text; however, CP affects the whole family and community. These relationships and how the CP affects families and communities are discussed in greater detail in this chapter.

The process of growing and developing involves many factors. One of the most important factors in children's long-term success is a family caretaker. Likewise, for children with CP, families may be impacted by the CP as much as the children with the physical problems. It is very important for medical care providers to see the problems related to CP as not only involving the children, but also involving the families. Society is realizing more that the education of normal children works best when the family care providers actively participate. Likewise, providing medical care for children with CP must consider their whole families. The outcome for these children will be determined largely by their families, just as the success of normal children's education is determined by their families. The importance of family does not provide an excuse for medical care providers or educators to become pessimistic if they do not perceive the family is doing its part. In this circumstance, professional care providers still must give as much as possible to each child but recognize their place and limits in the care of these children. Medical care providers who fail to recognize their own limits in the ability to provide care often will become overwhelmed by their sense of failure and will burn out quickly.

Family Impacts of the Child with CP

A healthy liaison should be developed between children with CP, the family unit, and the medical care providers. Cerebral palsy is a condition that varies extremely from very mild motor effects to very severe motor disabilities with many comorbidities. In addition, there are great variations among families. To provide proper care for children with CP, physicians need to have some understanding of the family structure in which the children are living. Because of time pressures, this insight is often difficult to develop. Families vary from young, teenage mothers who may have the support of their families, to single parent families, to families with two wage earners and other children. All the pressures of caring for a child with a disability are added onto the other pressures that families of normal children have. Because most children with CP develop problems in infancy and early childhood, families grow and develop within the context of these disabilities.

Often, the father and mother will react differently or come to different levels of acceptance. It is our impression that these different reactions may cause marital stress leading to high levels of divorce, most frequently when the children are 1 to 4 years old. Although this is our impression, there is no clear objective evidence that the divorce rate for these families is higher than in the normal population. Another high time of family stress is during the teenage or young adult years for those individuals with severe motor disabilities. Often, as these individuals are growing to full adult size and the parents are aging, it becomes very apparent to the parents that this is not a problem that is going away, nor are these young individuals capable of going off to college and making a life of their own.

The response of an individual family varies greatly with the wide variability of severity of CP. Many families develop a stable and very supportive structure for their disabled child. Physicians and other medical care providers may be amazed at how well these families deal with very complex medical problems. For many of these families, however, the medical complexities have accumulated slowly and are themselves a part of the growth and development phenomena. With multiple medical treatments often provided by many different medical specialists, a high level of stress develops in almost every family.

For the medical professional, continuing to be aware of this stress and listening for it during contact with families is important. Families with less education and limited financial resources may do remarkably well, whereas a family with more education and more financial resources may not be able to cope with the stresses of a child with a severe disability. It is extremely difficult to judge which family can manage and which family will develop difficulty, so it is important not to become prejudiced either for or against specific families. Medical care providers should continue to be sensitive to how the family unit is managing to deal with their stresses. Some families will be seen to be doing well and then suddenly will become overwhelmed in the face of other family stress. This stress may be illness in other family members, financial pressures, job changes, marital stress, and, most commonly, the effects of aging on the parents, siblings, and individuals with CP.

Care-Providing Community

Children with CP develop in supporting communities, which vary with each individual child. There are four general segments of these caring communities, with the family or direct caregivers being the primary relationship. This primary relationship is surrounded by community support services, the medical care system, and the educational system (Figure 1.1). The community support includes many options such as church, Scouting, camping,

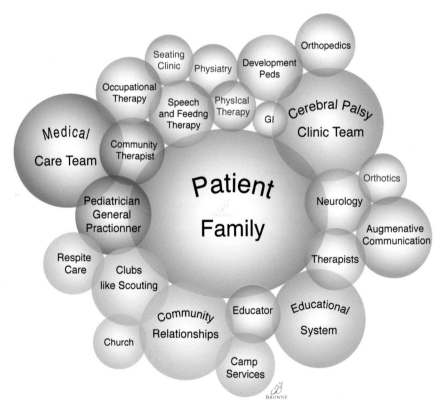

Figure 1.1. A large and extensive care team surrounds the family with a child who has cerebral palsy. These care providers are roughly organized around the educational system, primary medical care provider, the cerebral palsy specialized medical team, and community support services. Significant overlap and good communication provide the best resources to the child and the family.

respite services, and recreational programs. The educational system includes both educational professionals and therapeutic professionals, especially physical and occupational therapists. The focus of this text is to address the medical issues, so there will be no specific discussion of these support services, except to remind medical professionals that other services provide crucial roles in the lives of children and their families. The organization of the medical care system tends to organize around the general medical care and the specialty care for the problems specific to CP.

It is very important for families to have an established general medical care provider, either a pediatrician or family practice physician. Families must be encouraged to maintain regular follow-up with a primary care physician because very few orthopaedists or other specialists have the training or time to provide the full general medical care needs of these children. Standard immunizations and well child care examinations especially will be overlooked. However, most families see their child's most apparent problem as the visible motor disability and will focus more medical attention on this disability at the risk of overlooking routine well child care. The physician managing the motor disability should remind parents of the importance of well child care by inquiring if the child has had a routine physical examination and up-to-date immunizations. A physical or occupational therapist will provide most of the medical professional special care needs related to the CP. The specialty medical care needs are provided in a specialty clinic, usually associated with a children's hospital.

Cerebral Palsy Clinic

Another way to organize the management of these well child care needs is with a multidisciplinary clinic in which a primary care pediatrician is present. The administrative structure for setting up a clinic to care for children with CP is not as well defined as it is for diseases such as spina bifida. Spina bifida, meningomyelocele, or spinal dysfunction clinics are all well-established concepts and are present in most major pediatric hospitals. These clinics, which are set up to manage children with spinal cord dysfunction, have a well-defined multidisciplinary team. This team works very well for these children because they all have similar multidisciplinary needs ranging from neurosurgery to orthopaedics, urology, and rehabilitation. However, this model does not work as well for children with CP because their needs vary greatly. These needs range from a child with hemiplegia who is being monitored for a mild gastrocnemius contracture only to a child who is ventilator dependent with severe osteoporosis, spasticity, seizures, and gastrointestinal problems. It is impossible to have all medical specialists available in a clinic setting, especially in today's environment where everyone has to account for their time by doing productive work, described mainly as billable time.

There are two models currently being used in most pediatric centers for the care of children with CP. One model has a core group of clinicians who see the children, often including an orthopaedist, pediatrician, or physiatrist, social worker, physical therapist, and orthotist. The second model consists of families making separate appointments for each required specialist. The advantage of the first model is that it helps families coordinate their child's needs. The major disadvantage is that it is costly and not reimbursed by the fragmented American healthcare system. The advantage of the second system is its efficiency to healthcare providers; however, there is often no communication between healthcare providers, and the responsibility of coordinating care from many different specialists thus falls to families.

From a practical perspective, considering the cost restriction of the healthcare environment, the best system is some blending of the two clinic models. We use this blended model, and it works for many patients with CP and their families. We schedule outpatient clinics where an orthopaedist and pediatrician share the same physical office space; however, each child is given an individual appointment with each physician. If there are only musculoskeletal concerns, only the orthopaedist is scheduled to see the child. However, if a child also has additional medical needs, the pediatrician is seen before or after the orthopaedic appointment. Orthotics, rehabilitation engineering for wheelchair services, nutritionists, social workers, and physical and occupational therapy are available in very close proximity to this outpatient clinic. If a child had a recognized problem before the clinic visit, appointments would have been made to see any of these specialists. However, if the problem is found at the current visit, such as an orthosis that is too small, this child can be sent to the orthotist and be molded on the same day for a new orthotic. This clinic also has a special coordinator to help parents schedule appointments with other specialists such as dentistry, gastroenterology, or neurology.

This structure is most efficient for medical care providers; avoids duplication of services, such as having a physical therapist evaluate a child who is getting ongoing community-based therapy; and can potentially provide maximal efficient use of the parents' time. The main problem arising with this system is that it requires cooperation between many areas in the hospital. This model only works if the needed specialists are all working on the same day and are willing to work around each other's schedules. For example, holding the CP clinic on a day that the dental clinic is closed or the orthotist is not available does not work. Although individual appointments are made with specialists, schedules often are not maintained perfectly, so if the orthopaedic appointment is for 10 a.m. but the child is not seen until 11 a.m., the time of the next appointment with a neurologist, all the schedules are affected. Making this system work requires flexibility by all involved.

One area of efficiency that the medical care system pays little attention to is the parents or caretaker's time. Most caretakers have to schedule a whole day to take a child to a physician appointment because it means taking the child out of the school, usually driving some distance, seeing the physician, then returning home. This system of actively trying to schedule a number of appointments on the same day allows parents to make use of the whole day, avoiding more days out of work for the parent and out of school for the child.

Coordination between team members is accomplished by weekly team meetings where outpatient children with specific needs, along with pending and present in-hospital patients, are discussed. No matter what administrative structure is used for the outpatient management of children with CP, because of the diverse population and needs, there are always individuals who will not fit the structure. Therefore, an important aspect of providing medical care to this patient population is to have some flexibility in the delivery system.

Family Care Provider and Professional Care Provider Relationship

The specific organizational model for providing care is not as important as the fact that the medical care provided to the child with CP must always be provided to the family–child unit. This relationship may be somewhat different for educational professionals than for medical care professionals. This discussion focuses primarily on the medical care professional relationship, specifically on the care of the motor disabilities provided by a physician.

The first aspect of treating children with CP is ensuring that the families have heard and come to some level of acceptance that their child has a problem called CP, which is permanent and will not go away. Hearing and acknowledging a diagnosis is a process that requires families first to come to terms with hearing the words and, second, to internalize these words. This process may take many years, with families initially acknowledging that there is a problem, but still expecting a cure soon. In the initial session with families to discuss this diagnosis, it is important that physicians allow plenty of time to answer all their questions, do not demand that they immediately accept the physicians' words, and avoid definitive words that bring a sense of hopelessness to families. During this discussion with families, there is little role for the use of absolutist terms like "never," "will not," "cannot," "will die," or "will never amount to anything." These terms often strike families as extremely cruel and threaten to remove all their hope, which they desperately need. Having time to answer all a family's questions and allowing them to have their own doubts is important. As the physician relationship develops with a family, especially in the context of a clinic for CP, the families will slowly come to their own realization. However, this process of coming to terms with the diagnosis may be impacted by the circumstances and situations surrounding the etiology.

Family Response Patterns

All families come to terms with their children's problems in their own way; however, there are several problems that are based on mechanisms surrounding the inciting event or the time of the diagnosis. In general, most families struggle to understand why this happened to their children and who is at fault.

Obstetric difficulties surrounding delivery can be the clear cause of CP. However, many of these birthing problems are probably due to a fetus that was already sick. Nevertheless, the birthing problems often focus the parents on looking for someone to blame, frequently the obstetrician. Some families can come to the point where they can release this need to blame; for others, it may lead to finding a legal solution by way of bringing a legal suit against the individual or organization perceived to be at fault. These legal pursuits are often encouraged by lawyers, and for many families, this only leads to more disappointment when some of the legal efforts are unsuccessful. For families who win legal judgments, there may be some sense of justice; however, the difficulty of caring for a child with a disability continues, and the need to come to terms with why this happened does not disappear by receiving money from a successful lawsuit.

Some parents, who have difficulty dealing with why this happened to their child, will be very suspicious of the medical system and will be perceived as being very difficult. There is a tendency for medical care providers, doctors, nurses, and therapists to avoid contact with these families, which often leads to more stress because the families feel that they are being avoided. This kind of very suspicious family, especially with underlying unresolved anger related to the initial diagnosis, needs to be kept exceptionally well informed and have frequent contact with the senior attending physician.

When a child is hospitalized, it is important to have the attending physician meet with the family frequently and always keep them appraised of changes and expected treatment. This level of communication with families sounds very simple; however, we have seen many families who endured a series of terrible events in hospitals, such as oversights or staff failure to recognize an evolving event that the family already pointed out. When these situations are brought up with staff, such as nurses and residents, there is a tendency for the response to be "they brought it on themselves." This kind of thinking is unacceptable because lack of contact with the senior responsible medical staff is usually the main cause.

It is important for medical staff to recognize this pattern of behavior in families and respond very consciously by increasing communication and frequent contact. Again, the primary responsibility for this contact rests with the senior treating physician, who must display confidence, knowledge, and control of the situation to comfort the family. These families are very perceptive of physicians and care providers who do not have experience and confidence in dealing with their children's problems. Often, these families have considerable experience in hospitals and notice when things are overlooked or symptoms are not addressed in an appropriate time (Case 1.1).

Dealing with Blame

Medical care providers must not get into situations where they inadvertently inflame this need to blame someone for the cause of these children's CP. When parents give their perception of the history of the inciting event, it should be accepted as such without comment. Medical care providers should not tell parents how terrible the person they blame was or anything else that gives the impression that the CP could have been avoided if only this or that were done. This kind of postmortem evaluation of past medical events helps medical practitioners to learn; however, a detailed dissection of long-gone biomedical events to look for a person to blame seldom helps the families to come to terms with their children's disabilities. By far, most of these families' "need to find someone to blame" is a stable enduring part of their lives, and if the treating physician acknowledges this need and focuses their concerns on the children's current care and situation, the blame issue tends to fall to the background.

There is no need for the orthopaedic physician caring for these children's motor disabilities to get an extensive history of the birth and delivery directed at understanding the etiology of the CP from the families, so long as the diagnosis of CP is appropriate. Instead, the families' mental energies should be directed at the goal, which is to help their children be all they can be, given the current circumstances. However, trying to convince the parents that they have to give up looking for a cause or a person to blame is also futile. If the parents are totally immobilized and cannot move forward, arranging psychotherapy may be worthwhile; however, most parents will perceive this as another attempt to sweep away the problem of who is responsible.

Another common scenario for the diagnosis of CP is when a parent or grandparent recognizes some slow development in a child. This child was then taken to see the family doctor or pediatrician who reassured the family that they were overreacting. Often, these families end up going to their primary care provider two, three, or four times to hear the same response, that is, that they are just overreacting. The child is a little slow, but there is nothing to worry about. These families often want to lay the blame for the CP upon the

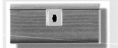

Case 1.1   Susan

Susan was born after a normal pregnancy and delivery at term and was discharged home from the hospital as a normal newborn. At 3 weeks of age, her grandmother thought that her head looked abnormal, and Susan was taken to a pediatrician where a workup revealed hydrocephalus. A shunt was placed at 4 weeks of age, followed by some complications. After this time, she was noted by her parents and grandmother to be less strong and less interactive. However, she did well, and by age 3 years was crawling, rolling, and talking. At age 3 years, she developed severe seizures and was hospitalized. During this hospitalization, she had a rather severe overdose of antiseizure medication along with other subsequent complications and lost the ability to crawl, roll, and talk. Her parents started patterning therapy when she did not rapidly regain these functions. She also started to develop increased spasticity and had more trouble with her trunk control.

By age 6 years, Susan had an adductor lengthening and was developing scoliosis. She was started in a body jacket to help control her scoliosis, and by age 8 years, she had a painful dislocated hip. After the family searched for several different opinions, they elected to go ahead and have the hip reconstructed. Because Susan had substantial complications with loss of neurologic function on several previous admissions, her parents were perceived as being extremely anxious during the hospitalization. The operative procedure and the recovery phase of the hip reconstruction went very well and the family was very gracious.

By age 9 years, she needed to have additional soft-tissue lengthenings of her right shoulder for a painful dislocation as well as for progressive varus deformity of the feet. The family was less anxious during this procedure than they had been with the prior procedure because they were more comfortable with the staff.

By age 12, the scoliosis had progressed substantially, requiring a posterior spinal fusion. The family was very anxious about this very large procedure. Their anxiety was perceived by some staff as being overreactive; however, considering the history of their experience with past medical treatment, we felt it was appropriate. At the time of the posterior spinal fusion, the shunt tubing was noted

to be broken; however, she was no longer dependent on her shunt so shunt repair was not performed.

By age 13 years, she developed more lethargy and a shunt revision was recommended. During this shunt revision, she had severe complications including an infection that required the shunt to be externalized. The external drainage was not controlled carefully enough and, as a consequence, the ventricles collapsed, causing intracranial bleeding. This episode caused substantial neurologic functional loss, so she was now less able to interact socially with her parents on top of her very severe spastic quadriplegic pattern motor disability. In addition, her seizures increased substantially. This episode made her parents extremely anxious about medical treatment, especially about the fear of developing complications and having functional loss.

Shortly after the shunt problems, she was noted on routine medical examination to have a retinal detachment requiring surgery. This surgery occurred without any complications. She continued to have problems with her seizures, and her parents were anxious to have control of the seizures, while at the same time to allow her to regain some of her alertness and contact with her parents, which they much enjoyed.

This family was often perceived by nurses and house staff as being exceedingly difficult to deal with because they were so anxious and always wanted to observe and understand specific treatments and know exactly which medications were being administered. This family was extremely dedicated to the care of their daughter, and the anxieties that they expressed were very understandable considering their history. Often, medical care providers, especially physicians and nurses, were not aware of this history and therefore did not understand the parents' anxieties. This anxiety tends to make nursing staff and medical staff try to avoid the parents, which just greatly increases their anxiety level. These parents had more than one hospitalization per year on average with their daughter and were very aware of what her proper medical management should be. They were very astute in picking up inexperience in both the nursing and medical staff and would become much more anxious when they sensed this inexperience or discomfort in dealing with their daughter.

physician, believing that this delayed diagnosis is why the child currently is so severe. There is almost no circumstance where a delayed diagnosis will be of any significance. It is important for these parents to have their concerns about the delayed diagnosis acknowledged, but then they must be reassured that this delay did not, in any way, cause their child to have a greater severity of CP. Some of these families will have difficulty developing other trusting relationships with physicians and may call, especially initially, for many minor concerns until confidence in their physician is developed.

Sometimes CP is the result of an accident or event in childhood, such as a toddler with a near drowning, or a child with a closed head injury from a motor vehicle accident in which the parent was the driver. In these situations, the parents often feel a substantial amount of blame for causing their child's disability. This self-blame and guilt may be even more difficult for a parent to come to terms with than blame focused outward. One response to the inwardly focused blame is to search for extraordinary cures, demand more therapy, or get more devices. This behavior seems to be one of "making it up to the child." It is helpful to reassure the family that things besides more therapy or more devices, such as maximizing the child's educational ability, will help the child.

Giving and Dealing with Prognosis

Another experience frequently reported by parents whose children were in neonatal nurseries is the comment that the children probably will not survive, and, if they do, will be vegetables. This comment has been reported to us by parents of children who end up with hemiplegia as well as children with quadriplegia. We believe this comment stems from the great difficulty of making a specific prognosis of outcome in the neonatal period. Also, some physicians tell families the worst possible outcome, believing that when the children do better, the families will be grateful for their good luck. However, this explanation almost never has the intended outcome, and much more commonly the families perceive these comments as the physician being incompetent or deceitful. Often, these families will interpret attempts by later physicians to discuss prognosis or expected results of surgery as being too pessimistic. For these families, it is important to be as realistic as possible; however, their optimism may cause some disappointment as their expectations of greater outcomes are not realized. Generally, these families do come to appropriate expectations, but continue to have some negative feelings about their neonatal experience.

An important aspect of giving prognosis or information that is requested by families is to always acknowledge that it is imperfect. Requests to know if a child will walk or sit should be answered as honestly as possible, always avoiding absolutist terms such as "never," "cannot," or "will not."

Giving the Diagnosis

Another common problem surrounding diagnosis of children with CP is failure to give the parents a diagnosis. A common example of this is a mother of a 5-year-old who is unable to sit and brings the child to see the orthopaedist to find out why the child cannot walk. The history reveals a normal pregnancy and delivery; however, by age 12 months, the child was not sitting, so the mother starting going to doctors to find out what was wrong with the child. She has seen three neurologists and a geneticist, has had skin biopsies, muscle biopsies, computed tomography (CT) scan, magnetic resonance imaging (MRI) scan, and many blood tests, but everything is normal. The mother hears from these doctors that they can find nothing wrong with her child; however, what the doctors probably told the mother is that the medical tests are normal and they do not know what caused the child's current disability.

Families need to be told what is wrong with their child. This type of family is easily helped by explaining that the child has CP. Physicians should clearly explain that even though they do not understand why the child has CP, it is the diagnosis, which they know exactly how to treat. Taking time and providing information to these families will stop the endless and futile search for "why" and allow them to focus on caring for and treating their children. This situation is caused almost entirely by physicians not being clear in communication with parents and the particular aversion by some physicians to giving a diagnosis of CP. This aversion is very similar to wanting to avoid telling a patient that she has cancer, and therefore telling her that she has a nonbenign growth whose cause cannot be explained. In this way, CP is like cancer in that a physician often cannot determine the etiology; however, the treatment options are well defined and should be started immediately.

Medical Therapeutic Relationship to Child and Family

There are many different types of therapeutic relationships that work for families and their children; however, there are some patterns that work better than others. These patterns each have their risks and benefits as well. The major therapeutic relationships in the treatment of motor problems of children with CP include the parents, the physical therapists, and the physicians. The parents will spend the most time with their children and will know them best. Often, the parents recognize developmental gains and day-to-day variability in their child's function first. Physical therapists will spend the most therapeutic time during treatment with children and will bring the experience of similar children. This in-depth experience with similar children allows therapists to help parents understand the expected changes as well as teach parents and children how to maximize their function. The orthopaedist treating the motor disability will have the least experience with an individual child, but will have the broadest experience with many children to understand the expectations of what will occur. The physician's experience with each child, however, will be much more superficial and the physician depends on the parents' and therapists' observations of the children's function over time and the variability of function during the day. Recognizing these individual strengths will allow the parents', therapists', and orthopaedists' perception of individual children to be combined to make the best therapeutic judgment.

The Physical Therapist Relationship

The role of the primary treating physical therapist, especially for the young child between the ages of 1 and 5 years, will incorporate the typical role that the grandmother and the general pediatrician play for normal children. In addition, the therapist fulfilling this role must have knowledge and experience in dealing with children with CP. This role model involves time spent teaching the parents how to handle and do exercises with their child. This role also involves helping the parents sort out different physician recommendations, encouraging the parents, and showing and reminding parents of the positive signs of progress in the child's development. When this role works well, it is the best therapeutic relationship a family has. The positive aspects of this role are providing the parents with insight and expectations of their child, reassuring the family that they are providing excellent care, and being readily available to answer the family's questions.

The "grandmothering" role of the therapist has associated risks. One of the greatest risks in our current, very unstable medical environment is that a change in funding or insurance coverage may abruptly end the relationship. An abrupt change can be very traumatic to a family. The therapist must be careful not to be overly demanding of the family, but to help the family find what works for them. Occasionally, a therapist may be fixated on a specific treatment program and believe that it is best for the child; however, the parents may not be in a situation to follow through with all this treatment. The parents feel guilty, and the therapist may try to use this guilt to get them to do more.

The physical therapist in this role as a therapeutic "grandmother" can help parents sort out what medical care and choices are available. The therapist can help parents by attending physician appointments and making the parent ask the right questions, which is often not possible because of funding restrictions. The physical therapist must not give specific medical advice beyond helping parents get the correct information. Therapists with extensive experience should recognize that they have great, detailed, and deep experience with a few children and that generalizing from the experience of one child is dangerous. We have heard therapists tell parents on many occasions that their child should never have a certain operation because the therapist once saw a child who did poorly with that surgery. This type of advice is inappropriate because one child's experience may have been a rare complication of the operation. Also, there are many different ways of doing surgery. This would be like telling someone to never get in a car again after seeing a car accident. A more appropriate response to the family would be giving them questions to ask the doctor specifically about the circumstance with which the therapist is concerned and has experience.

Another physical therapist therapeutic relationship pattern is the purely clinical relationship in which the therapist thinks the family is incompetent, unreliable, or irresponsible and only wants to deal with the child. Almost invariably, this same therapist next will complain that the family and child never do the home exercise program or that the child is not brought to therapy regularly. This relationship may work for a school-based therapist or a therapist doing inpatient therapy, but it leads to great frustration for both the therapist and family when it is applied to an outpatient-based, ongoing developmental therapy. In this environment, the therapist must try to understand and work within the family's available resources.

The Physician Relationship

Families of children with CP often have a series of physician relationships and tend to choose the physician with whom they are comfortable, who responds to their needs, and who is able to help them with their child's problems. As pediatric orthopaedists, many of our patients will report to their schools and emergency rooms that we are their child's doctors. We strongly encourage families to have family doctors or general pediatricians to care for well child care needs and minor illnesses. With the changing healthcare payers, some families have changed family doctors every year or two and the physician who cares primarily for the musculoskeletal disabilities of a child often becomes defined as the child's doctor.

The musculoskeletal problems of CP are well known and are relatively predictable; therefore, a major part of the treatment is educating the family of what to expect. For example, a nonambulatory 2-year-old child who is very spastic has a high risk of developing spastic hip disease. This risk needs to be explained to parents so they know that routine follow-up is important and that, if spastic hip disease is found, there is a specific treatment program. At each visit, this plan is reviewed again. Diligent attention to this individual education process gives parents a sense of confidence about the future and helps prevent the development of a nihilistic family approach that nothing can be done for their child.

Because families usually start to see the CP doctor when the children are about age 2 years, and in our clinic stay until age 21 years, a long-term relationship is developed. Keeping a healthy therapeutic relationship, understanding and taking into consideration the family's strengths and limits, is important. In addition to helping the family understand what to expect with their child, continuing to support the family as much as possible is very important. One easy way to give the family positive feedback is to focus on the positive things that the child has accomplished, such as better physical functioning, good grades, good behavior, gaining weight, growing taller, and being nicely dressed. There is a tendency for parents to only hear negative things from doctors, such as a catalog of all the things the child cannot do.

Another aspect of the therapeutic relationship is recognizing that this is not a family relationship. Many of our patients are very happy to see us and we enjoy seeing them; however, as they grow and develop, their doctor should be a positive influence but not their main adult role model. These children should not be seen more than every 6 months unless there is an active treatment program such as one following surgery. One goal of the medical treatment of these children should be to have as little direct impact as possible on their normal lives so that they grow up having experiences similar to normal children. To this end, medical intervention should be limited as much as possible and should be episodic so that it more closely mimics normal childhood medical experiences, such as fractures or tonsillitis. Frequent trips to a doctor's office or to a clinic are also very time consuming for families. There are almost no musculoskeletal problems that need to be monitored more than every 6 months.

Recognizing the strengths and weaknesses in families and trying to work within their limits to provide medical care for children with motor disabilities is important. The medical system is limited to working within the confines of what the families and school environment can provide, especially for children with severe physical disabilities. The state social service protection agencies seldom get involved or are very helpful to families, except in rare dire circumstances.

When the Doctor–Family Relationship Is Not Working

Medical care providers need to understand that personalities are such that one individual can never meet everyone's needs. This does not mean that as soon as the doctor therapist family relationship becomes difficult, it is not working. At this time, the relationship needs to be discussed and the physician or therapist should be open about giving the family permission to go to another doctor or therapist. Some families will just leave without saying anything and others will feel guilty about wanting to leave. Physicians and therapists must be honest with themselves because this situation tends to make them feel like a failure. There may be a combined sense of relief that the family left and a sense of failure and anger that the family does not trust their physician or therapist. These are normal feelings that the physician or therapist should acknowledge and not place blame on themselves or the family.

When the Family Chooses Medical Treatment Against the Physician's Advice

Families may seek a second opinion for a specific treatment recommendation. This desire to get a second opinion should not be seen by the primary treating physician as a lack of faith or confidence. The family may require a second opinion for insurance purposes or, for many families, they just want to make sure they are getting the correct treatment. Usually, getting a second opinion should be viewed as a very prudent move on the family's part and should be encouraged. Families should be given all the records and support that are needed for them to get a meaningful second opinion. If this second opinion is similar to that given by the primary physician, the family is often greatly comforted in moving ahead. However, there is still variability in medical treatment for children with CP, so depending on the family's choice of opinions, the recommendations may be slightly to diametrically opposed.

In a circumstance where the recommendation of another physician differs significantly, the primary physician must be clear with the family and place the second opinion in the perspective of their recommendation. Sometimes the words used may sound very different, but the recommendations are very similar. In other circumstances, the recommendation may be diametrically opposed and the primary physician must recognize this and explain to the family the reasons for their recommendation. When recommendations are diametrically opposed, clear documentation, including the discussions concerning the other opinion, is especially important. This situation has a high risk for disappointment. Often, families have great difficulty in choosing between divergent opinions, even when one opinion is based on published scientific data and the other opinion is completely lacking in any scientific basis (Cases 1.2, 1.3). Therefore, a family may base their decision on other family contacts, a therapist's recommendations, or the personality of the physician.

Physicians must understand that it is the family's responsibility and power to make these choices; therefore, with rare exception, no matter how medically wrong the physician believes these decisions are, the family must be given the right to choose. Only in rare, directly life-threatening circumstances will a child protective service agency even consider getting involved, and then this involvement is usually very temporary. With a long and chronic condition such as CP, temporary intervention by a child protective agency generally is of no use in interacting with families. With clear documentation of the recommendations, the physician must let the family proceed as they choose; however, we always tell them that we would be happy to see them back at any time. When they undergo treatment against their primary physician's advice and return, usually after several years, the physician should not make the previous situation a conflict. The family usually feels guilty and may not want to discuss past events. Occasionally, they will come back and

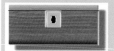

Case 1.2   Judy

Judy was born premature as one of twins and weighed 1300 g. She was in the neonatal nursery for many weeks. Her development was noted to be significantly delayed early on, and her CP was recognized within the first 2 years of her life. By school age, Judy was not able to walk, but was able to do some speaking, and there was concern about her educational ability. At age 7 years, she was seen by a developmental pediatrician for an educational assessment. This pediatrician thought that she had excellent cognitive ability, but also noted that she was developing significant contractures, and recommended follow-up with a pediatric orthopaedist. However, she was not seen by a pediatric orthopaedist until age 10 years, when she started to develop some pain in the right hip. At this point, she was in a regular school and was complaining of pain in the hip during the school day. An evaluation demonstrated a completely dislocated right hip and severe subluxation of the left hip; however, this hip was an excellent candidate for reconstruction because, at age 10 years, she had substantial growth remaining. Hip reconstruction was recommended to the family and details were given. For reasons that were never quite clear, this family pursued many other options in trying to deal with their daughter's painful dislocated hip and eventually decided on a treatment that they had located through unknown sources, which consisted of having a spinal cord stimulator implanted in her spinal cord. In addition to the spinal cord stimulator, other alternative medicine treatments were pursued. The hip pain would get better intermittently and then would flare up, requiring her to be in bed for several days. By 14 years of age Judy had periods of relative comfort between bouts of severe pain, until age 15 when the pain became more constant and severe. By age 15 years, as she entered high school with normal cognitive and educational achievements, the pain got so severe that she could no longer sit during the school day. At this point, her parents kept her home in bed and gave her a variety of different pain medications. She was out of school for 1 year, spending most of her time in bed, when her parents finally came back with a request to have her hip reconstructed because they now perceived she could no longer deal with the pain.

At this point, except for getting a brief history, her parents were told simply that reconstruction was no longer possible, and she now required some palliative treatment. Her parents were assured that good treatment was available to get rid of her pain; they were informed of the treatment options, and it was strongly recommended that these options be pursued. Surgery was scheduled emergently and was completely successful in alleviating her pain.

This is an example of a family who for unknown reasons chooses alternative medical treatments instead of well-recognized appropriate medical treatment. This type of behavior may be very difficult for a physician to accept. This family only saw us once when their daughter was 10 years old, and then did not come back for more treatment. In these situations a physician can only make the recommendations, but cannot force the families to follow through with treatment. This girl clearly would have been much better served by a reconstruction at age 10 years; however, the family had complete control. This family's choice of treatment was not inappropriate enough legally whereby the physician would have gained anything by reporting the family to child protective services or making any other efforts to try to force them to have treatment. There are many different types of alternative medical treatments that families may pursue, some of them performed by a physician, such as spinal cord stimulators, which provide absolutely no benefit to this kind of spasticity or pain. There is nothing that the primary caring physician can do except try to persuade the family and then accept their decisions. However, it is very important to always leave the family the option of coming back when they are ready and then provide appropriate treatment, as was done in this situation.

Six weeks after this girl's surgery, at which point all her hip pain was gone, the family noted that she was having difficulty sitting because of her scoliosis. They were now very keen on moving ahead and having the scoliosis corrected. This is a circumstance where although the family feels extremely guilty and are often very hesitant to return because of fear that the physician will be angry with them, once the appropriate treatment has been performed and is successful, the family will become very committed to continuing with appropriate medical care.

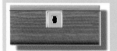

Case 1.3   Rhonda

Rhonda was born following a normal pregnancy and normal delivery. She was perceived to be normal until 18 months of age when her development was noted to be substantially slow and a full evaluation demonstrated an infantile cytomegalovirus (CMV) infection. She continued to make progress and by age 3 years had started walking independently and was speaking. She had low muscle tone with some difficulties with balance. She was doing well in a special education class environment until age 9 years, when she had sudden complete loss of hearing in both ears. An evaluation demonstrated that this hearing loss was in response to the CMV infection. By age 13 years, she had developed severe scoliosis that was making her ambulation difficult. At this point she was quite healthy, and although she had not regained any hearing, she was a full community ambulator. The posterior spinal fusion was performed without difficulty, and the family was told that based on her excellent general health, a fairly quick recovery was anticipated, with her being ready to leave the hospital in approximately 7 days.

However, in the intensive care unit (ICU), on the first day following surgery she became quite hypotensive, requiring a substantial bolus of fluid as well as a dopamine for blood pressure support. Blood pressure support was required for 5 days, and she then developed respiratory problems and was on ventilator support for 5 days. Following extubation, she continued to have pulmonary problems needing positive pressure respiratory support at night. In the meantime, she also developed a mild pneumonia requiring antibiotic treatment. Instead of being discharged from the hospital in 7 days, she was discharged from the ICU to the floor 13 days postoperatively.

During this time, the family became anxious because it was medically difficult to make specific predictions about what to expect. The family was kept informed and, overall, they were able to relax as slow progress was made in the ICU. Each day, the family saw that she was stable or slightly better. Gains were made, such as discontinuation of the dopamine for her blood pressure support, then discontinuation of the ventilator. This progress was followed by needing fewer respiratory treatments as her pulmonary status gradually improved. Being able to see these gains, although slow, gave the family hope and understanding that things were progressively improving.

By postoperative day 10, she had developed some superficial wound separation and very minimal drainage; however, she was afebrile because she was being treated by antibiotics for her pneumonia. The family was informed that this wound opening was not uncommon, especially after having been extremely edematous, and the mild wound drainage was not a concern.

By postoperative day 17, this wound drainage was not decreasing and instead was increasing. The patient was still afebrile, was continuing to make good progress with her respiratory status, and was able to be up walking in physical therapy. However, based on the amount of drainage and the appearance of the wound, it was possible that this could be a deep wound infection. The family was told that the wound did not look good, and that if after 2 more days the drainage did not substantially decrease, a more vigorous exploration would be done. On postoperative day 19, the drainage increased slightly; therefore, a more detailed digital inspection, trying to determine the depths of the wound, was undertaken. The deep fascia was noted to be open at the far superior aspect of the wound, and the family was informed that this was a deep wound infection. The girl needed to be returned to the operating room, and the wound surgically cleaned out, then treated with open packing and dressing changes. At this time the family was told that she would now be in the hospital for an additional 4 weeks on intravenous antibiotics and wound dressing changes, followed with probably 2 weeks of home intravenous antibiotics. The family was already very anxious about all the complications in the ICU, and now the deep would infection was another major setback. However, after the parents went home and discussed the significance of this new problem with an understanding of the exact timetable that was required, they were able to make family plans. They came back to the hospital the following day and had more discussions concerning details about the planned treatment. After making plans with the specific information they were given, they shared that they had made arrangements for their other children and were comfortable and relaxed with the plan. They were prepared for the 4 weeks, and the remainder of the treatment was very uneventful.

This case demonstrates how important it is to keep the family well informed as complications are occurring. To give the family the information, the physician has to recognize the complication and develop a clear treatment plan. There is a tendency, especially in situations where there have been multiple complications and the family is very anxious, for the physician to not want to give the family more bad news. Ignoring problems like deep wound infections will not make them go away, and the problem will continue to be frustrating. When a clear treatment protocol with the expected outcome is outlined, and the family is informed that although this is a substantial setback, it should not compromise the long-term outcome of their child's treatment in any way. In this specific case, it was equally important to reassure the family that the spine fusion was successful in spite of the current problem and that the rod did not need to be removed.

blame the physician for the problems because they have transferred the blame for the recommendation (Case 1.4). Nothing will be gained by bringing up these past problems with the family, and the focus should be to move on with the problems at hand as they present themselves.

Recommending Surgery

For children who have had regular appropriate medical care, the need for specific orthopaedic procedures is usually anticipated over 1 to 2 years, and as a consequence is not a surprising recommendation. We prefer to have these discussions in the presence of the child. For young children, there is no sense that something is being hidden from them. Children in middle childhood and young adulthood can take in as much as possible, allowing us, as their physicians, to directly address their concerns as well. For younger children, those under age 8 years, their main concern is that they will be left alone. We reassure them that we make a major effort to allow the parents to stay with them during preinduction in the surgical suite and again in the recovery room. We also reassure children that their parents will be with them throughout the whole hospitalization. As children get older, especially at adolescence, there is often an adult type of concern about not waking up from anesthesia or having other severe complications leading to death. These individuals may have great anxiety, but have few of the adult coping skills that allow the rationality to say that this surgery is done every day and people do wake up. Some of these adolescents need a great deal of reassurance, most of which should be directed at trying to get them to use adult rational coping skills. If adolescents are having problems with sleeping or anxiety attacks as the surgery date approaches, treating them with an antianxiety or sedative agent is very helpful.

Some adolescents and young adults with mental retardation develop substantial agitation over surgery. Parents of such children are usually very aware of this tendency and may wish to not tell them about having surgery until the day before or the day of surgery. Although this is a reasonable practice for individuals with severe mental retardation who are not able to cognitively process the planned surgery, approaching children who are cognitively able to process the event in this way is only going to make them distrustful of their parents and doctors.

In preparing children and families for surgery, it is important to discuss the expected outcome of the surgery with them. Part of this discussion must focus on what will not happen, specifically that their child will still have CP after the surgery. If the goal is to prevent or treat hip dislocation, showing radiographs to the families helps them understand the plan. They also need to be told what to expect of the procedure from a functional perspective, such as "Will the child still be able to stand? Will the child be able to roll? Will the child's sitting be affected? Will the child's walking ability be affected?" For children in whom the surgery is expected to improve walking, showing families videotapes of similar children before and after surgery helps them get a perception of what level of improvement is anticipated.

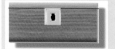

Case 1.4 Patricia

Patricia was born at 35 weeks weighing 2250 g. She had a relatively normal postnatal course except that she was noted to be very good and slept a lot, even requiring awakening occasionally to eat. However, by 19 months of age, she had significantly decreased tone in her lower extremities and trunk, but had increased tone in her right upper extremity with some spasticity and was diagnosed as a right hemiplegic pattern CP. By age 4 years, she was able to sit but had very spastic lower extremities, which caused scissoring and equinus when she was standing. She was able to sit on a tricycle and pedal. At this time, the parents first heard about dorsal rhizotomies and were very interested in pursuing this method to decrease the spasticity. By age 5 years, she was walking handheld, but scissoring substantially, and the parents were pursuing various opinions concerning the dorsal rhizotomy. By age 6 years, the parents had gotten a recommendation to use a transcutaneous nerve stimulator on the upper right, very spastic extremity. A course of this stimulation was undertaken even though the child objected because of the discomfort, but the parents persisted for several months until it was clear that there was no benefit.

At age 7 years she was able to stand but could not do independent transfers, although she was doing standing transfers with considerable scissoring. She was not able to walk independently without someone guarding her. The parents continued to get various conflicting opinions on the merit of a dorsal rhizotomy from several dorsal rhizotomy evaluation programs. Finally the family decided to have the child undergo a dorsal rhizotomy at age 7 years. After 1 year of intense rehabilitation, the mother was very depressed and angry with herself and with the physicians. After an extensive discussion, the mother volunteered that she was blaming herself and also the physicians, both those who recommended for and against the procedure, for her daughter having undergone a dorsal rhizotomy. She believed the rhizotomy caused her daughter to lose function in spite of an extremely intense amount of physical therapy work and stress over the year following the surgery.

After further discussion, the mother was encouraged and began to see this experience as an attempt by herself and her husband to choose what was right for their daughter. The mother was slowly able to acknowledge how difficult it is for a family to make decisions when there are varying medical opinions about a procedure, especially a new procedure where there are few data available, such as the dorsal rhizotomy in the late 1980s. The mother was able to come to terms with feeling badly about her daughter having the surgery, and she stopped blaming herself and the physicians because she understood that everybody was trying to do what they thought was best with the knowledge they had available at the time. The mother was encouraged to focus forward because, following dorsal rhizotomy, some of the spasticity does return and her daughter probably would slowly regain some of the lost function. The functional loss was specifically identified as the inability for independent stance, for good assisted transfers, and for household ambulation while being held by her hands.

Over the next 3 years, some tone did return and this girl was able to do some minimal standing transfers; however, she has become very heavy, making it difficult for her and her family. She underwent reconstructive surgery of her right upper extremity, which improved her ability to use the right extremity to hold on and assist with transfers. Seven years after the dorsal rhizotomy, she developed a severe kyphosis at the site of the rhizotomy that required a posterior spinal fusion. This development caused her parents some renewed agitation about their daughter having undergone a procedure that they still felt was very detrimental. This combination of the family struggling to deal with their daughter's disability as she is becoming full adult size, and trying to find past blame for the cause of some of the disability, has made it somewhat difficult for the girl to come to terms with her own disability.

After the posterior spinal fusion, she developed a substantial depression and anxiety syndrome with a period of pain, difficulty with sleeping, and poor appetite. Initially, she was started on amitriptyline to help with the poor diet and sleep. This medication helped by substantially improving her diet; however, she continued with significant amounts of anxiety and the amitriptyline had to be increased over a 2- to 3-month period instead of being decreased. She was referred for a psychiatric consultation for better pharmacologic management of her depression and anxiety. The improved pharmacologic management, as well as some counseling with the parents, has greatly assisted this young woman in making the transition to young adulthood.

This case is an example of parents who try very hard to find the latest and best treatment, and after extensive consultation with conflicting opinions, make a decision that does not turn out well. This decision-making process can inflame the process of coming to terms with the child's disability further, making the parents feel that they are themselves partially to blame. This concept of who is to blame and why this has happened seems to get magnified at adolescence, especially with development of major deformities and surgery, such as a posterior spinal fusion. These issues often lead to family stress, including depression in both the child and family members and marital stress, and may aggravate substance abuse. It is important in such families that the family stresses are identified and that good psychiatric consultation be obtained for both psychologic and pharmacologic management.

A Plan for Managing Complications

Discussion of possible complications is also important; however, the expected outcome should be honestly approached. Some surgeons tend to have very pessimistic expectations with regard to expected outcome and complications. Surgeons with this approach soon overwhelm themselves and their families with their assessment of the poor balance between the expected outcome and the possible complications. Most surgeons who have a large CP practice tend more toward the overly optimistic approach in which the outcomes clearly will be worth the risk of the complications. The risk of an overly optimistic approach to families occurs when there are complications. These families may be surprised and angry and find it difficult to deal with the unexpected. It is difficult for physicians to have the perfect balance, but each physician should be aware of their own tendency. Usually, an honest assessment and feedback from partners will identify which personality trait, either optimistic or pessimistic, a physician tends to use when approaching families. By recognizing this tendency, surgeons can be more sensitive to what families are hearing and make suggestions to moderate this perception.

There are families who for some reason or another have not been obtaining appropriate orthopaedic care for their children. Then, when these children are adolescents, they may come to see a CP surgeon with a painful hip dislocation, severe scoliosis, or other deformities that are in a severely neglected state. Some of these families are surprised to hear that only a surgical procedure will be the appropriate treatment. Some families may be very resistant to surgery and will want to try everything else. These families must understand that only surgery will correct the problem, but the surgery seldom has to occur on an emergency basis. If a surgeon perceives a family's hesitancy, and attempts to mollify them by suggesting that a brace, injections, or some other modality be tried even though it will provide no long-term benefit, the family will likely hear uncertainty in the physician's approach. Families may miss the message completely that only surgery will address the problem when they are appeased by nonsurgical treatment. Giving children temporizing measures to provide relief of pain is appropriate; however, doctors must be clear to families that these measures are only providing temporary pain relief and are not treatments. By giving families a little time with the use of these temporary measures, physicians can develop a relationship with the families. There are situations where medical and psychiatric treatment may be required before the surgical treatment can occur. For all these reasons, it is important to be clear about the required treatment, its expected outcomes, and then to outline the full treatment plan. As this treatment plan is undertaken, the relationship a physician has developed with children and families will allow them to be confident that the recommended treatment can occur in a safe and effective way.

When Complications Occur

When treatment of a child does not go well, the orthopaedist must first recognize this as a complication. The judgment of recognizing a complication is one of the most difficult to develop and some physicians may never do it well. Many complications, especially in orthopaedics, do not present with the drama of a cardiac arrest. In orthopaedics, a more typical example is the presentation of a deep wound infection. Every wound with a little erythema and a mild superficial drainage is not a deep wound infection. However, when a deep wound infection is present, it should be acknowledged as such. These families should be told of the complication and a definitive treatment plan should be described (Case 1.3). For this process to work, physicians first have to acknowledge the complication to themselves. We have seen many physicians who cannot bring themselves to acknowledge the magnitude of the complication. Likewise, we have seen physicians who overreact to relatively minor problems that will resolve if left alone.

Finding a balance requires physicians to be honest with themselves and be aware of their own tendency toward optimistic or pessimistic ends of the spectrum. The optimist tends to see the complication as minor variance of normal, whereas the pessimist tends to be overly concerned that any wound change may be a deep wound infection. By being aware of one's own tendency, as experience is gained, an approach to diagnosing and acknowledging complications and then making specific treatment plans will be developed. Complications tend to make physicians feel like failures, and a good retrospective evaluation of the treatment course may demonstrate errors of judgment or execution. These errors should be viewed as learning experiences and opportunities to teach oneself as well as others.

A significant number of the case histories in this book are careful analyses of complications that have occurred in our practice. It is important that the approach to analyzing a complication is to determine the exact cause of the complication when possible so that it may be avoided in the future. Saying that "I will never do that operation again" is an inappropriate response to complications. This response comes very close to that of people who say they will never get in a car again after they have had a car accident. Our goal is to always have a complication-free treatment and recovery for every patient; however, we learn the most from careful analysis of our complications and poor outcomes.

Once physicians acknowledge the complications to themselves, the families then need to be told. Families may react with quiet acceptance, frustration, or anger. These feelings are often the same feelings that physicians have about the same complication. If physicians are willing to share some of their frustration and concern about the complications, it often helps families to put the problem in perspective. It is very important to explain to families what to expect from a complication. This explanation should include a detailed outline of the expected treatment plan. If a complication arises that physicians are not comfortable treating, getting a second opinion from, or seeking the help of, another physician is very important. This step should be explained carefully to families. Frequent contact with families is very important, especially if they develop considerable anger and anxiety, because if they feel that the doctor is trying to avoid them, these feelings often increase.

Complications should be managed very much like the initial decision to have an operation. First, specific problems should be carefully defined to families. Next, the range of options and expected outcomes, with respect to the short- and long-term implications, should be placed forward as specifically as possible. As much as possible, families should be told the detailed expected timeline and exact treatments. For instance, if repeat or additional surgery is expected in the future as a consequence of a complication, this should be laid out for families. If antibiotics are to be used, families should be told for how long and what factors will be monitored to determine a good outcome. This kind of detail gives families a sense that there is someone in charge with experience in dealing with these complications and helps them deal with the fear of the unknown, which the complications often bring to the foreground.

Complications need to be recorded in detail in the medical record and should reflect all the objective observations and alternatives that were considered. This record is not the place where blame should be directed. What is observed to have occurred should be documented objectively without rewriting history. For example, if the toes are found to be insensate and without blood flow in a child who has had a cast on a foot following surgery, this should be reflected in the medical record, followed by a recording of the immediate action taken, such as removing or opening the cast, and the outcome of that action, such as the improved and returned blood flow to the toes. There is no reason to speculate that the cast was applied too tightly, or that the nursing staff failed to elevate the cast, and so forth. This kind of analysis is important, but should be done after the patient is treated appropriately and there has been time to reflect on the whole situation. Often, these initial assessments are incomplete and wrong and most frequently are written to protect the writer. Later, during a more thorough investigation or legal action, these assessments only make it appear as if the writer was trying to cover up or shift blame to someone else.

During stressful treatment periods, especially when dealing with difficult complications, it is very important to ask partners and other colleagues to evaluate the patients and give unbiased opinions. A treating physician can develop a biased view, especially in the face of complications where one would not like to acknowledge personal culpability. Involving other colleagues also gives families the sense that their physician really is trying to keep all options open. If these consultants do have different opinions, these opinions should be discussed between the physicians first, then the options should be outlined for families with a unified recommendation wherever possible. Giving families different treatment recommendations and expected treatment outcomes from several different consultants should be avoided.

The Final Goal

The goal in treating children with CP is for them to grow and develop within the context of a normal family. Their medical treatment and medical condition should be an experience just as a normal part of who they are. For example, a 6-year-old child who fractures her femur will have a 6-month treatment course until most of the rehabilitation is completed. This occurrence will remain a definite event in the child and family's growth and development; however, when she is graduating from high school and going off to college, this medical event probably will have faded into many other growing-up experiences. This is the pattern that we want to try to mimic in children with CP (Case 1.5).

In the past, children might have spent 30% to 50% of their growing-up years in hospitals having and recovering from surgeries trying to make them walk better or to make them straighter, which was very detrimental. Mercer Rang termed this the "birthday syndrome," in which children were in the hospital for most of their birthdays, and nurses were baking their birthday

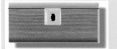

Case 1.5   Emily

Emily was born premature at 28 weeks weighing 1500 g. She was in the hospital for 2 months following birth. Following her discharge, she was recognized to have increased tone in her lower extremities with some developmental delay early on. By age 4 years, she was developing substantial contractures and had an adductor, hamstring, and tendon Achilles lengthening. She was noted to have rather severe neural deafness. In addition, several eye surgeries were performed in childhood. She started school with some educational support and special treatment for the deafness, but was noted to have excellent cognitive functioning. She succeeded in school with assistance of special support for her hearing disability. At one point, she was sent to a boarding school specializing in teaching children with hearing disabilities. However, after 1 year, she missed interaction with her family and returned to the normal school setting.

She had two additional medical treatments, one at age 10 years for additional muscle lengthening, and one at age 13, which consisted of a triple arthrodesis of her feet, hamstring lengthenings distally, and a rectus transfer at the knee. She continued to walk in the community with a combination of Lofstrand crutches and a walker. Around the house, she would walk holding on to furniture. During her high school years, she developed a mildly increased crouching gait pattern and was placed in a ground reaction ankle foot orthosis (AFO), which she disliked. However, she acknowledged that the braces allowed her to walk easier so she would use them for ambulation in the community. In high school, she did very well both academically and socially. By age 16 years, she was working as a camp counselor for children with hearing disabilities during the summer; at age 18 years she obtained a driver's license. At age 18, following graduation from high school, she entered college. Her goal on entering college was to become a teacher; however, after a little over 1 year in college, she became tired of the college scene and was interested in going to work and being closer to her family and community.

In her high school years, her crouching gait pattern increased slightly during the adolescent growth spurt but then leveled off as her growth completed. On several occasions, we had recommended additional muscle lengthening and realignments to assist her in having a more upright posture. She was always clear that she was not having any pain with walking, she was doing well walking, and she herself was not interested in any more surgery. At the time of these discussions, she would always listen carefully to the recommendations. Because she perceived herself as doing well, she could see no benefit in having surgery.

Emily, in spite of having two substantial disabilities, the diplegic pattern CP, and a significant hearing disability, was able to have a childhood and adolescent experience very similar to her age-matched peers. She is an excellent example of success in reaching our real goal of treatment, because she has responded to many of the stresses of growth and development similar to her age-matched peers, even to the point of dropping out of college and deciding that she would rather go to work. It is especially significant that after she dropped out of college, she has worked for several years now as a teacher's aide, a job she greatly enjoys. She continues to have the goal of returning to college and becoming a teacher. We are quite confident that in time she will accomplish this goal because she has a strong sense of who she is and a strong sense of what she wants to do. Most of this has come from an excellent family environment in which she was given strong structure but also allowed to express herself. She is an example of an individual who did not end with the ideal medical treatment because the crouched gait pattern she currently has as a young adult could probably be improved; however, it has been her choice to not pursue further treatment. The positive assessment we can make as physicians is that the medical care that was provided has not interfered with her growth and development as a competent functioning adult.

---

cakes and having birthday parties for them rather than their families at home.[1] Many of these children came to see the hospital staff as a second family (Figure 1.2). This seldom happens currently because of greatly shortened hospital stays and improved diagnostic abilities. For most children with CP, all orthopaedic management should ideally be done with only two major surgical events during their growth and development. This ideal is not possible

Figure 1.2. The typical approach to the surgical treatment of children with CP was to perform a surgery almost every year. This concept often led to children spending a great deal of time in the hospital, to the point where the nursing staff would become "pseudo-parents," more often celebrating birthdays with the children than the children's own families.

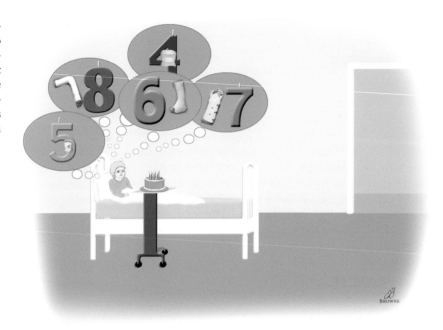

to achieve in all children but should continue to be the goal. Striving for decreasing the number of orthopaedic operative events in children's lives and moderating the amount of other medical treatments to only those that will have definite and lasting benefit should be continued. For example, an ambulatory child with normal cognitive function should not be having physical or occupational therapy at any time that interferes with their education. Therapeutic goals should be planned during summer months or in ways that do not interfere with education.

Twenty years ago, the use of inhibition casting was popular. It was believed that this technique decreased contractures and managed spasticity. These children were in leg casts for 8 weeks, often requiring trips to the clinic to change the cast every 2 weeks. After 2 or 3 months, the whole process would have to be repeated. If families could tolerate the stress, although few did, these children would be in a cast for 30% to 50% of their growing years. The time and behavioral stress placed on these families meant that a large part of their lives revolved around their children's medical treatments. When these children graduated from high school, they tended to see all these casting events as a major focus of their growing-up experience instead of the more normal childhood growing experiences, such as going to the beach, going to Disney World, or other parties and events.

In young adulthood, the success of the whole individual with CP is determined much more by the family and the individual's educational experience than by the activities of the medical treatment. The medical care system can help children and families cope with the disability and allow individuals with CP to function at their maximum ability. However, the medical care system also must recognize that too much focus on perfection of function may cause damage to the growth and development of the children and family unit, especially in the social, psychologic, and educational domains. Achieving this balance varies with each child and family. For example, many successful young adults without disabilities do not have the ideal maximization of their physical function because the focus of their interests is sedentary activities. Just as with these nondisabled young adults, there is great variation in how important maximizing physical function and appearance is to each individual with CP. When young adults are truly able to make informed and well-articulated decisions, then they have arrived at a level of success in young adulthood. Just as with nondisabled adolescents and young adults, the medical care providers should stress the importance of good physical conditioning; however, trying to enforce a specific level of physical activity against the person's wishes tends not to be very productive. Individuals with disabilities should be allowed to make these decisions in the same way that individuals without disabilities are allowed to decide, even if their physician thinks it is not in their best interest. Therefore, the final goal is to encourage the development of individual adults who are as competent as possible to make their own decisions, who develop the confidence to make those decisions, and are then willing to make decisions and live with the consequences. Always in the context of this final goal, we as therapists and physicians want the individual's physical impairments minimized as much as technically possible.

Reference

1. Rang M. Cerebral palsy. In: Morrissy R, ed. Lovell and Winter's Pediatric Orthopedics, Vol. 1. Philadelphia: Lippincott, 1990:465–506.

Etiology, Epidemiology, Pathology, and Diagnosis

Cerebral palsy (CP) is a static lesion occurring in the immature brain that leaves children with a permanent motor impairment. The lesion may occur as a developmental defect, such as lissencephaly; as an infarction, such as a middle cerebral artery occlusion in a neonate; or as trauma during or after delivery. Because brain pathology in all these etiologies is static, it is considered CP. Many minor static lesions leave no motor impairment and do not cause CP. Many pathologies, such as Rett syndrome, are progressive in childhood, but then become static at or after adolescence. These conditions are not part of the CP group, but after they become static, they have problems very similar to those of CP from the motor perspective. Other problems, such as progressive encephalopathy, have very different considerations from the motor perspective.

Saying a child has CP only means the child has a motor impairment from a static brain lesion, but says nothing about the etiology of this impairment. Some authors advocate using a plural term of "cerebral palsies" to imply that there are many kinds of CP.[1] There is some validity to this concept, similar to the term "cancer," in which many specific pathologic types of cancer, each with a different treatment, are recognized. Although applying this concept to CP is appealing from the perspective of determining etiologies and understanding the epidemiology, it provides very little help in actually managing the motor impairment. From the cancer analogy, for example, the specific cellular type and stage of breast cancer are important to know to prescribe the correct treatment. With CP, knowing the cause does not help treat a child who has a dislocated hip. The treatment is based on the diagnosis of CP, as opposed to a muscle disease, spinal paralysis, or a progressive encephalopathy. The original cause of the CP does not matter. Therefore, the concept of "cerebral palsies" is not used in the remainder of this text, and the term cerebral palsy will not carry any information on specific etiology. Although the etiologic information has little relevance in the management of motor impairments, it is of limited importance in some children for giving a prognosis. The etiology can be important to families in terms of genetic counseling with respect to the risks of future pregnancies, and it is important as an outcome measure for nurseries and epidemiology.

Physicians who manage the motor impairments must always maintain a healthy suspicion of the diagnosis of CP, as sometimes a dual diagnosis may be present or the original diagnosis may be wrong. When progression of the impairments and disability, along with a child's maturity, do not fit the usual pattern of CP, more workup is indicated. For example, a child may be diagnosed with diplegia because he was premature and had an intraventricular hemorrhage, but, by age 6 years, the physical examination demonstrated very large calves with much more weakness and less spasticity than would usually be expected. This child would need to be worked up for muscle disease with the understanding that he can have both Duchenne's muscular dystrophy and diplegic pattern CP. Alternatively, the child's history may have been a red herring and he does not have CP, but does have Duchenne's muscular dystrophy. There are children born prematurely who have intraventricular hemorrhages but are completely normal from a motor perspective.

Etiology of Cerebral Palsy

As noted previously, there are many causes of CP, and knowing the exact etiology is not very important for a physician managing the motor impairments. The etiology may be important when considering whether a child is following an expected course of maturation and development. Also, parents find the etiology important because it is part of coming to terms with the larger question of why the CP happened. Many etiologies can be separated into a time period as to when these insults occurred. For more detailed information on the etiologies of CP, readers are referred to the book *The Cerebral Palsies* by Miller and Clarke,[1] which provides much greater detail on this specific topic.

Congenital Etiologies

A whole group of congenital developmental deformities lead to CP. These deformities result from defects that occur in normal development and follow patterns based on failures of normal formation (Figure 2.1). A defect of the neural tube closure is the earliest recognized deformity leading to survival with motor defects. The most common neural tube defect occurs in the spine and is known as meningomyelocele. However, this lesion typically does not cause CP, but instead causes spinal-level paralysis. In the brain, the neural tube defect is called an encephalocele, and may be anterior, with a major midface or nasal defect. Anterior encephaloceles occurs most commonly in Asia, whereas posterior encephaloceles most often occur in Western Europe and America and affect the posterior occiput.[1] The cause of this regional difference is unknown; however, just as folate used during pregnancy has been found to protect against myelomeningocele development, it is believed to protect against the development of encephalocele as well.[1–3] Some encephaloceles are related to larger syndromes, such as Meckel's syndrome.[4] This syndrome includes encephalocele with microcephaly, renal dysplasia, and polydactyly and is due to a defect on the 17th chromosome, specifically in the homeobox gene (HOX B6). This information suggests that many of these deformities may have unrecognized genetic causes. Most children with significant encephaloceles have very significant motor impairments, usually quadriplegic pattern involvement with more hypotonia than hypertonia.

Segmental defects in the brain are called schizencephaly, meaning there is a cleft in the brain.[5] These schizencephalies vary greatly, from causing minimal disability to causing very severe quadriplegic pattern involvement, usually with spasticity and mental retardation. Several patients with severe forms have genetic defects in the homeobox genes.

Primary proliferation defects of the brain lead to microencephaly. However, there are many causes of microencephaly, most involving toxins or infections, which are discussed later. Conditions in which the brain is too large are called megaloencephaly, which should not be confused with macroencephaly, meaning a head that is too large. Megaloencephaly is caused by

A

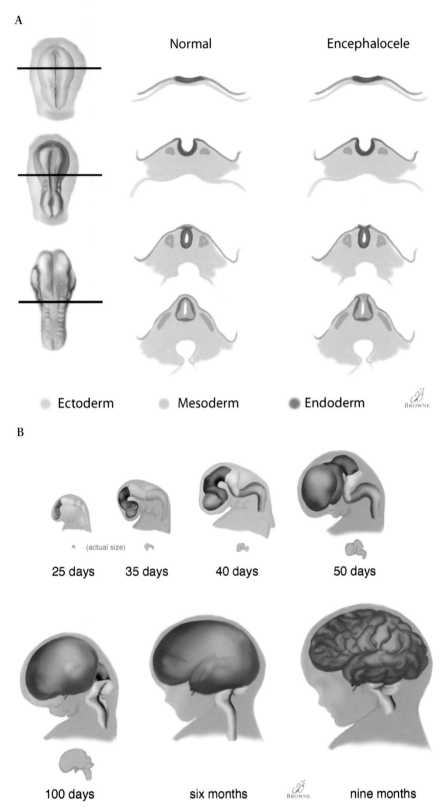

Normal　　　　　Encephalocele

Ectoderm　　Mesoderm　　Endoderm

B

25 days　　35 days　　40 days　　50 days

100 days　　six months　　nine months

Figure 2.1. In the earliest stage, the neural plate differentiates from the ectoderm, then enfolds to create a neural tube. Failure of this enfolding causes neural tube defects (A). During the embryonic stage, this neural tube develops complex folding with the formation of flexures. During the period of 30 to 100 days of embryonic life, the brain demarcates and develops the cerebral hemispheres. During the rest of gestation, there is a large growth of mass and cell specialization (B).

Figure 2.2. As the brain matures, the cells proliferate centrally and migrate toward the cortex. During this migration, trailing connections remain to the deep layer. This migration is an important element in the formation of the gyri of the cerebral cortex. Defects in the migration lead to a smooth brain surface called lissencephaly.

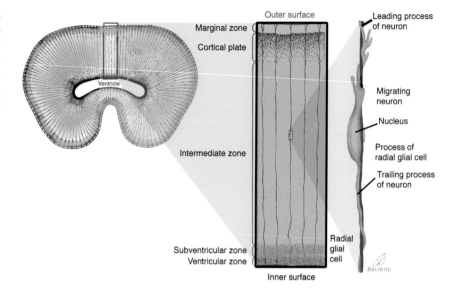

cellular hyperproliferation, usually in syndromes such as sebaceous nevus syndrome, whereas macrocephaly most often is due to hydrocephalus.

During development, the neurons migrate toward the periphery of the brain, and a defect in this migration pattern leads to lissencephaly, meaning a smooth brain, or a child with decreased cerebral gyri. Lissencephaly usually leads to severe spastic quadriplegic pattern involvement, but there is a significant range of involvement. Lissencephaly is X-linked in a few cases. The opposite of too few gyri seen in lissencephaly is polymicrogyria, in which there are too many small gyri (Figure 2.2).[1]

A large and variable group of children have differing degrees of cortical dysgenesis, which is a disorder of brain cortex formation. This disorder may be called focal cortical dysplasia and presents mainly with seizure disorders. The motor effects may vary from none to very severe and from hypotonia to hypertonia.

Another part of normal development of the brain in the neonatal and prenatal period requires formation of the synapses and then subsequent remodeling of this neuronal synapse formation. As the cells migrate into the correct position and initially form their synapses, many of these premature synapses need to be remodeled through the influence of external stimuli for normal function to develop. The classic demonstration of this principle was shown in the experiment in which eyes of kittens, one each kitten, were sewn closed at birth. The eye that was denied light stimulation became cortically blind; however, the opposite eye that did get light and normal stimulation became overrepresented in the cortex of the brain.[6] This experiment has become the basis for treating and understanding amblyopia, or lazy eye, in children. The synaptic remodeling and formation, also called synaptic plasticity in older ages, continues throughout life and is the basis for much of learning. The nature of this synaptic remodeling potential changes with age as demonstrated by the example with the kittens. If the kitten whose eye was sewn shut is denied light stimulation until a certain age, it can no longer recover the ability for sight in that eye.[6]

This concept of synaptic formation and remodeling has been the basis of some therapy programs, specifically the patterning therapy proposed by Doman and Delacatta.[6-8] There is no scientific evidence to suggest that the human gait generator can be accessed and impacted in the same way one can treat lazy eye at an early age in children. However, there is a general understanding that significant seizure activity in a young child may prevent synaptic remodeling through excitotoxic injury, which leads to CP. Inappropriate synaptic formation and remodeling, or remodeling alone, has been implicated as the major neurologic anatomic pathology in Down syndrome, Rett syndrome, autism, and fragile X syndrome as well as many cases of ataxia, idiopathic spasticity, and mental retardation in which there is no other recognized etiology.[1]

Neonatal Etiologies

Neonatal and prenatal causes of CP are mainly related to prematurity and birthing problems, which lead to various injury patterns. However, the immature brain has much more equipotentiality or plasticity, both of which are terms used to define the much greater ability of an uninjured part of the immature brain to assume the function of an injured part. This potential of the immature brain to reassign function makes the response to injury much different than in the mature brain.

Prematurity and brain hemorrhages are much better understood since the widespread use of cranial ultrasound, in which the infant brain can be imaged through the open anterior fontanelle. This image provides an excellent view of the ventricles and the periventricular white matter. This is the area where hemorrhages occur, and major risk factors for developing hemorrhages are younger gestational age and mechanical ventilation. Bleeding in the ventricle is called intraventricular hemorrhage (IVH), and bleeding in the periventricular area is called germinal matrix hemorrhage (GMH), or it may be combined in a term called periventricular-intraventricular hemorrhage (PIVH). A common grading system for the severity of these hemorrhage patterns includes grade I with germinal matrix hemorrhage only, grade II with hemorrhage in the lateral ventricle and dilation of the lateral ventricle, grade III with ventricular system enlargement, and grade IV with periventricular hemorrhage and infarctions (Figure 2.3). Reported prognostic significance of these grades varies greatly, and the general consensus is that premature infants with no PIVH have a better survival prognosis than those with PIVH.[1] Also, in group studies, the more severe the grade, the higher the risk of developing CP, as demonstrated in a study that reported the risk of CP was 9% in grade I, 11% in grade II, 36% in grade III, and 76% in grade IV.[9] However, different studies vary significantly, so good consensus values are not currently available.

These cerebral hemorrhages evolve from GMH and IVH, which develop in the first 72 hours after birth. The brain bleeds then resolve, and periventricular leukomalacia (PVL) develops 1 to 3 weeks after birth in some children. Periventricular leukomalacia in the form of periventricular echogenicity (PVE) may be seen on ultrasound, but does not develop cysts. If cysts develop, it is called cystic periventricular leukomalacia (PVC). In general, infants with PVC have the highest risk of developing CP and infants with PVE have the lowest risk.[10] In one study, 10% of children developed CP if they had PVE; however, 65% developed CP if they had PVC.[9] Again, these numbers vary between studies. The general trend is that premature infants with more severe bleeds have a worse prognosis for survival and a higher risk for developing CP; however, there are no specific parameters that fully predict risk of developing CP or, much less, predict the severity of CP in an individual child.

Hypoxic events occurring around delivery, usually in full-term infants, also lead to disability. These events have been termed hypoxic-ischemic

Figure 2.3. Bleeding in the immature brain occurs primarily around the ventricles, which have many fragile vessels. Intraventricular hemorrhage (IVH) means bleeding into the ventricles. Germinal matrix hemorrhage (GMH) means bleeding into the tissue around the ventricles. Periventricular intraventricular hemorrhage (PIVH) means bleeding into both areas. Periventricular cysts (PVC) form in these same areas as the acute hemorrhage resolves.

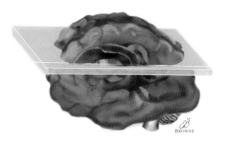

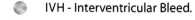 IVH - Interventricular Bleed.

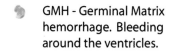 GMH - Germinal Matrix hemorrhage. Bleeding around the ventricles.

PIVH - Periventricular and Interventricular hemorrhage.

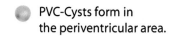 PVC-Cysts form in the periventricular area.

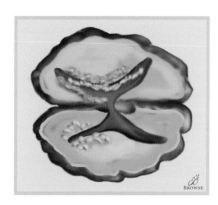

encephalopathy (HIE). The causes of this hypoxia may vary from obstetric dystocias to other anoxic and low-flow states in the neonate. In severe cases of HIE, subcortical cyst formation develops and is called multicystic encephalomalacia. In general, when this cystic pattern forms, the prognosis for good function is poor, with most of these children developing severe quadriplegic pattern involvement with severe mental retardation. Some of these children develop cysts in the thalamus and basal ganglia, which may lead to dystonia.[1]

Neonatal stroke occurring in the preterm or full-term infant usually involves the middle cerebral artery and presents as a wedge-shaped defect in one hemisphere. These defects may develop as cysts, which, if very large, are called porencephaly or porencephalic cysts. In general, if these wedge-shaped defects are small, the children may be normal; however, a significant defect especially with a cyst usually presents as hemiplegic pattern CP. Even with large cysts, these children's function, especially cognitive function, may be quite good.

Postnatal Causes of Cerebral Palsy

Postnatal causes of CP may overlap somewhat with the prenatal and neonatal group; however, postnatal trauma, metabolic encephalopathy, infections, and toxicities are considered as etiologies in this group. Although the data are difficult to assimilate, between 10% and 25% of CP cases have a postnatal cause.[11,12]

Child abuse or nonaccidental trauma causing brain injury in a young child may be due to blunt trauma with skull fractures or fall into the pattern of shaken baby syndrome. Shaken baby syndrome occurs usually in a child less than 1 year of age when a caretaker shakes the baby back and forth to quiet the crying. This vigorous shaking causes stretching, shearing, and tear-

A   B

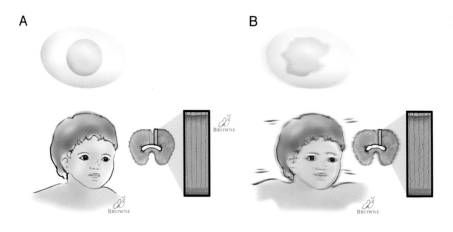

Figure 2.4. Shaken baby syndrome creates an injury in which axons are disrupted by the shear forces created from the violent shaking of the head. The brain of the baby is like an egg in which the liquid center is enclosed in a solid outer shell. By vigorous shaking, the egg yolk can be broken without breaking the shell of the egg. In the same way, vigorous shaking of a baby's head can cause tissue disruption. This shearing stress disrupts brain tissue, especially the long migrating axons of the cerebral cortex. The trauma of the shaken baby does not usually cause a skull fracture and may not even cause intracranial bleeding, but it often causes severe long-term neurologic impairment because of the cellular disruptions.

ing of the long axons and capillaries in the cortex of the brain (Figure 2.4). If these babies survive, they often have a severe spastic quadriplegic pattern involvement with a poor prognosis for improvement.[5] Even children with less severe motor involvement often have a concomitant profound mental retardation.

Blunt head trauma may also occur from child abuse, falls, or motor vehicle accidents, and it involves the direct injury as well as the secondary injury from brain swelling. Most children with blunt trauma recover and have no motor defects.[13] However, if there is a unilateral bleed, these children are often left with a hemiplegic pattern motor disability. The more severely involved children are usually left with a severe quadriplegic pattern involvement and do not become functional community ambulators. Many children with motor impairments from closed head injuries have ataxia as a major impairment.

Children with closed head injuries will make substantial improvement for 1 year after the injury and only in rare severe cases should surgical treatment of secondary problems, such as contractures, be considered during this year. Also, many children continue to improve even through the third year after injury; therefore, it is probably best not to consider the lesion static until 3 years after the injury.[14] Even then, these lesions continue to evolve in some individuals, with the well-recognized syndrome in which early spasticity resolves but then dystonic movements later develop in the previously spastic limb. This syndrome has been reported to occur up to 9 years after closed head injury, even when it seemed that all the spasticity had resolved.[15] We have seen recurrent dystonia become most severe during and after puberty, as the hormonal surge somehow makes it worse.

Metabolic encephalopathy has a wide variety of causes, most extremely rare. It is impossible to give a comprehensive review in this text, and when specific cases are encountered, it is important to obtain disease-specific up-to-date recommendations from the subspecialized expert who is managing the care of the child. Also, the neuro-orthopaedist should have a good reference text available, such as the Aicardi text *Diseases of the Nervous System in Childhood*.[16] The metabolic disorders can be divided into storage disorders, intermedullary metabolism disorders, metallic metabolism, and miscellaneous disorders (Table 2.1).

It is extremely important for physicians caring for children's motor problems to understand the expected course of the disease. For example, many of the storage disorders are progressive and these children have limited life expectancy, which limits attempts to correct motor impairments that are not

Table 2.1. Metabolic neurologic diseases.

Name	Primary defect	Typical course	Significance for surgical management
Storage diseases	intercellular accumulation	Most of these have no treatment and are progressive	
Gangliosidoses	Hexosaminidase defect, multiple types	Each type has its own course	
Tay–Sachs disease	HexA and HexB nonfunctional due to chromosome 15 defect	Short-term survival in childhood	
Sandhoff's disease	Type O gangliosidosis	Clinically like Tay–Sachs	
GM1 gangliosidosis	Multiple subtypes, beta-galactosidase deficiency	Rare cases and variable effects	
Gaucher's disease	Multiple types, beta-glucocerebrosidase deficient	Outcome is variable, based on the subtype, from rapid course with death in early childhood to relatively mild involvement	Most patients have hepatosplenomegly Be especially aware of significant splenomegly Also, bone lesion from the storage disease may be present
Niemann–Pick disease	Sphingomyelinase deficient, multiple subtypes	The more severe types have rapid degeneration and death; some mild types may have minimal involvement and life into middle adulthood	Bone marrow may be involved, and some patients develop a peripheral neuropathy
Fabry's disease	Sex-linked deficiency of ceramide trihexoside	Foam cells with vacuolated cytoplasm develop in muscles, nervous system, kidneys	Death is usually from cardiac or renal failure Females are less affected May begin as severe muscle pain Renal failure may occur
Metachromatic leukodystrophy	Cerebroside sulfatase deficiency, multiple types	Often presents as a gait disorder in childhood May initially look like a neuropathy Adult forms present as behavior problems	
Krabbe's disease (globoid cell leukodystrophy)	Beta-galactocerebrosidase deficiency	Age of onset, and survival, are variable	May present with slow-onset hemiplegia or diplegia
Mucopolysaccharidosis	All have deficiencies of lysomal glucosidase or sulfatase	Often the neurologic problems are less severe than the systemic ones	Bone marrow transplantation is used to treat a number of these conditions
Hurler's syndrome	—	Severe neurologic retardation	Severe dwarfism Cervical instability
Scheie's syndrome	—	Types, very mild to minimal problems	Hydrocephalus may develop
Hunter's syndrome	—	Severe dwarfism	Mild to moderate neurologic involvement
Sanfilippo's syndrome	—	Severe progressive neurologic involvement	Minimal skeletal problems
Morquio's syndrome	—	Variable forms but marker bone involvement	Cervical instability may cause spinal cord compression
Maroteaux–Lamy's syndrome	—	No neurologic involvement Severe dwarfism	Nerve entrapment syndromes are common Mild to severe bone and neurologic involvement
Sly's syndrome	—	Very variable	Mild to severe bone and neurologic involvement
Mucolipidosis, sialidosis, glycoprotein metabolism deficiency	—	Many types, all very rare	
Sialidosis type one	Also called cherry red spot myoclonus syndrome	Slow progression No other involvement	Late onset Has a pure intention myoclonus that slowly gets worse with age
Mucolipidosis IV	—	Failing vision and mental delay after normal infancy	May develop dystonia

Table 2.1. Continued.

Name	Primary defect	Typical course	Significance for surgical management
Mannosidosis	Alpha-mannosidase deficiency	Several types, usually with cognitive limits and minimal progression	
Fucosidosis	Fucosidase deficiency	Progressive mental retardation	Develop significant spasticity
Galactosialidosis	Neuraminidase and beta-galactosidase deficiency	Develops progressive myoclonus and extrapyramidal signs	Thoracolumbar spinal deformity may be present
Salla disease	Sialic acid transport deficiency	Mental and motor retardation, progressive	Course varies
Aspartylglycoaminuria		Has mental deterioration in late childhood or adolescence	Causes bone deformities, mitral valve insufficiency
Pompe's disease		Hypotonia	Severe mental retardation Early death
Batten disease (infantile form)	Neuronal ceroid-lipofuscinosis	Severe brain atrophy	Anxiety and autistic behavior Death after a prolonged vegetative state Has repetitive hand movements that may be confused with Rett syndrome
Spielmeyer–Vogt–Sjogren (juvenile form)		Condition starts in middle childhood	Slower course Death in 15–30 years
Kufs' disease (adult form)		Present with behavioral changes and dementia	
Amino acid metabolism	Many causes, only those more relevant included		
Phenylketonuria (PKU)	A defect in the hydroxylation of phenylalanine to tyrosine; the defect may occur in one of two enzymes or two required cofactors	Untreated children develop severe mental retardation and self-abuse	With early dietary treatment most of the symptoms can be avoided Requires treatment until age 4–8 years
Hyperphenylalaninemia (HPA)	Same as PKU		
Maple syrup urine disease	Organic aciduria; many subtypes	Disease varies from rapid progression to later onset or minimal progression	May cause acute coma Treatment varies by the specific defect Most of these conditions cause most of the problems during periods of stress when the body may depend on protein metabolism for energy source; this is especially true during major surgical procedures and can usually be avoided by using high-glucose infusion such as a 10% glucose solution intra- and postoperatively Blood pH level needs to be monitored and urine should be monitored for ketosis If proper precautions are not taken, ketoacidosis, hyperammonemia, and hyperlacticemia may develop and cause cerebral edema with further neurologic injury
Glutaric aciduria	Glutaryl-CoA dehydrogenase deficiency	Several types	Untreated neurologic effects leave the child with severe dystonia Cognitive process more preserved Stress causes a ketoacidosis, which causes brain injury Neurologic effects can be avoided with early dietary treatment Must take all the same precautions as noted for maple syrup urine disease

(continued)

Table 2.1. Continued.

Name	Primary defect	Typical course	Significance for surgical management
Homocystinuria	Cystathionine beta-synthase deficiency	Cause mental retardation and spasticity	Develop dislocated lens Also have thromboembolic disorder May present with a Charlie Chaplin-like walk Other common bone deformities include pectus, genu valgum, biconcave vertebra, epimetaphyseal widening Because of the thromboembolic problems, even children should probably have anticoagulation during surgical procedures
Sulfite oxidase deficiency		During infancy children have poor feeding, severe seizures, and present with quadriplegic pattern motor involvement Usually die in early childhood	
Tyrosinemia		Present with liver failure and neuropathy	Also often complain of severe leg pain Course is variable
Tetrahydrobiopterin deficiencies ("malignant HPA")	Same pathway as PKU and HPA	Children have progressive deterioration even with appropriate dietary treatment Children have progressive spasticity and limb rigidity Sometimes with dystonia or athetosis	Clinical course is variable
Nonketotic hyperglycinemia	Glycine accumulates because it cannot be metabolized	Course is usually with severe seizures and short-term survival, although some develop a more typical spastic CP pattern	
4-Hydroxybutyric aciduria	GABA neurotransmitter metabolism error	Presents with a static hypotonia and ataxia	
Urea cycle disorders	Ammonia accumulation causes brain injury	There are a number of different deficiencies, all with a similar presentation, but with varying severity	These conditions are like maple syrup urine disease in that during stress periods, such as acute sepsis or major surgical procedures, patients must be protected from high protein metabolism, which will cause the ammonia level to raise, running the risk of developing cerebral edema; this can be prevented with high-glucose fluid infusion, usually using 10% dextrose
Citrullinemia			Hepatomegly common
Argininosuccinic aciduria			Often have brittle hair Hepatomegly common
Arginase deficiency			Usually presents as a quadriplegic pattern CP with progressive spasticity
Vitamin metabolism disorders	Many are autosomal dominant inherited		
Multiple carboxylase deficiency	Impairment of the biotin recycling pathway	Skin rash, hypotonia, seizures, ataxia	Symptoms improve with high-dose biotin treatment
Vitamin B_{12} metabolism defect		Anemia, seizures, mirocephaly, pancytopenia, malabsorption Variable presentation	
Folate metabolism defect		Similar to B_{12} deficiency	

Table 2.1. Continued.

Name	Primary defect	Typical course	Significance for surgical management
Lactic acidosis (respiratory chain disorders)	Defect in the terminal step of the energy production cycle		The workup and diagnosis of many of these conditions require a skeletal muscle biopsy because the muscle is often involved This biopsy is also how to study mitochondrial function
Mitochondrial cytopathy		Usually presents in early infancy or early childhood with delayed motor skills, fatigue, muscle pains	The response is variable, from long static period to spontaneous improvement to sudden deterioration
Multisystem disorders			
Kearns–Sayre syndrome		Normal at birth	Develop headaches, mental retardation, peripheral neuropathy
Mitochondrial myopathy	Ragged red muscle fibers	Often present with stroke-like symptoms between childhood and young adulthood	High incidence of heart block and, if surgery is planned, the team needs to be prepared to insert a cardiac pacemaker
Alpers syndrome	Many different defects are probably causing this clinical syndrome	Autosomal recessive condition of progressive spastic quadriplegic pattern CP syndrome	
Leigh syndrome	Syndrome defined by necrotizing encephalomyelopathy Probably has multiple molecular causes	Course is extremely variable but usually progressive, although there may be long static periods	
Lactic acidosis			
Pyruvate dehydrogenase deficiency	Defect of pyruvate entry to mitochondria	Presents with highly variable hypotonia, seizures, failure to thrive	Some die in early childhood and others survive long term with a severe quadriplegic CP pattern
Mitochondrial fatty acid defects		Very variable with muscle weakness, cardiomyopathy, seizures	
Carnitine deficiency	Because of inability to metabolize protein, depends on glucose for energy	Presents in childhood with muscle weakness and cardiomyopathy	Under stress, such as major surgery, must give high-glucose infusion or there will be no energy even for the heart to function
Peroxisomal disorders	All have autosomal recessive inheritance		
Zellweger syndrome		Hypotonia	Poor swallowing Failure to thrive Develop severe equinovarus feet and flexion contractures Stippled calcification in the bones, especially the patella
Adrenoleukodystrophy		Same as Zellweger but milder form	
Refsum's disease		Similar but is the mildest form	
X-linked adrenoleukodystrophy		Variable, but males are always more affected than females	
Rhizomelic chondrodysplasia punctata		Rhizomelic dwarf with joint contractures	Calcification in the epiphysis and soft tissues Also with mental retardation
Wilson disease	Disorder of copper metabolism	Early on have facial masking, then develop tremor	Later develop a Parkinson-like presentation with psychiatric problems Have hepatic dysfunction When giving medication, must consider liver function
Lesch–Nyhan syndrome	X-linked	Very variable course and usually presents with hypotonia, torsional dystonia, mental retardation, self-abuse	Develop gouty arthritis
Enzyme defect allowing			

seriously disabling. Alternately, many disorders of intermedullary metabolism have acute insults during toxic events before the diagnosis has been made. With proper management, these disorders become static and mimic similar children with CP.

These metabolic disorders often require very specific management protocols during surgery. An example of such a condition is glutaric aciduria type 1, which presents with infants who are normal. When an infant experiences a stress, such as a childhood illness with a high fever, an acidosis develops that causes damage to the brain, especially the putamen and caudate areas. This insult leaves the child with a wide range of spastic and movement disorders, often with significant dystonia.[17] This neurologic disorder is static if the proper dietary management is carried out; therefore, the orthopaedist can approach this child similarly to a child with CP. However, these children must be prevented from becoming acidotic during operative procedures by infusing high levels of glucose, usually using a 10% dextrose solution as the intravenous fluid.

A wide variety of infections leave children with permanent neurologic deficits. Most of these deficits are static and therefore definitely fall into the CP diagnosis group. Prenatal and neonatal viral infections are the most common infectious cause of CP. Cytomegalovirus (CMV) leaves 90% of children with mental retardation and deafness, but only 50% develop CP or motor defects. Children who develop congenital rubella infections very commonly will have mental retardation; however, only 15% develop CP.[1] Neonatal herpes simplex infection has a high mortality rate, and 30% to 60% of survivors have some neurologic sequelae, although CP is not common. In utero varicella zoster infection causes high rates of CP. This same high rate is seen in lymphacytic choriomeningitis, which is a rodent-borne arenavirus. All these conditions cause neurologic insults that are static and should be treated as CP. Infections with human immunodeficiency virus (HIV) may cause neurologic sequelae; however, this is a progressive encephalopathy and these children should be treated anticipating a very short life expectancy. The most common parasite is *Toxoplasma gondii,* which is an intracellular parasite whose most common host is the household cat. With aggressive medical treatment, the infection can be eradicated, and approximately 30% of children are left with CP and mental retardation. Neonatal bacterial meningitis may be caused by many organisms and may be very severe, with as many as 30% to 50% of survivors having CP.[1] In our experience, most of these children who survive bacterial meningitis and have CP will have very severe spastic quadriplegic pattern involvement.

Temporary neurologic deficits are caused by many toxic agents, with alcohol being the most commonly encountered. Alcohol almost never causes a static neurologic deficit. Also, children with prolonged anoxic events, such as near drowning, near hanging, or near asphyxia, can make remarkable recoveries. However, when these children do not recover completely, they are usually left with extremely severe neurologic deficits and are among the most neurologically disabled individuals in our practice. These children tend to be relatively healthy and, in spite of severe neurologic deficits, tend to grow and thrive physically with good nursing care. One child in our practice has been ventilator dependent for 10 years from an anoxic event at age 9 months.

As noted in the beginning of this chapter, knowing the exact etiology is not always important to care for children's motor disabilities; however, it is important to understand whether these lesions are static or not. Also, parents may be more relaxed if physicians and therapists have some understanding of the specific etiology, if known, of their children's problems.

Epidemiology

Because of the wide variety of causes of CP, the exact numbers from different studies do not completely agree. However, there is remarkable similarity in the prevalence across the world, from Sweden in the 1980s with a prevalence of 2.4 per 1000[18] and 2.5 per 1000 in the early 1990s,[19] 2.3 per 1000 from Atlanta,[11] and 1.6 per 1000 in China.[20] Considering the difficulty in making specific diagnoses, and especially finding mild cases, these numbers probably reflect much more variation in counting than clear differences in prevalence. A report from England, which is representative of many studies, shows that there has not been much change in prevalence over the past 40 years. However, the patterns of CP have shifted more toward diplegia and spastic quadriplegia and away from hemiplegia and athetosis.[21] This change probably reflects increased medical care with better obstetric care and some increased incidence from survivors of neonatal intensive care units. Also, multiple births have increased with increasing maternal age,[22] and these multiple births have a substantially higher risk of developing CP. The reported prevalence rate per pregnancy for singles is 0.2%, for twins 1.5%, for triplets 8.0%, and for quadruplets 43%.[23]

Terminology and Classification

Although understanding the specific etiology of CP is not very helpful for physicians treating motor problems, by segmenting this very diverse condition by cause, patterns that are useful in planning treatment can be identified. There are many ways of classifying CP, one of which is by etiology. However, for the treatment of motor disabilities it is much more important to classify children by anatomic pattern and specific neuromotor impairments than by the cause of the CP. Classifying CP in this way provides a framework in which to discuss the functional problems of individuals in their whole environment.

A framework for understanding individuals with limited motor function has been agreed to at an international forum held in 1980, organized by the World Health Organization (WHO). The report is entitled "Classification of Impairments, Disabilities and Handicaps."[24] In this report, the term "impairment" defines the primary lesion and pathology, such as the problem with the brain that caused the spasticity, and includes the direct effects of the spasticity, such as the dislocated hip caused by the spastic muscles. "Disability" is used to mean the loss of function that individuals experience because of the impairment; therefore, the inability to walk or sit well is a disability arising from the impairment. The "handicap" is the result of limits in the environment and society, which limit individuals as a result of their specific disability. Therefore, an individual who uses a wheelchair has a handicap if he wants to visit a friend and the only way into the house is up a long flight of stairs. This inability to socialize is the handicap and, for many adults, is what impedes them from being integrated into full society of jobs, friends, and social entertainment.

In 1993, the National Center for Medical Rehabilitation Research (NCMRR) added to the WHO classification by dividing impairments into "pathophysiology" and "impairment." In this classification, "pathophysiology" refers to the primary problem, such as the brain lesion, and "impairment" refers to the secondary effects, such as spasticity and the dislocated hip. "Functional impairment" was added to reflect the inability to do activities

Figure 2.5. The WHO initially developed a model for disability that was later expanded by the USA National Center for Medical Rehabilitation Research. The concepts of both models are similar, with a focus that expands the understanding that problems of function are related beyond the isolated anatomic problem of an individual person.

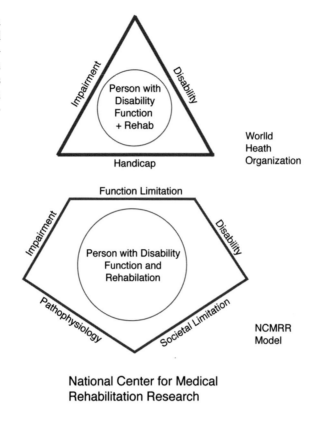

National Center for Medical Rehabilitation Research

such as walking that is a direct result of the impairment. "Disability" has retained almost its original meaning, and "handicap" has been renamed "societal limitations" to clarify where the problem of the limitation arises.[25] Although there are some merits to the changes NCMRR made to the WHO report for research purposes, the complexity does not work well in thought of daily practice; therefore, in the remainder of this text, the WHO definitions and terminology are used (Figure 2.5).

Anatomic Classification

The most useful primary classification for children with CP is based on the anatomic pattern of involvement. This involvement is the first classification used by physicians treating motor impairments, as it gives a very general sense of severity and a general overview of what patients' problems likely are. Classification into hemiplegia, which involves one half of the body; diplegia, which involves primarily the lower extremities with mild upper extremity involvement; and quadriplegia, which involves all four limbs, is most useful. In general, individuals with hemiplegia and diplegia can walk, and those with quadriplegia use wheelchairs as their primary mobility device. For patients who do not clearly fit these patterns, many other names have been suggested. Double hemiplegia has been suggested for children with upper and lower extremity involvement that is much more severe on one side than the other. Triplegia has been suggested for individuals who have a hemiplegic pattern on one side and a diplegic pattern in the lower extremities. There are rare children who appear to have hemiplegia and diplegia, which would make anatomic sense, so this term triplegia has some merit; however, it does not aid in treatment planning.

Monoplegia is used when one limb is primarily involved; however, from a motor treatment perspective, these children are treated as if they had mild hemiplegia. In North America, the term paraplegia implies a pure lower extremity paralysis and is used only for spinal cord paralysis because almost all children with brain origin disability will also have some upper extremity involvement, although it may be very minor. Pentiplegia is occasionally used to define the most severely impaired individuals who have no independent head control. This term adds little over the use of quadriplegia in planning motor impairment treatment; therefore, it has not gained widespread use.

Evolutionary Pathology

Even though there are many causes of CP, there are few recurring anatomic patterns of involvement because damage to specific areas, regardless of how the damage occurs, creates similar patterns of impairment. However, a specific region of brain injury can cause variation in the impairments because the initial injury also overlies normal development, which continues after the injury. Because all these injuries occur in the young and immature brain, growth and development over time affects the impairment. A brain injury occurring in early pregnancy, meaning most congenital syndromes, has a different presentation than an injury occurring in a 4-year-old child.

The first aspect of this pathology is to understand the presence of very early primitive reflexes that should disappear as normal children grow. The cutaneous reflexes, mainly finger and toe grasp, occur with stroking of the skin on the palm or on the sole. The sucking and rooting reflexes are similarly initiated with stroking of the face and lips (Figure 2.6). The labyrinthine reflex is a response to the inner ear being stimulated by changing a child's position (Figure 2.7). When held prone, a child will flex, and when placed supine, a child will extend. The proprioceptive reflexes are initiated by stimulating the stretch receptors in the muscles and the position sensors in the joints. This reflex creates the asymmetric tonic neck reflex (ATNR) such that when the head is turned to one side, the leg and arm on that side extend (Figure 2.8). The symmetric tonic neck reflex (STNR) causes the arms to flex and

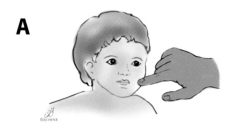

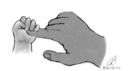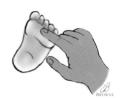

Figure 2.6. The most primitive reflex is the sucking reflex, which is stimulated by contact of the infant's perioral area (A). The hand (B) and toe grip (C) grasp reflexes are also present at birth and are stimulated by stroking the palm or plantar surfaces. Babies' early lives are dependent on the sucking reflex and, before high-level medical care, babies who lacked the sucking reflex always died.

Figure 2.7. The tonic labyrinth reflex shows the baby with abducted shoulders, flexed elbows, adducted extended hips, and extended knees and ankles. This posture primarily occurs with the baby in the supine position.

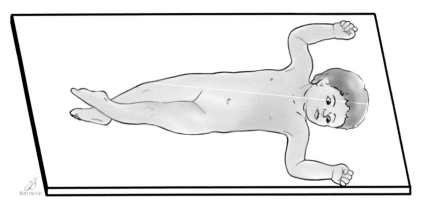

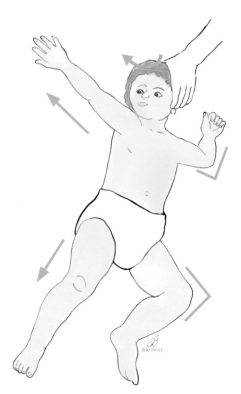

Figure 2.8. The asymmetric tonic neck reflex is activated by turning the child's head. The side to which the face turns causes the shoulder to abduct with elbow and hand extension. The leg on the same side also develops full extension. On the opposite side, the shoulder is also abducted but the elbow and hand are fully flexed and the leg is flexed at the hip, knee, and ankle. By turning the head to the opposite side, the pattern reverses.

the legs to extend when the neck is flexed, and the opposite happens when the neck is extended. Both the ATNR and the STNR are suppressed by age 6 months.[26] The moro reflex is a sudden abduction and extension of the upper extremity with finger extension when a child is lifted, followed by shoulder adduction, elbow flexion, and closing of the hand as the child becomes comfortable again (Figure 2.9). Usually, this reflex is absent by 6 months of age. The parachute reflex occurs when a child is held upside down and lowered toward the floor. If the response is positive, which should occur by age 12 months,[26] the child should extend the arms in anticipation of landing on the hands (Figure 2.10). The step reflex, also known as foot placement response, occurs when the dorsum of the foot is stimulated; the child will flex the hip and knee and dorsiflex the foot in a stepping response. Usually, this reflex is suppressed by age 3 years (Figure 2.11). It is important to separate this reflex stepping, which some parents occasionally discover, from volun-

A

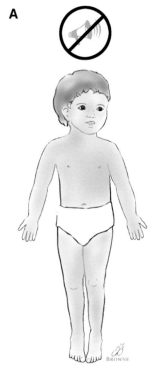

B

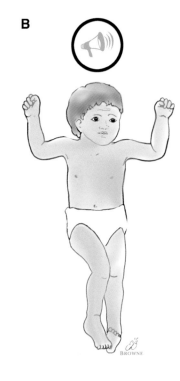

Figure 2.9. The Moro reflex is initiated with a loud noise, such as a hand clap, that causes the child to have full extension of the head, neck, and back. The shoulders abduct and the elbows extend. The legs also have full extension. After a short time, the pattern reverses and the head, neck, and spine flex; the arms are brought to the midline; and the legs flex.

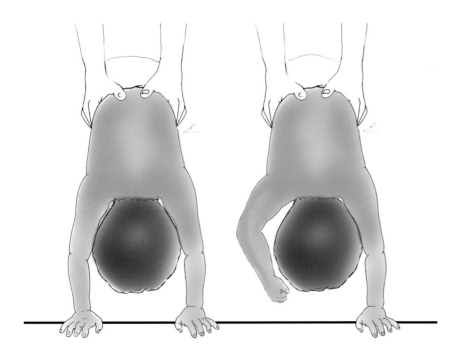

Figure 2.10. The parachute reaction is initiated by holding the child at the pelvis and tipping him head down. As the child is lowered toward the floor, he should extend the arms as if he were going to catch himself with his arms. This self-protection response should be present by 11 months of age. If the child has hemiplegia he will often only reach out with the extremity that is not affected. The affected extremity may remain flexed, or will extend at the shoulder and elbow but with the hand kept fisted.

tary step initiation. So long as a child's only stepping is the step reflex, the prognosis for achieving full gait is limited.

Although the presence of these reflexes after they should have disappeared is a negative neurologic sign, we have not found them helpful in making a specific prognosis as outlined by Bleck, who reported that the presence

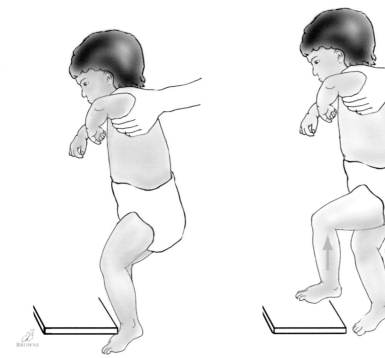

Figure 2.11. The foot placement reaction or step reflex is initiated with the child held under the arms or by the chest. When the dorsum of the foot is stimulated at the edge of a table, the child will flex the hip and knee, simulating a stepping action.

of two or more abnormal reflexes at age 7 years means a child has a poor prognosis to walk 15 meters independently. If one abnormal reflex is present, prognosis is considered guarded, and if no abnormal reflexes are present by age 7 years, the prognosis for walking is good.[26] Clearly, the absence of a parachute reflex at 18 months of age with persistent ATNR is not a good combination; however, it is not an absolute bad prognosis either. The presence of significant hyperextension reflex response, demonstrating opisthotonos, is a bad prognosis for functional gain because learning control to overcome this extensor posturing is very difficult. Instead of using these rather poorly defined abnormal reflexes at age 7 years, we have found that children who are walking at age 7 should continue to walk equally as well after completion of growth; therefore, if one desires to know how well a child will walk, look at the child walking, not his abnormal reflexes. Only a minimal improvement in ambulatory ability can be expected after age 7 years in children who have had appropriate therapy and orthopaedic corrections and have the musculoskeletal system reasonably well aligned. There are exceptions to the rule that gait function has plateaued by age 7 to 8 years, and these are usually seen in children with severe cognitive deficits. The most significant exception to this rule we have seen is a 12-year-old child with severe mental retardation who refused to weight bear before age 12, then started independent ambulation at age 12.5 years.

Deviation from Normal Development

As children mature from infancy to adolescence, there are many factors occurring in tandem, all of which come together in full-sized and normal motor functioning adults. To help develop a treatment plan for children with CP, it is important to have a concept of normal development. All innate normal motor function, such as sitting, walking, jumping, running, reaching, and speaking, is a complex combination of individual motor skills that allow development of these activities of daily living. Other activities, such as playing a piano, dancing, gymnastics, and driving a car, require much more learning and practice to remain proficient. These motor activities all include volitional motor control, motor planning, balance and coordination, muscle tone, and sensory feedback of the motion.

As babies mature from infancy to 1 year of age, neurologic maturity develops rapidly from proximal to distal. To demonstrate, children first gain head control, then develop the ability to weight bear on the arms, followed by trunk control and the ability to sit, then develop the ability to stand (Table 2.2). This progressive distal migration of maturation includes all the parameters of the motor skills. An early sign of abnormalities may be the use of only one arm for weight bearing, different tone in one arm, or a different amount of muscle tone between the arms and the legs. Children who move everything randomly, but are not doing volitional movements at the age-appropriate time, may be cognitively delayed. Children who show an early preference for one side or mainly use one side will probably develop hemiplegic pattern CP. Children who do not develop distal control for standing or sitting will probably develop quadriplegic pattern CP. These deviations in normal developmental milestones are usually the first signs of neurologic problems. Each individual child has their own rate of development; therefore, when contemplating the diagnosis of CP, it is important to consider the upper range of normal instead of the mean, which is quoted in most pediatric books (see Table 2.2).

Table 2.2. Normal developmental milestones.

Gross motor skill	Mean age of development	Abnormal if not present by:
Lifts head when prone	1 month	3 months
Supports chest in prone position	3 months	4 months
Rolls prone to supine	4 months	6 months
Sits independently when placed	6 months	9 months
Pulls to stand, cruises	9 months	12 months
Walks independently	12 months	18 months
Walks up stair steps	18 months	24 months
Kicks a ball	24 months	30 months
Jumps with both feet off the floor	30 months	36 months
Hops on one foot with holding on	36 months	42 months

Source: Adapted in part from *Standards in Pediatric Orthopedics* by R.N. Hensinger.[27]

Patterns of CP can be categorized further by using the elements of motor function required for normal motor task execution. This categorization has direct implications for treatment. All mature motor activities should be under volitional control with a few exceptions of basic responses, such as the fright response or withdrawal from noxious stimuli (e.g., burning a finger). Motor activities that are not completely under volitional control are termed "movement disorders" and can be separated into tremor, chorea, athetosis, dystonia, and ballismus. Tremor, a rhythmic movement of small magnitudes that usually involves smaller joints, is not a common feature in children with CP. Chorea involves jerky movements, most commonly including the digits, and has varying degrees of magnitude of the range of motion. Athetosis is large motions of the more proximal joints, often with an extensor pattern predominating. Fanning and extension of the digits is included as a part of the proximal movement. Each patient has a relatively consistent pattern of athetosis. Dystonia is a slow motion with a torsional element, which may be localized to one limb or involve the whole body. Over time, the motions vary greatly, and the pattern may completely reverse, such as going from full-extension external rotation in the upper extremity to full flexion and internal rotation. Dystonia can be confused with spasticity because, within a very short time period, if the changes are not seen, the dystonic limb looks very similar to a spastic contracted limb. Ballismus, the most rare movement disorder, involves random motion in large, fast patterns focused on the whole limb.

Motor control and planning of specific motor patterns requires a combination of learning to plan the motor task and then execute the functional motor task. This concept is best visualized in the context of a central motor program generator, which suggests that, like computer software, there is a program in the brain that allows walking. For the more basic motions such as walking, the central program generator is part of the innate neural structure, but for others, such as learning gymnastic exercises, it is a substantially learned pattern. Children who do not have function of this basic motor generator for gait cannot walk, and there is no way to teach or implant this innate ability. If there is some damage to the brain involving the central motor generator, gait patterns such as crouched gait more typically develop, which probably represents a more immature version of bipedal gait. These gait problems are discussed further in the chapter on treating problems of gait in children with CP (see Chapter 6).

Figure 2.12. A normal child will demonstrate equilibrium reactions such that they will respond by extending the arms in the direction of the expected fall to catch themselves or by flexing forward into a ball if they are falling backward (B1). By an automatic reflex, the child will move the head in the opposite direction of the fall to prevent striking the head as the primary area of contact. A child lacking these equilibrium responses will fall over like a falling tree with no protective response when given a small push (B2). This is a very poor prognostic sign for independent ambulation, although some children can learn to control this response with appropriate therapy.

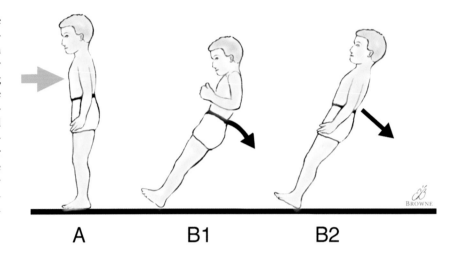

Balance, which means the ability to maintain one's position in space in a stable orientation, is required for normal motor functioning. A lack of balance causes children to overcompensate for a movement and be unable to stand in one place. Ataxia is the term used to mean abnormal balance. Also, feedback to the motion and position in space is important for maintaining motor function. In children with CP, sensory feedback may be considered part of the balance spectrum as well, but the problems that are usually considered in this spectrum do not typically come under the umbrella of ataxia. For example, when a child stands and starts to lean, the lean should be perceived and corrected. Children with ataxia often overrespond by having excessive movement in the opposite direction. Additionally, there are children who do not recognize that they are falling until they hit the floor, and as a consequence, they tend to fall like a cut tree (Figure 2.12). This pattern of sensory deficiency makes it extremely dangerous for affected children to be upright and working on walking because of the risk of sustaining an injury from a fall.

Figure 2.13. The control of human gait is very complex and poorly understood. There is some combination of feed-forward control, in which the brain uses sensory feedback and prior learning to control movement, with a closed-loop feedback system in which the brain responds by altering the control signal based on the sensory feedback of how the anticipated movement is progressing. Many movements probably use a combination of feed-forward control and feedback control.

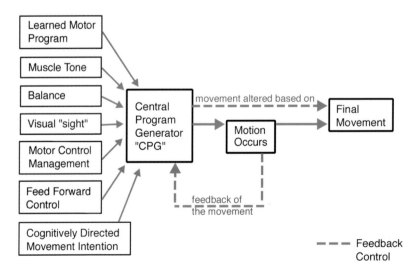

Another important aspect of normal function is muscle tone. Muscles can respond appropriately only when they generate tension; therefore, their ability to function properly requires that this tension be carefully controlled. Based on increasing understanding of controller theory developed in the field of robotics research, the inherent stiffness that adds resistance to motion is important in developing fine motor control. Motor control is a very complex area involving learning and sensory feedback with several different patterns (Figure 2.13). Normal muscle tone is probably a key element of motor functioning. Abnormalities in motor tone are the most common motor abnormalities that occur in children with CP. Increased motor tone is called spasticity. A more complete, classic definition of spasticity is a velocity-dependent increase in resistance to motion or clasp-knife stiffness, such that the tension releases with a constant torque. Usually, hyperreflexia is part of this syndrome. The opposite end of spasticity is hypotonia, which means decreased muscle tension when the joint is moved.

Making the Diagnosis

There are no agreed-upon diagnostic criteria to make the diagnosis of CP in individual children. When a child is not meeting developmental milestones, has persistent primitive reflexes, or has significant abnormalities in the elements of motor function, a diagnosis of CP can be made. The history should clearly demonstrate that this is a nonprogressive lesion and is nonfamilial. If abnormalities in developmental milestones are marginal, the term developmental delay is the appropriate diagnosis. This diagnosis implies that these children will likely catch up with their normal peers. The diagnosis of developmental delay is not appropriate for a teenager who has mental retardation and cannot walk. Developmental delay typically does not refer to major abnormalities involving elements of motor function.

Making the diagnosis of CP in a very young child may be risky unless the child has severe and definitive disabilities. There is a well-recognized phenomenon of children occasionally outgrowing CP. For this reason, we prefer to make the diagnosis in young children only when it is clear and without doubt, but wait until at least age 2 years for children who have more mild and questionable signs. Making the diagnosis is important from families' perspectives so they know what is wrong with their children; however, making the diagnosis usually does not affect treatment.

Often, how much workup should be done before the diagnosis is made is questionable, with no definitive answer. In a premature child who has been following an expected course, no workup is indicated. If a child has hemiplegia with no recognized cause, but has a typical course, it is very unlikely that a magnetic resonance imaging (MRI) scan will show anything that will impact the child's treatment. The imaging study is obtained to rule out other treatable causes such as tumors or hydrocephalus, and the imaging studies are of very little use in making a prognosis or definitive diagnosis (Case 2.1). An aggressive workup of a child may be indicated when parents are interested in knowing the risk of recurrence in another baby. These children need a full neurologic workup, sometimes including skin and muscle biopsy, to rule out genetic diseases. A referral to a knowledgeable geneticist is recommended because there is some increased risk of a second child also having neurologic problems, even if no definitive diagnosis can be made. This increased risk is probably related to an as yet undiagnosed chromosomal anomaly that causes the CP in many children.

The difficulty in making predictions extends to medical imaging, such as MRI or CT scans, during childhood. In a population, statistically more severe structural changes mean more severe motor and cognitive neurologic disability, as demonstrated by this MRI of Shawn, a boy with severe mental retardation and spastic quadriplegic CP (Figure C2.1.1). Other individuals may have equal cognitive and motor severity with a near normal MRI (Figure C2.1.2). There are also many individuals with severe structural changes on the MRI who are similar to Lauren, who is cognitively normal and has a triplegic pattern CP but ambulates using a walker (Figure C2.1.3). These cases demonstrate how important it is for physicians caring for children not to develop prejudices concerning an individual child's function based on imaging studies.

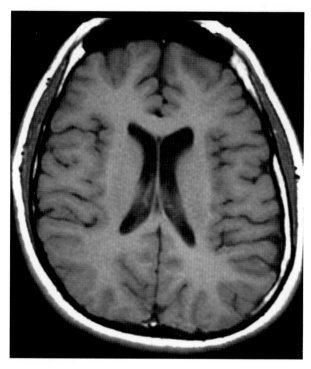

Figure C2.1.2

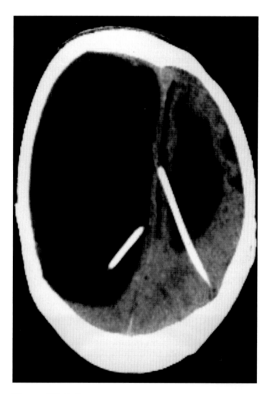

Figure C2.1.1

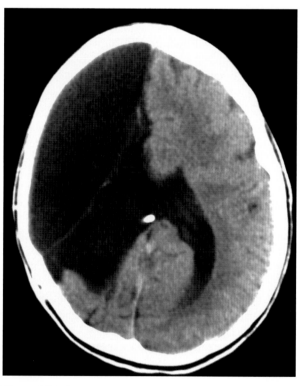

Figure C2.1.3

References

1. Miller G, Clark GD. The Cerebral Palsies: Causes, Consequences, and Management. Boston: Butterworth-Heinemann, 1998.

2. Use of folic acid for prevention of spina bifida and other neural tube defects—1983–1991. MMWR Morb Mortal Wkly Rep 1991;40:513–6.

3. Prevention of neural tube defects: results of the Medical Research Council Vitamin Study. MRC Vitamin Study Research Group [see comments]. Lancet 1991; 338:131–7.

4. Salonen R, Paavola P. Meckel syndrome. J Med Genet 1998;35:497–501.

5. Lindenberg R, Freytag E. Morphology of brain lesions from blunt trauma in early infancy. Arch Pathol 1969;87:298–305.

6. Hubel DH, Wiesel TN. The period of susceptibility to the physiological effects of unilateral eye closure in kittens. J Physiol (Lond) 1970; 206:419–36.

7. Jurcisin G. Dynamics of the Doman–Delacato creeping-crawling technique for the brain-damaged child. Am Correct Ther J 1968;22:161–4.

8. Kershner JR. Doman-Delacato's theory of neurological organization applied with retarded children. Except Child 1968;34:441–50.

9. de Vries LS, Eken P, Groenendaal F, van Haastert IC, Meiners LC. Correlation between the degree of periventricular leukomalacia diagnosed using cranial ultrasound and MRI later in infancy in children with cerebral palsy. Neuropediatrics 1993;24:263–8.

10. de Vries LS, Regev R, Dubowitz LM, Whitelaw A, Aber VR. Perinatal risk factors for the development of extensive cystic leukomalacia. Am J Dis Child 1988;142:732–5.

11. Murphy CC, Yeargin-Allsopp M, Decoufle P, Drews CD. Prevalence of cerebral palsy among ten-year-old children in metropolitan Atlanta, 1985 through 1987. J Pediatr 1993;123:S13–20.

12. O'Reilly DE, Walentynowicz JE. Etiological factors in cerebral palsy: an historical review. Dev Med Child Neurol 1981;23:633–42.

13. Jaffe KM, Polissar NL, Fay GC, Liao S. Recovery trends over three years following pediatric traumatic brain injury. Arch Phys Med Rehabil 1995;76:17–26.

14. Mahoney WJ, D'Souza BJ, Haller JA, Rogers MC, Epstein MH, Freeman JM. Long-term outcome of children with severe head trauma and prolonged coma. Pediatrics 1983;71:756–62.

15. Lee MS, Rinne JO, Ceballos-Baumann A, Thompson PD, Marsden CD. Dystonia after head trauma. Neurology 1994;44:1374–8.

16. Aicardi J. Diseases of the Nervous System in Childhood. Oxford, England: Cambridge University Press, 1992.

17. Baric I, Zschocke J, Christensen E, et al. Diagnosis and management of glutaric aciduria type I. J Inherit Metab Dis 1998;21:326–40.

18. Hagberg B, Hagberg G, Olow I, van Wendt L. The changing panorama of cerebral palsy in Sweden. VII. Prevalence and origin in the birth year period 1987–90. Acta Paediatr 1996;85:954–60.

19. Hagberg B, Hagberg G, Olow I. The changing panorama of cerebral palsy in Sweden. VI. Prevalence and origin during the birth year period 1983–1986. Acta Paediatr 1993;82:387–93.

20. Liu JM, Li S, Lin Q, Li Z. Prevalence of cerebral palsy in China. Int J Epidemiol 1999;28:949–54.

21. Colver AF, Gibson M, Hey EN, Jarvis SN, Mackie PC, Richmond S. Increasing rates of cerebral palsy across the severity spectrum in north-east England 1964–1993. The North of England Collaborative Cerebral Palsy Survey. Arch Dis Child Fetal Neonatal Ed 2000;83:F7–12.

22. Keith LG, Oleszczuk JJ, Keith DM. Multiple gestation: reflections on epidemiology, causes, and consequences. Int J Fertil Womens Med 2000;45:206–14.

23. Yokoyama Y, Shimizu T, Hayakawa K. Prevalence of cerebral palsy in twins, triplets and quadruplets. Int J Epidemiol 1995;24:943–8.

24. World Health Organization. Classification of Impairments, Disabilities, and Handicaps. Geneva, Switzerland: WHO, 1980.

25. National Institutes of Health. Research Plan for the National Center for Medical Rehabilitation Research. NIH Publication Vol. 93-3509. Bethesda, MD: NIH, 1993.
26. Bleck E. Orthopedic Management in Cerebral Palsy. Oxford: Mac Keith Press, 1987:497.
27. Hensinger RN. Standards in Pediatric Orthopedics. New York: Raven Press, 1986.

Neurologic Control of the Musculoskeletal System

Children with cerebral palsy (CP) have a large variety of motor impairments, all of which are secondary to the encephalopathy. These impairments, which directly emanate from the encephalopathy and the disability that results, are well recognized as specific problems; however, the pathophysiology connecting the encephalopathy to the impairment and the disability is not well defined. The treatment goal of children with CP is to allow them to function in their environment, ideally the larger society, to the best of their abilities. These children continue to have CP, and the changes made by the medical treatment are directed at decreasing these disabilities by altering the secondary impairments. To alter the impairments in ways that decrease the disability requires that the interaction of different impairments in a given individual must be well understood. An understanding of the neurologic control of motor activity is required to place a construct around these impairments.

Controlling the Motor System

One of the most basic functions of living organisms is the ability to control and move the body in space. After cognitive and reasoning abilities, motor function is what most defines an individual as a human being. There are wide variations of motor function in which some individuals, such as athletes, focus most of their activity on motor skills and others focus more of their attention on cognitive skills. However, even individuals such as writers who are primarily engaged in cognitive activity still depend on motor function to relate and transmit their cognitive achievements. In children with CP, loss of motor function is a major part of the disability. Motor function involves almost all tasks of living including speech, swallowing, upper extremity function, and all mobility. It is helpful to have some conceptual construct of how control of the motor system works to develop treatment strategies.

A common framework for understanding motor control is learning the anatomic structure and function of each part of the nervous system. Most physicians will remember this approach from their medical school classes. This system is too complex to yield an understanding of how the neurologic system really controls motion in a way that can be applied usefully to treat a child. This anatomically based approach aids understanding the difference between spinal cord injury and brain injury in a few children. This approach also helps explain the difference between hemiplegic and diplegic pattern CP involvement. With the anatomic approach, the nervous system can be divided into central and peripheral. The central structures include the spinal cord and brain, and the peripheral system includes the peripheral motor, sensory nerves, muscles, bones, and joints.

Anatomic Motor Control Structure

Central Motor System

Cerebral palsy, by definition, requires that the pathologic lesion be in the brain. Therefore, the spinal cord presumably does not have a primary lesion, although there are children in whom this may not be true. The control of motion is either volitional or automatic. Most activities are volitional; however, reflex responses, such as withdrawal after accidentally touching a hot stove, are automatic responses. This type of automatic response occurs as a relatively simple neuronal reflex at the spinal cord level. All volitional motion initiates in the cerebral cortex and is transmitted to the peripheral motor nerves through the cortical spinal tracts traversing the internal capsule and the spinal cord. These transmissions are not simple commands but are highly modulated based on inputs from many other areas. The components that make up the basal ganglion are extremely important modulators of motion. The cerebellum also monitors sensory input and further modulates motion, especially smoothing the motion pattern. The relative function of each of these structures has been somewhat defined by classic lesioning experiments in animals and close observation of naturally occurring lesions in humans.[1, 2] The very complex modulation occurring in the brain is not well understood in a way that can help explain the problems in children with CP. Some problems of movement disorders have specific patterns that can be linked to specific problems in the basal ganglion[3]; however, even these are usually complex and not focal isolated lesions (Figure 3.1). The spinal cord is not only a series of connecting ascending and descending tracts like a telephone cable, but it also has a very important modulating layer of interconnecting neurons in the motor control system. Some of these interconnections are modulated by descending tracts and others are modulated by interconnections within the spinal cord. For example, when the plantar flexors are stimulated to contract during the simple Achilles tendon reflex, another interconnection in the spinal cord suppresses function of the dorsiflexors, causing them to remain quiet. The specific role of these rather simple connections in complex activities such as walking is not well defined, and the pathologic role of these reflexes in CP is even more difficult to understand.

Peripheral Motor Control

The peripheral motor system includes the nerves and musculoskeletal system. The peripheral motor nerves carry the impulses that cause muscles to contract and the sensory nerves carry this information to the central system. The sensory information includes tendon tension, muscle length, joint position, and cutaneous sensation. In children with CP, there is no primary lesion in any of these peripheral systems; however, the effects of the central pathology cause these systems to develop in abnormal ways. These abnormal changes, such as lack of muscle growth, in the peripheral motor system can be positively affected. These secondary responses to the primary central nervous system defect are the cause of many problems in children with CP.

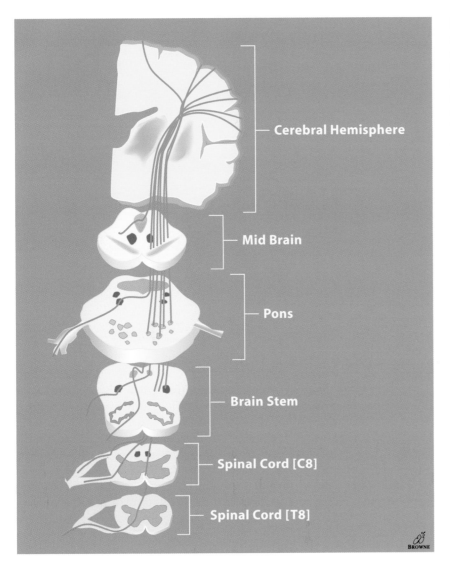

Figure 3.1. Although the cerebral spinal tracts transmit information from the cerebral cortex to the peripheral muscles to cause motion, there are many modulating influences especially from the basal ganglion, cerebellum, and spinal cord. These modulating influences are not well defined as to the specific changes that occur in children after different brain lesions.

Development of the Anatomic Structure

Central Nervous System

The early development of the central nervous system begins with the neural tube structure, which folds and then is followed by development of the anterior part of the brain. By 9 to 17 weeks of gestation, interconnections from the brain to the muscles have developed and the fetus is beginning to make flexor movements. By 18 to 30 weeks, extension movements are routinely seen.[1] By the time the baby is born, she has vigorous kicking and sucking movements and hand and toe grasp. During this time, the anatomic synapses are undergoing considerable remodeling, which is best understood in the development of sight where external light stimulation is needed to develop a normal central neurologic system. The role of external musculoskeletal movement on the maturation of the central nervous system is unknown. Maturation of the central nervous system motor skills, especially in areas such as balance and the ability to learn complex motor skills, are not complete until middle childhood.

Figure 3.2. The H-reflex is initiated by low-level electrical stimulation of the afferent muscle spinal fiber in the same muscle. The H-reflex has the same pathway as the stretch reflex and causes a contraction in the same muscle that was stimulated; however, it is easier to control the timing and quantity of the stimulation.

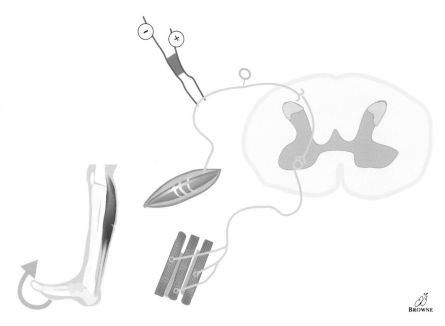

Peripheral Motor System

The peripheral motor system has some primitive function by the ninth week of gestation; however, at birth this system is a long way from being mature. The nerve conduction velocity at birth is 28.5 m/s and by adulthood it reaches 82 m/s. However, because of the large amount of length growth, the H-reflex at the ankle still goes from 15 seconds at birth to 28 seconds at adulthood, even though there is increased velocity (Figure 3.2). Also, skeletal muscle fiber types change to a more mature mix and the whole system has to increase greatly in size. Abnormalities in this growth and development will be considered when the specific pathologic patterns are evaluated.

Controller Mechanisms and Theory

As was already noted, it is quite easy to understand the concept of simple nerve reflexes, such as the knee reflex; however, this concept has not led to an understanding of how the central nervous system controls human gait. New understanding of ways to conceptualize the neuromotor control come from computer sciences and mathematics. The role of these theories, and the benefit they provide, is in helping to place the function of a child with CP in a context that can be understood clinically as the child is growing and continuing with neurologic maturation.

Sensory System Feedback Versus Feed-Forward Control

To conceptualize how the central nervous system controls motor function, a framework of what is possible needs to be considered. Either the system can alter function in response to the sensory information it receives, or it can cause a motion and then learn what has occurred from the sensory feedback system. Constantly changing the motor instructions based on sensory feedback is called feedback control, and ordering a muscle activity and then receiving the effect of that activity from a sensory perspective is called feed-forward control. These two models are important aspects of control theory

Feed-Forward Control

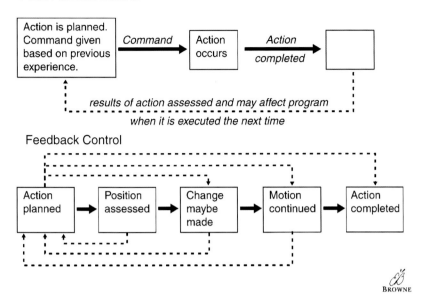

Feedback Control

Figure 3.3. Feedback control depends on constant sensory input, which directly modulates the action in progress. Feed-forward control uses the sensory information to learn and calculate how much muscle activity is needed to make a specific movement occur. The sensory feedback cannot alter the activity in progress but is added to the learning progress for the next activity cycle.

to understand how sensory information is processed and incorporated (Figure 3.3). Other terms that are very similar are closed-loop control, which is almost the same as feedback control. Open-loop control means there is no control once the activity is initiated, which is slightly different from feed-forward control in which a delayed reaction can cause impact on the activity. Firing a bullet from a gun is open-loop control because the shooter has no ability to impact the path of the bullet after it is fired.

Another example of this concept is demonstrated best by the control system present in driving a car or firing a rocket. The control primarily used in driving a car is feedback control in which the driver, when going around a corner, will steer into the corner and constantly correct the turn based on sensory feedback received of how the car is progressing. With this type of control, if the car is going too far to the left, the driver turns more to the right and if the car is going too far to the right, the driver turns back to the left. In this way, the activity of driving around the corner can be accomplished with minimal prior experience and knowledge about the specific corner; appropriate adjustments are made as the task progresses. Launching a rocket is an example of feed-forward control in which the engineer knows where the rocket is to go, then calculates a trajectory. From the knowledge of the trajectory, and the rocket's weight, a calculation of how much fuel is needed and the angle of launch can be made. After all the calculations are completed, a program is given to the rocket's engines. Then, when the rocket is started, it will execute this program to follow the predetermined course based on the programmed engine thrust and angle of launch. There is minimal feedback or ability to change directions 2 seconds after launch if it is determined that the rocket is going in the wrong direction. There is, however, usually the ability to explode the rocket if it is perceived to be going off target. This rocket launch is an example of feed-forward control.

Neurologic control uses both feed-forward and feedback control. An example of feed forward is jumping, where a determination is made similar to a rocket launch in which the brain calculates the amount of muscle force needed and then orders the muscles to contract, generating the required force. Many aspects of walking are feed forward in pattern, although this is less clear at times. Feedback systems are predominantly used for activities with which one has little experience and wants to make changes as the activity is progressing, such as drawing a picture or painting. Many functions probably contain some mix of feed-forward and feedback control.

Understanding feedback mechanisms is somewhat difficult, especially because the concept of muscles is that they are either activated or not activated. Based on the understanding of neural anatomy, all feedback is similar to the knee reflex where the threshold of sensory of stimulus is reached and a fixed contraction occurs. However, staying with this concept makes it difficult to understand how complex feedback would work as feedback is experienced in a much more controlled response than the single synapse reflex. From the area of computer engineering, this feedback can be conceptualized in terms described as fuzzy feedback. This description uses a mathematical concept of fuzzy logic based on graded response options.[4] When a stimulus is received, the response does not need to be all or none, but is chosen rather from a gradiation of options; for example, five options of muscle activation. These options might be a maximum contraction, a moderate contraction, an average contraction, a low contraction, or no response. Although it is hard to relate this type of fuzzy control directly to the neuroanatomy, it is functionally a better conceptual model to understand feedback control in the motor system than the all-on or all-off concept that simple neuroanatomy would suggest. This fuzzy control, or rheostatic-type control, is developed through the multiple levels of modulation and with many muscle fibers in each muscle. Variable whole-muscle activation can be obtained by firing varying numbers of muscle fibers.

Controller Options: Maturation Theory

In considering neurologic control theory, motor activities that most people experience in daily life can be understood in a simplistic way similar to the function of a computer. In this context, it seems natural to think about the computer as a model for the nervous system. For example, in this model the hardware is the anatomic structure in which a software program is placed. Using this analogy, the software program for the brain is called a motor engram[2] or a central program generator (CPG).[1] The term central program generator is used here because it is more descriptive of the motor control concept. The CPG would be equivalent to a word processing program, which has complex but fixed responses to all inputs. Some of these responses are direct, such as the keyboard response occurring when a specific key is pushed and commanding the word processing program to place a specific letter where indicated. Other instructions are more complex responses, such as a predetermined series of steps when a macro in the word processing program is executed. Using the analogy of the computer in understanding motor control, it is also presumed that most of these movement responses are remembered by either the genetic encoding of a motion, such as sucking or stepping, or are developed through a learning response, such as learning to ride a bicycle. The CPG is developed in a process of maturation by a combination of genetic encoding and direct learning. This understanding of the function of the CPG is called the maturation theory of motor control.[1]

Controller Options: Dynamic Systems Theory

The concept of dynamic systems self-organization has arisen from many disciplines of natural science, and has more recently been applied to understanding human motor control. An example of this application of dynamic

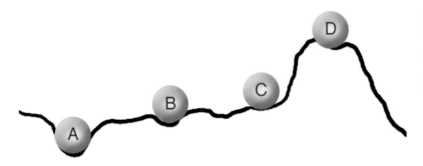

Figure 3.4. The concept of chaotic attractors is easy to visualize as a landscape over which a ball is rolled. There may be many areas where the ball could stop and be stable; however, a relatively small force would dislodge the ball and start it rolling again. There are a few deeper valleys in which the ball might roll and require a lot of force to start it rolling again. Each of these landscape depressions simulates a chaotic attractor of varying strengths.

systems theory is the understanding of the flow of fluids, such as the flow of a river or the flow of fluids through a pipeline. As the speed and pressure of the liquid flow changes, the flow pattern reorganizes itself from a smooth laminar flow where the center of the water column has the highest velocity to the slowest velocity at the periphery, which is in contact with the immobile walls. At some point, this flow reorganizes into turbulence. This turbulence looks totally disorganized; however, in dynamic theory, it has reorganized itself into another control system, which is responding to demands placed on the structure. This changing state from nonturbulent to turbulent is highly nonlinear and is a transition from one state to another, both of which are stable.

Understanding this kind of system reorganization required the development of a new branch of mathematics called chaos theory.[5] In chaos, there are attractors, which are defined as regions or states that are stable or relatively stable (Figure 3.4). For example, there is a rapid transition in fluid flow between turbulent and nonturbulent flow. The fluid does not like to remain a mix of the two states; in other words, the fluid is attracted to one state or the other with varying strengths. This concept of attractors can be used to understand motor control. An example in human gait is walking speed, in which not all velocities have equal preference from standing to maximum running. The chaotic attractor of normal adult walking velocity tends to be strong, between 100 and 160 cm/s. If a person cannot walk close to 100 cm/s, they will often walk at a comfortable speed, then stop and wait for a while, then walk at a natural speed, then stop again. Standing and not moving is another velocity attractor. On the other hand, if an individual has to go faster than 160 cm/s, they typically break into a running gait pattern with a preferred comfortable speed between 250 and 300 cm/s. For speeds around 200 cm/s, most individuals alternate between running and walking because these speeds are more comfortable than trying to stay at an in-between level of not quite walking and not quite running comfortably. Most adults experience and respond to these velocity attractors by altering their speed to be in one of the three stated gait patterns.

Another feature of these attractors is that they may be very stable or somewhat unstable. An example of an unstable attractor is the body position taken in the middle of a jump. This position is an unstable attractor because the body cannot stay this way for long before it has to move to the next attractor, which is the response for landing. Understanding and defining these attractors in motor control can be very helpful in understanding response to growth and development as well as responses to treatment. To clarify the understanding, the term chaotic attractors is used in the remaining text to define these attractors, although the more classic mathematical term used in chaos theory is strange attractors.[5] In medicine, the area where chaotic theory has been applied most is in understanding variability of heart rate.

This principle is demonstrated especially well by the change from a variable heart rhythm to ventricular fibrillation. These two states of heart rhythms are both stable because they are not easily changed without significant external force.

The concept of dynamic systems theory for motor control also aids understanding of how individuals end up doing similar tasks with variable but similar patterns. For example, if a walking child is asked to pick a cookie up off the floor, the pattern used likely will be either predominantly bending at the hip and spine with the knees straight, or flexing the hips and knees keeping the spine straight. With all the muscle and joints available, there are almost endless variations of how a task can be accomplished; however, there is a chaotic attractor toward two or three patterns of motion to accomplish a given task.

The Cause of Chaotic Attractors

Understanding the anatomic or mechanical origin of these chaotic attractors is very difficult, and based on chaos theory, there are too many variable inputs to the system to specifically define these attractors; therefore, they are usually defined as a region. For example, a chaotic attractor draws normal human walking velocity to a relatively stable attractor of around 100 to 160 cm/s. The strength and definition of this attractor are related to the length and mass of the legs, the speed of muscle contraction, the speed of nerve conduction, and the environment. It is impossible to define the exact center of this chaotic attractor because it is based on many things, from the environment to the individual's behavior and mood. Using this concept of dynamic systems theory, a framework exists for understanding why different movement patterns develop in children with CP. For example, children with diplegic pattern involvement frequently develop a crouched gait at adolescence. Depending on what treatment is chosen, the child may continue in the crouched pattern or may revert to a back-kneeing pattern. This gait change is an example of the chaotic attractor organizing the child's motion. The important thing for the surgeon to understand is that the system does not want to organize around normal knee extension, which is the physician's treatment goal.

Another important concept arising from dynamic systems theory is that the control system is self-organizing and there is no need for a CPG or genetic encoding or learning. The example from physics is that the fluid does not need genes, learning, or software to decide to reorganize from turbulent to nonturbulent flow. Another area where dynamic systems theory is widely used is in understanding weather patterns. The weather patterns organize systems, such as high-pressure areas with sunny days or severe storms, in patterns that can be explained with dynamic systems theory, again all without learning, genetic code, or software programs. This organization develops around chaotic attractors, each of which can be characterized somewhat; however, all the inputs and impacts to define this attractor cannot be described. Because dynamic systems theory requires no encoding program, such as a CPG, it is directly opposed to the maturation theory of motor control. Reports of the ability of mechanical robots to self-organize around movement patterns and studies with animals suggest that dynamic theory has some basis as an organizational structure of motor control.[1]

A Unified Theory of Motor Control

The goal of having a concept of motor control is to help in treatment of children with motor control problems, and perhaps to develop a conceptual context to test theories in an experimental format. There is a need to combine both the maturation and dynamic systems theories. One way of combining them is to separate the functions of the motor control system into subsystems. There is a subsystem for balance that includes the sensory feedback areas, another system for controlling muscle tone, and a third system for motor pattern control. Other aspects of these subsystems might include sight, oral motor function, and hearing. The three defined subsystems having the most direct impact on the motor systems related to the musculoskeletal system are our focus, although sight is clearly a very important aspect of motor control by providing feedback to the motor control system.

With each of these subsystems, there is a basic level of organization programmed by genetic encoding and learning. Above some level of basic function, dynamic systems theory best explains actions. Some of the patterns coming out of dynamic systems theory may be further refined through learning, especially activities that depend heavily on feed-forward control. An example is an athlete's activity, such as learning to broad jump. After middle childhood, with a fully mature neurologic system, maturation to execute the concept of jumping has developed. When a child is asked to jump as far as she can, the natural general pattern, which is probably determined by dynamic control organizing the activity around the chaotic attractor or series of attractors that are not very stable, will be used. However, if the individual wants to become a champion broad jumper, they must work on a specific pattern and be able to execute this pattern consistently within a very narrow range. This part of the activity now becomes a maturation activity around defining a specific CPG, which helps to explain why the basic pattern is seen, but also allows for refinement. Also, much more energy is required to change the basic pattern than to refine the current pattern.

When considering individual pathologic problems, the neurologic aspects of the motor impairments can be separated into abnormalities of the three subsystems of motor control. These subsystems are muscle tone, motor planning, and balance The variety of abnormalities in these three subsystems leads to almost all the motor problems in children with CP. Some children have impairments in only one area, such as a spastic gastrocnemius in child with a hemiplegic pattern involvement. Others, such as children with severe quadriplegic pattern involvement, have significant abnormalities in all three subsystems.

Disorders of Muscle Tone

Muscle tone is defined as the stiffness of the muscles or the limb as one tries to passively move the limb. This stiffness has a spring characteristic, which is stiffer with small movements than with large movements and is defined as a nonlinear response to movement.[6] The exact origin of this tone comes from the passive stiffness emanating from the shape of the soft-tissue envelope, friction in the joint and soft tissue, and may also have an undefined active neuronal element. In studies using the leg drop test, a difference has been seen between an awake and alert child compared with the same child under neuromotor blockade anesthesia. In normal individuals there is less muscle tone under anesthesia than when they are awake, which strongly suggests that there is an active stiffness in the muscle that is not due to contraction induced by the motor neuron, as this stiffness is occurring with a silent electromyogram (EMG) (Miller et al., unpublished data, 2001).

In addition to nonlinear passive and active spring stiffness, tone in the limb also has a component of viscoelastic dampening, which is velocity-dependent resistance to movement. This dampening effect works very similar to a shock absorber in a car. The dampener also has a nonlinear response to varying velocity and position of the limb. The function of the viscous dampener is to provide passive tone in the normal motor system so the movement is smoothed. Muscle tone here is defined as some tension in the muscle while it is not actively contracting. This tone probably provides an important functional factor to the muscle. If the muscle is completely loose, without tension, it would have a slower response and the fine control would be lacking.

Also, there is some undefined important aspect of this tone in allowing the muscle to maintain its strength and to regulate its growth in childhood. A second major aspect of muscle tone is the motion-induced stretch reflex, which is commonly known as the knee or ankle jerk reflex. This is a monosynaptic reflex induced through stretch reception of the receptors in the muscles. The stretch reflex synapse can be modulated from the brainstem and cerebral white matter by the vestibulospinal and reticulospinal pathways.[7] It is through these spinal pathways that monosynaptic reflexes are modulated through a large variety of experiences, such as changes in the person's mood, environment, and the activity being performed.

Motor Tone

Normal motor tone has many important but poorly defined functions in the control of the motor system. Most of these functions are defined by problems caused when the motor tone is too high or too low. In general, high tone is called spasticity or hypertonicity and low tone is called hypotonia. The classic definition of spasticity typically includes an increased sensitivity of the normal stretch reflex in addition to a velocity-dependent increase in resistance, which initiates a muscle contraction to resist the motion.[8] This widely reported and often-repeated description of spasticity, which includes the velocity-dependent feature, sounds like a definition of an increase of the viscous dampening of normal muscle tone, but it is not. This description is typically used as another definition of hyperreflexia, which is part of the syndrome. There are no reports documenting that spasticity is related to velocity of angular joint motion in the mechanical sense of the change of the joint angle over time. The term velocity is used in a general way to mean movement. Also, there is a variability to spasticity that has been defined as a clasp-knife, release, and catching characteristic. Spasticity is difficult to explain, and it is not clear if all the characteristics used to describe it are different aspects of the same response or totally different responses occurring in the same muscle. The syndrome of altered muscle tone is extremely easy to recognize but much harder to define. In this way, spasticity is like pornography, which has been described by a supreme court justice as "hard to define but easy to recognize when you see it." Movement patterns, especially dystonia, may be difficult to differentiate from spasticity when the child is seen for only a short time; however, the presence of the secondary changes, especially in the muscle, usually allows the differentiation to be easily made.

Measuring Muscle Tone

Muscle tone is such a basic aspect of motor control that there have to be ways for it to be quantified. The most common method has been the use of the Ashworth scale.[9] This scale is a manual scale that evaluates resistance to motion of a specific joint; however, it only considers hypertonicity. The scale has been modified to include more levels and to allow assessment of hypo-

Table 3.1. Ashworth scale and modified Ashworth scale.

Ashworth Scale:

Score	Description of the muscle tone
1	No increase in normal tone
2	Slight increased tone with a catch with rapid joint motion
3	Increased tone but the joint is still easy to move
4	Considerable increase in tone making passive movement difficult
5	Limb is rigid, movement is difficult

Modified Ashworth Scale:

Score	Description of the muscle tone
00	Hypotonia
0	Normal tone, no increase in tone
1	Slight increase in tone manifested by a slight catch and release or minimal increased resistance to joint range of motion
1+	Slight increase in tone manifested by a slight catch and minimal increased resistance to joint range of motion for more than half the joint range
2	More marked increase of tone through most of the whole joint range, but the affected joint is easily moved
3	Considerable increase in muscle tone; passive movement difficult but possible
4	Affected joint is stiff and cannot be moved

Hensinger RN. Standards in Pediatric Orthopedics. Lippincott Williams and Wilkins, 1986.

tonia in a scale called the modified Ashworth scale (see Table 3.1). This scale is the most widely used scale for assessing spasticity; however, it is very subjective and at times difficult to separate limb stiffness resulting from muscle stiffness as opposed to the stiffness induced by spasticity.

Other methods for assessing spasticity include the leg drop test in which the leg is allowed to swing over the edge of a table and the oscillations and magnitude of the movement are measured. This test only works in a child with mild to moderate spasticity and requires excellent cooperation from the individual being tested. Many mechanical movement devices have been designed to move and measure the torque generated by the movement as methods for measuring spasticity. None of these systems has gained wide acceptance for clinical use.[1] Many people have tried to record the EMG activity; however, it is impossible to determine any force data from electromyography. Another very old technique is to measure the H-response, which is a nerve potential recorded in the motor neuron that occurs when a sensory nerve in close proximity is stimulated. The amplitude of this H-wave is thought to reflect the excitability of the alpha motor neuron (Figure 3.5). This measurement has been correlated to hyperreflexia, but does not correlate well with the Ashworth scale[7, 10]; therefore, we still are using the modified Ashworth scale for clinical evaluation of spasticity.

Spasticity

Spasticity is the most common presentation of all neurologic alterations in children with CP. Increased muscle tone expressed as spasticity must be a very strong chaotic attractor to the organization of residual activity in a child with a central neurologic injury. It is very difficult to understand what the components of the system are that make this spasticity such a strong attractor. Because it has persisted in humans but is seldom seen in animals, this

Figure 3.5. The effect of spasticity on the growth and development of skeletal muscle results in a muscle that has fewer muscle fibers, shorter fiber length, and a longer tendon. This aberration results in a muscle that is weaker because of decreased cross-sectional area and has less excursion, resulting in decreased joint range of motion because of the shorter fiber lengths.

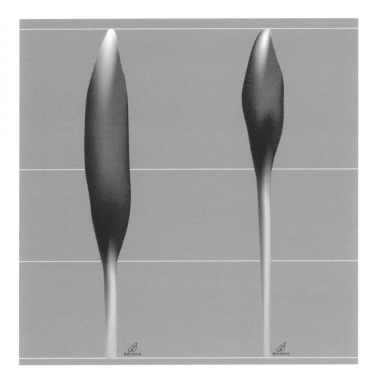

suggests that there is a functional benefit to spasticity. Even though spasticity is a strong chaotic attractor, any judgment about its benefit or harm to an individual cannot be made. From modern robotic research, it is known that adding stiffness to joints helps improve fine motor control; and also everyone has experienced a tendency to stiffen when wanting to do very fine delicate movements with their hands. It seems most conceivable that, on the whole, when the neurologic system loses some function but its organization still has the ability, muscle tone will increase to allow function with a lower degree of neurologic control. Therefore, when treating children with spasticity, the basic supposition is that muscle tone is good and the amount of muscle tone should be modulated for their maximum benefit.

Effects of Spasticity on Nerves

Because the lesion in CP is central, all other more distal changes are presumed to be secondary. The best recognized change in spasticity is hyperreflexia, which occurs because of a decreased inhibition from the cortical spinal tracts. As a normal child grows, the rate of muscle contraction and the ability to increase power by cerebral cortex modulation continues to increase until the child is approximately 10 years old.[1] Although this change has been well documented by studying the ability of increased rapid alternating movements in children and adults,[11] it is not clear where these changes occur. In CP, this more immature pattern of slow corticospinal and pyramidal tract potentials persists.[1] There is an increased latency and a decreased ability to recruit large numbers of motor fibers at the same time.[12] Some of this activity is modulated through changes in the excitability of the spinal motor neurons, which are also sensitive to joint position or, probably more specifically, muscle length. The strength of the ankle reflex is very sensitive to ankle joint position as measured by the H-reflex, which is initiated through stimulation of a peripheral sensory nerve. This change is much greater than can be explained by mechanical positioning.[1] As noted earlier, there has to be some tension in the muscle while the muscle is at rest for it to function properly. Some of this tension seems to disappear when the individual is under neuromotor blockade anesthesia. It has been postulated that active neuronal stimulation is required to maintain this muscle tone[1]; however, no direct evidence of this has been found. It is this element of increased neurologic stimulation not generating an active EMG that seems to increase most when tone increases in CP. Because many of these children also demonstrate abnormalities in temperature regulation and blood flow in the extremities, some regulatory abnormality in the sympathetic nervous system may be involved. At this time, however, there is no direct evidence to support this theory.

Effects of Spasticity on Muscles and Tendons

Hypertonia and hypotonia have the most dramatic secondary effects on the muscle. The well-observed effects of spasticity on skeletal muscle include decreased longitudinal growth of the muscle fiber length, decreased volume of the muscle, change in motor unit size, and change in the fiber type and neuromotor junction type. In the mouse model, the spasticity causes loss of approximately 50% of the longitudinal growth of the muscle fiber, resulting in contractures.[13] Muscles in children with CP are always very thin in addition to being short, which means that these muscles are also weak, as a muscle's strength is related to its cross-sectional area. Understanding strength has been an extremely confusing topic in spastic muscle evaluation. The mechanical definition of strength is defined by how much load a structure can support. When discussing strength of a limb, such as the strength of plantar flexion at the ankle, the strongest ankle tends to have a severe fixed flexion contracture, but this is not the strength for which most clinicians are looking. Usually, the term strength is used to describe the ability to move a load or to do work, which is called active strength, whereas the contracture is a passive strength. By creating a significant contracture, the spastic muscle has great passive strength but low active strength compared with normal muscles. Active strength is altered more in spastic children because of the difficulty of avoiding co-contraction, as there is less antagonist inhibition in spasticity. Motor units tend to get larger and have slower responses with longer latency periods combined with a large shift to the slow-twitch type 1 fibers.[12, 14] All these changes mean the muscle responds slower during contraction, and combined with the changes in the nerve, has a longer latency period. Children with spasticity were recently found to be resistant to succinylcholine, and on further investigation, it was found that the neuromotor junction contains immature subunits. The effects of spasticity on skeletal muscle are pervasive and often experienced by neuro-orthopaedists; however, a physiologic explanation of how increased tone causes all these changes is still unknown.

There is a grave need for basic research and understanding of muscle response to spasticity. In a major textbook containing 1936 pages of descriptions related to muscle embryology, physiology, and muscle diseases, not one mention of the impact of spasticity on muscle was found.[15] Yet, surely more people have myopathic changes secondary to spasticity than all the other primary muscle diseases combined. In the context of dynamic control theory, these changes seem to be revolving around a strong, stable attractor whose basic factor seems to be a damaged motor control system, which is slowing the response time, stiffening the system, and providing passive strength in the face of absent active strength. This stable chaotic attractor may also be organizing around the functional benefit of the organism, which can now support weight in stance and is able to move in space, although at a slower rate than normal. Although there are no good detailed explanations at this time from the maturation perspective of exactly what determines these changes, they all make sense in the dynamic control model. The major problem of this chaotic attractor is that it seems too stable and there is an overreaction in many children, with the changes in themselves becoming functionally limiting and causing problems.

Effects of Spasticity on Bones

Changes in the bones caused by spasticity are modulated by muscular changes. The most common effects are dislocated hips; scoliosis; foot deformities, such as planovalgus feet or equinovarus feet; bunions; knee contractures; and elbow, shoulder, and wrist joint contractures. Torsional malalignments of the femur and tibia are common as well. A major part of this text discusses the management of these deformities. These secondary deformities, such as dislocated hips, have been very well defined and have clear mechanical etiologies.[16] These deformities all have clear and strong pulls to develop toward easily understood chaotic attractors. In the hip, on one side the muscle will become contracted causing adduction, and on the other side, it will become contracted in abduction. Therefore, both hyperadduction and hyperabduction are stable attractors. With a decreased level of fine motor control and spasticity, the neutral position of the hip is not a stable region. This concept also applies to other affected joints.

Functional Effects of Spasticity on Sitting, Gait, and Activities of Daily Living

There are many functional effects of spasticity, some of which help children and some of which cause major problems. For children who are ambulatory, the spasticity causes typical spastic gait patterns. These gait patterns are discussed in Chapter 6. Children who are able to do minimal weight bearing for transfers or household ambulation are often greatly aided in these activities by the spasticity, which provides the strength and stability for weight bearing. These same children may have problems relaxing in seating positions and therefore are difficult to seat. They may also have so much spasticity that activities of daily living, such as dressing and toileting, are difficult. Each child requires a careful assessment of the specific problems and benefits caused by the spasticity. There is a tendency for family members and some clinicians to equate the spasticity to CP. It is often difficult for them to see the benefits provided by the spasticity.

Treatments

When planning for treatment of the spasticity, the benefits and problems should be carefully considered. Everyone must realize that no matter how successful the treatment of the spasticity is, the child will still have CP. It should always be kept in mind that the goal in treating spasticity is to never remove all muscle tone. It is much better to conceptualize spasticity treatment similar to treating hypertension. Clearly, the treatment of hypertension would not be successful if all the blood pressure were removed. There is considerable similarity between no blood pressure and no muscle tone. The ideal treatment of spasticity would be a situation where the tone is decreased only at the time and in the anatomic area when and where it causes problems. The spasticity would then be preserved in all situations in which it is helping the child. It is also important to remember that some of the secondary effects in the muscle noted above may also have direct effects from the primary lesion. For example, the strength of a muscle contraction is mediated by the cerebral cortex impulse. Therefore, in a child with CP, this ability to modulate strength may be a primary deficiency due to the brain lesion. After the child has been evaluated with an assessment of the specific benefits and problems of spasticity, available treatment options should be considered.

The treatment of muscle tone may be applied at different locations in the neuromuscular system. Treatment options start in the central nervous system with the use of medications, electrical stimulation, or surgical ablation. In the peripheral nervous system to the level of the muscle, medication and ablation are the main choices. At the muscle level, medication, electrical stimulation, or surgical lengthening are the treatment options.

Oral Medication Affecting the Central Nervous System

Oral medication treatments tend to impact both the spinal cord and brain where gamma-aminobutyric acid (GABA) receptors are the main inhibitory receptors of the motor control system (Table 3.2). The two major drugs are diazepam and baclofen. Both these drugs block GABA at the main point of action. Baclofen is an analog of GABA and binds to the receptors but does not activate GABA. The activity of diazepam is more diffuse. Baclofen has poor absorption across the blood–brain barrier. Both drugs have a very high rate of accommodation, meaning they are effective initially but lose their effectiveness over several weeks. This accommodation effect can be overcome with larger doses; however, the use of higher doses makes the complication rate higher. The use of both these drugs orally for chronic control

Table 3.2. Spasticity medications.

Drug	Trade names	Benefit for spasticity	Side effects
Baclofen	Lioresal	Useful in some patient groups; in CP seldom has a lasting benefit when given orally, but very effective by intrathecal administration	Causes sedation, sudden withdrawal, psychosis; rapid drug tolerance develops in the oral doses
Diazepam	Valium	Very useful for acute postoperative spasticity management, little use for chronic management Oldest effective antispasticity drug	Has long and somewhat variable half-life, very sedating; tolerance develops with chronic use
Chlorazepate	Tranxene	Little use in CP; is an active metabolite of diazepam; may have less sedation but no other demonstrated benefit for spasticity management	Same as diazepam
Clonazepam	Klonopin, Rivotril	Has a quick absorption and an 18-hour half-life; may also be less sedating than diazepam; is useful for single-dose nighttime treatment of complaint-related sleep difficulty due to spasms	Same problem of drug tolerance as diazepam
Ketazolam	Loftran	New shorter-acting benzodiazepine, no CP data	Claimed to have less sedation
Tetrazepam	Myolastin	New drug, no CP data	Claimed to be less sedating
Dantrolene	Dantrium	Works by decreasing muscle fiber excitability; has no effective use in children with CP	Is hepatotoxic so liver enzymes must be monitored; causes muscle weakness
Tizanidine	Zanaflex, Sirdalud	Blocks the release of neuroexitatory amino acids; no CP data; personal experience is that there is rapid tolerance, similar to baclofen	Causes dry mouth, sedating; may cause drop in blood pressure
Clonidine	Catapres, Dixirit, Catapresan	Blocks alpha-agonist activity in the brainstem and spinal cord; no data in CP spasticity	Causes a drop in blood pressure and heart rate
Cannabis	Cesamet, Marinol	Effective to reduce adult spasticity but no data in children	Significant psychotropic effects and is addictive
Cyclobenzapine	Flexeril	Widely used to treat back muscle spasm, but studies have shown no effect on spasticity	Not indicated because it is not effective

of spasticity has not been successful in children with CP. The acute use of diazepam in the postoperative period is very useful and safe. Alpha-2-adrenergic receptors have primarily agonist function in the spinal and supraspinal regions. Tizanidine and clonidine hydrochloride are drugs that block these receptors. Although there is some evidence that this type of drug is effective in decreasing spasticity of spinal cord origin,[17] their use in children with CP has little or no experience and no published data. Personal experience with tizanidine suggests that it has very similar problems as the other oral antispasticity medications, which are a significant rate of sedation and a high accommodation effect. Other drugs acting at other sites in the central nervous system have the potential for decreasing spasticity. There are only incidental reports of use of these drugs and no documentation of their use in children with CP. Blockade of voltage-sensitive sodium channels can be done with lamotrigine and riluzole. Serotonin antagonists such as cyproheptadine decrease tone. Glycine is an inhibitory neurotransmitter that can be given orally and is absorbed by the brain. Cannabis has been shown to decrease spasticity through an unknown mediator.[18]

Intrathecal Medication Administration

Over the past 20 years, an interest in administering medication directly into the intrathecal space, especially in the spinal canal, has developed. Because there is a general perception that spasticity originates in the spinal segments, a high dose of drug concentrated in this region of the nervous system should be given. This route was initially developed to administer morphine[19] but was quickly applied to administer baclofen.[20] The intrathecal pump is battery powered and implanted in the abdomen, and an intrathecal catheter is introduced into the intrathecal space in the spine. This catheter is tunneled subcutaneously around the lateral side of the trunk to the anterior implanted pump site and connected to the pump. The pump is controlled with an external radiowave-mediated controller, and the pump reservoir is filled by direct injection through the overlying skin (Case 3.1). The primary medication used to manage spasticity by intrathecal pump administration is baclofen. The administration may be continuous, or the pump can be programmed to have higher doses over a short time, then be turned off for a period of time, and go to lower doses.

The use of intrathecal administration of baclofen is very new, having only been approved by the FDA for use in children in 1997. At the time of approval, there were fewer than 200 children with implanted pumps. In the past 4 years, these pumps have become much more common. These pumps have the great advantage of being adjustable and can be discontinued if the results are not thought to be worth the trouble. Usually, a careful assessment with a listing of the caretakers' concerns is made. If the child has not had a spinal fusion, a trial dose may be done with 75 to 100 μg injected as a bolus dose in the intrathecal space. Then the child is monitored by caretakers and the medical team and a joint decision is made as to the benefits. For especially difficult cases, an indwelling catheter, which can be left in place for several days, may be used so the dose can be adjusted. This implanted catheter is used for children with greatly variable tone, or individuals in whom adjustable doses of baclofen are to be monitored.

The initial recommendation was to do a series of three injections on consecutive days starting with 25 μg, then 50 μg, then 100 μg on the third day.[21] We have not found this algorithm very useful and prefer to give 75 to 100 μg or use the inserted catheter.[22] Children either respond or do not respond, and the small dose differences in the prior recommendation add little to understanding their effect. Also, the recommendation that children be tried

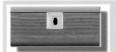

Letrisha, an 8-year-old girl with severe spastic quadriplegia and mental retardation, was totally dependent for all care needs. Her mother's complaint was that she had difficulty with diapering, dressing, and bathing her. Sometime she did severe extensor posturing that made seating difficult. She slept well, was fed by gastrostomy tube, and had seizures several times a day, which were felt to be in good control for her, and weighed 16.7 kg. A baclofen trial was given with 75 µg injection of baclofen, which provided excellent relief of the spasticity. A pump was then inserted with good spasticity relief. (Figure C3.1.1, C3.1.2). Over 6 months, she continued to have rapid accommodation to the drug; however, a plateau dose of 650 µg was reached that continued to control her spasticity. After having the pump for a year, her mother still noted that diapering was difficult because of contractures of the hip adductors. She then had an open adductor tenotomy. She had little body fat and the pump was prominent on her abdomen but caused no problems (Figure C3.1.3).

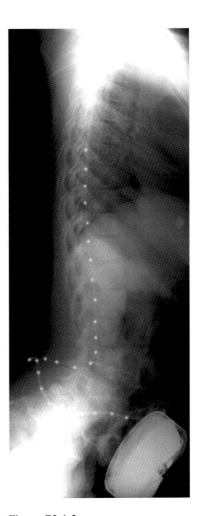

Figure C3.1.2

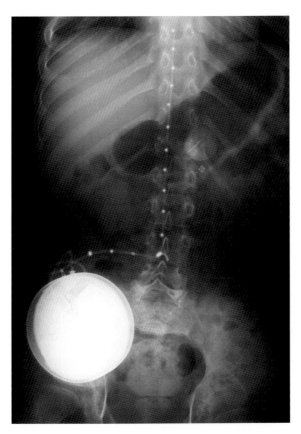

Figure C3.1.1

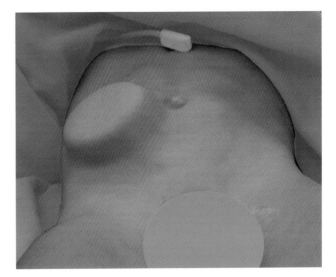

Figure C3.1.3

on oral baclofen[21] has little merit, as there are no data suggesting that it is helpful in children with CP. Our experience has been that oral baclofen is almost never of any benefit. The algorithm our colleagues and we use for intrathecal baclofen is to do a clinical evaluation, followed by one injection trial, then implant the pump and adjust the dose to the child's needs. We never use the small 10-ml pump because it is only minimally smaller than the 18-ml pump but has a capacity that is almost 50% less. This capacity becomes very significant when the child requires a high dose of baclofen, such as 1000 μg per day. If the 10-ml pump is used, it must be filled every 20 days if the 2000 μg/ml concentration for baclofen is used. This type of dose is not uncommon, and the size of the child is in no way related to their baclofen needs.

The outcome of administering baclofen via intrathecal pump is a clear reduction in spasticity in most children. After the initial implantation, it may take 3 to 6 months before a constant level of drug that will keep the spasticity decreased is found. The drug accommodation effect is well known in the oral use of baclofen and happens with intrathecal dosing as well; however, when a certain dose is reached, this accommodation effect no longer occurs. The required dosing for individual children varies greatly and is not related to body size. The dose requirements vary from 100 μg to 2000 μg per day. The correct dosing can be determined only by slowly increasing the dose and evaluating the effect on the child. After spasticity reduction has been accomplished, the functional gains are extremely variable, with the clearest gains occurring in children with quadriplegic pattern involvement based on subjective reports from caretakers. These caretakers report improved ease of dressing and other activities of daily living.[23, 24] Improved sleeping has been noted in many of our patients, as well as behavior improvements. Improved sitting and upper extremity use is also reported by families.[25, 26] All these functional gains are subjective reports that usually make the families very happy with the device. The use of intrathecal administration of baclofen in ambulatory children has very minimal experience and is used mostly in older children with severe gait disturbances.[26, 27] To date, none of these reports has included any quantitative gait evaluation. Our experience as well as the experience reported to us from a few other laboratories suggest that children's speed is not changed much; there may be some increased range of motion at the knee, but there is a tendency to drift into more of a crouched position. All these results are based on isolated cases and are very dependent on the dosing amount.

Complications with the use of the intrathecal pump vary; however, the rate is significant. Incidence of infection has been reported as between 0% and 25%.[23, 25, 28] Mechanical catheter problems have been reported as well, including catheter breakage, disconnections, and kinking.[20, 23, 25] Pump pocket effusion and persistent cerebrospinal fluid (CSF) leakage have also been reported.[25] The acute withdrawal of baclofen, if it is given either intrathecally or orally, may cause children to have hallucinations and acute psychosis.[29] The complications of the baclofen pump are generally easy to treat and do not have permanent consequences. Most infections that involve the pump require that the pump be removed and the infection cleared; then the pump can be reinserted. We have been able to treat an infection in one child without removing the pump, and there is one report in the literature where intrathecal vancomycin hydrochloride was used and the pump was saved.[30]

An important technical detail that will avoid wound problems over the pump in thin children is to make sure the incision used to insert the pump is very proximal so none of the scar resides over the pump or catheter after implantation. This means that the incision to insert the pump may be at the level of the lower ribs. All wound problems we have encountered have been

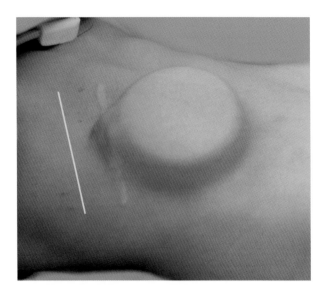

Figure 3.6. The incision for the baclofen pump should be higher than the expected placement site of the pump. When the incision runs across the connectors of the pump, as shown in the this picture, there is a higher risk of wound breakdown. Ideally the incision should be well away from the pump pocket, as shown by the *yellow line*.

in cases where the incision ended crossing the underlying pump, usually at the junction where the catheter inserts into the pump (Figure 3.6). Inserting the pump under the external oblique fascia is another option that will help with soft-tissue coverage. The major problem with catheter complications is diagnosing the problem. Sometimes children are not responding as expected, or suddenly stop responding, to the baclofen. If this occurs, there may be a possible catheter problem. The first study should be a radiograph to evaluate the catheter. Sometimes the radiograph will be able to visualize catheter discontinuity. If the pump inserted has a side port for catheter injection, an attempt can be made to aspirate from the catheter, or inject a radiopaque material, and get a radiograph. We almost never use this pump in children because it is too prominent. The pump can be emptied and injected with indium and then scanned after the indium is calculated to have reached the spinal fluid. If this is not positive and there is a serious concern, the child should be taken back to the operating room, the anterior catheter pump connection exposed, and the catheter removed. It should now be possible to obtain CSF from the catheter. If not, the posterior catheter has to be exposed, disconnected, and whichever section is not patent should be replaced.

Another complication that may occur is in a child who maintains a CSF leak after insertion of the catheter. The initial treatment is to leave the child in a supine position for up to 2 weeks to see if this leak resolves. The primary symptom from this CSF leak is a severe headache and nausea. Most of the time the leak stops. We had two children who continued to leak. One of these children had a posterior spinal fusion in which the fusion mass had been opened. This wound again was opened, and the fascia was placed over the dura with closure of the bone defect with methyl methacrylate. If an opening in the fusion mass is done to insert the catheter, the bone defect is now routinely closed with cranioplast. If the child has not had a spinal fusion, an epidural blood patch may be tried. This patch works well if a leak occurs following a trial injection; however, it has not been successful in stopping leaks around inserted catheters. In this situation, the insertion site may also need to be exposed and the catheter insertion site covered with a fascial patch.

If there is a sudden malfunction of the implanted pump, it will stop functioning instead of pumping too much. This safety feature of the pump has not been reported to fail. In this circumstance, if there is a question of pump function, the pump needs to be replaced. The battery that powers the pump has an implanted life ranging from 3 to 5 years. When the battery loses power, the whole pump has to be replaced. The catheter does not need to be replaced. If there is any question as to whether a child's pump is functioning or there is a catheter malfunction, the child should be placed on oral baclofen to prevent the withdrawal psychosis that occurs in some children. Baclofen also has an antihypertensive effect[31]; however, this is seldom a significant problem. There may be a sympathetic blockade-type effect decreasing the overreacting peripheral basal motor response that creates blue feet when the feet get cold.[32]

Another well-documented effect of baclofen in rats is a decrease in the number and frequency of penile erections.[33, 34] There is one report involving adult males with spinal cord injury-induced spasticity treated with intrathecal baclofen. In this report, a significant number of men reported a decreased time and rigidity of erections, and two men reported losing the ability to ejaculate.[35] One of our patients was a young man whose main complaint with intrathecal baclofen was a decreased quality of his erection and a prolonged latency period between erections. This complication should be mentioned to patients for whom it might be a concern.

A small group of children require a very high dose of intrathecal baclofen, sometimes 2000 to 3000 mg per day. Also, some children who are on a lower dose suddenly need increased doses if their spasticity is increasing 6 months to 2 years after the implantation. If a child has had an increasing need for baclofen, or is requiring a sudden increase in baclofen after having been stable, catheter malfunction should be considered. After the full workup for catheter malfunction, or after demonstration that the catheter is functioning, another option for dosing is to use a drug holiday. In this treatment, the intrathecal baclofen is reduced and then slowly decreased to zero to avoid a withdrawal psychosis. The pump may be left in the turned-off position for 1 month and then the drug slowly reintroduced. This drug holiday should allow the nervous system to redevelop a sensitivity to the drug. Another way to use this concept of a drug holiday is to give large intrathecal boluses several times a day instead of continuous dosing. Therefore, instead of giving a continuous dosing rate of 2000 mg, the child may be given 1000 mg just before bedtime, and then another 1000 mg over a 30-minute period the first thing in the morning. These different dosing regimens may provide a better benefit in some children compared with continuous administration.

The current role of intrathecal baclofen in the treatment of children with severe spasticity is primarily in nonambulatory children. From a theoretical standpoint, this treatment should also be ideal for the 3- to 8-year-old spastic ambulatory child for whom a rhizotomy could be considered. The size of the pump and the need for long-term maintenance, with filling at least every 3 months, has made it difficult to convince parents and physicians that this is a good treatment option. Also, there are no objective published data that allow one to develop confidence. This question would be an excellent project for a well-controlled study similar to the randomized rhizotomy studies.[36, 37] The other problem is the current pump has very poor design features, such as having a very superficial catheter connection site, making it a site for skin pressure, and the pump is much more bulky than is really necessary. As better engineered pumps are designed and medication that has more stability is found, so that the pump only needs to be filled every 6 months to 1 year, the intrathecal pump will become an even better option, especially for high-functioning children. Also, there are other medications that may be even better choices than baclofen; however, each of these needs to be trialed and tested in children with spasticity.

Rhizotomy

Central nervous system surgical approaches to reducing spasticity are most commonly done at the spinal cord level, with posterior dorsal rhizotomy being the most widely used procedure. This procedure involves cutting the dorsal sensory nerve rootlets, which contain the afferent sensory nerves, from the muscle spindles as well as other sensory nerves. By using peripheral motor stimulation and recording the electrical activity in the proximal sensory nerves, abnormal rootlets are identified and then sectioned. Many rootlets are not quite normal or not very abnormal, which makes choosing the abnormal ones very subjective. Evidence exists that there is no difference between selective nerve sectioning based on electrical stimulation and just random sectioning.[38–40] Also, the number of rootlets that are cut is very important, so there usually must be a decision on what percentage of the rootlets will be sectioned based on the child's general level of spasticity. The operative procedure may be done as popularized by Peacock et al.,[41] in which laminectomies are done from L1 to L5 and the rootlets identified at each level where they exit. The other technique, advocated by Fazano et al.,[42] consists of a laminectomy only performed at T12 and L1; then the rootlets are separated just below the conus (Figure 3.7). There is no apparent difference between outcomes of the two procedures based on published reports; however, the Peacock technique is more popular in North America. Cervical

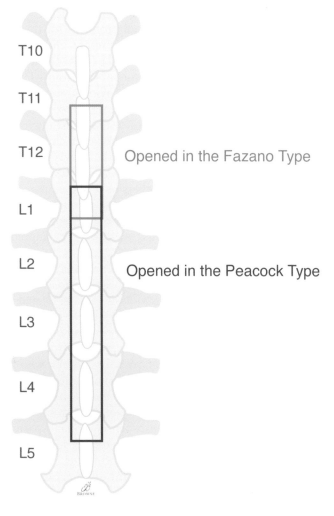

Figure 3.7. The Fazano technique involves doing only a T12–L1 laminectomy in which the rootlets are separated at the end of the conus. This exposure may lead to thoracolumbar kyphosis as a late spinal deformity. The Peacock approach involves a laminectomy from L1 to L5 with separation of the rootlets as they exit the spinal canal. The long-term spinal deformity, which occurs as a consequence of the Peacock technique, is progressive lumbar lordosis.

rhizotomy has also been promoted by some authors,[43–45] but has never become popular except for in a few isolated centers. Rhizotomy has been described for 100 years, and has had a series of advocates and periods of popularity, but has never developed a stable level of acceptance in medical practice.

Outcome of Rhizotomy

Since the modern popularization of rhizotomy by Fazano and Peacock in the 1980s, there have been many reports in the literature of its use in children with CP. A search at the time of this writing revealed 111 citations, the majority reporting small, individual surgeon's experiences. There seems to be a universal agreement that spasticity is reduced acutely after the dorsal rhizotomy procedure. There are no studies with good follow-up to maturity; all the long-term studies consider 5 to 10 years as long term.[46, 47] Most studies report outcomes at 1 to 3 years after the index procedure. Also, the majority of the studies have no controls with respect to other treatments or for the effects of growth and development. There are two well-designed studies that are very short term, 1 year or less, which randomized the children to a physical therapy-only group or a physical therapy and rhizotomy group.[36, 37] Both these excellent short-term studies confirm the generally well-recognized fact that spasticity is reduced; however, one[37] reported no significant functional gains with rhizotomy whereas the other reported some functional gain.[36]

The net result of these studies is that the functional problems of CP are not all, or maybe not at all, due to spasticity, which most people who work with children with CP have known for a long time.[48] There is a strong sense among parents and clinicians with little experience managing children with CP that spasticity is the root of all problems for these children during the growth and development period. Therefore, the general feeling is if spasticity were removed, everything would be better, which is the general tone of many articles reporting the outcomes of rhizotomy. There are no direct comparisons of rhizotomy to intrathecal baclofen, except for cost comparison.[49] One nonrandomized study compared orthopaedic surgery alone with rhizotomy.[50] Over a follow-up of 1 to 7 years, this study found the improvement in joint range of motion to be equal; however, children made better progress toward independent gait with orthopaedic surgery than with dorsal rhizotomy. Although there may be less need for orthopaedic surgery after a dorsal rhizotomy has been performed, others have shown that there definitely is still significant skeletal deformity occurring throughout development, possibly necessitating more orthopaedic surgery.[51] Also, some new deformities are created, such as lumbar lordosis[52–55] and a very unpredictable effect on hip subluxation.[56, 57]

Complications from dorsal rhizotomy may include hip dysplasia and spine deformities including kyphosis, lordosis, spondylolisthesis, and spondylolysis.[54, 55] This spondylolysis may be related to the postoperative back pain some children develop 6 months or more following rhizotomy.[58] It has been suggested that laminaplasty instead of laminectomy may be a way of reducing these abnormalities; however, there currently is no evidence that this makes a difference.[59] We have seen children who have the same problems after laminaplasty as laminectomy (Figure 3.8). Other reported complications following dorsal rhizotomy include heterotopic ossification of the hip if the rhizotomy is done concurrently with hip surgery.[60] Also, typical postoperative CP complications, such as bronchospasms, urinary retention, ilius, and aspiration pneumonia are reported.[61] Decreased sensation and dysesthesias are also well-recognized problems.[58, 61] Bowel and bladder dysfunction is related to cutting too many distal nerves and is a well-recognized complication.[58, 61]

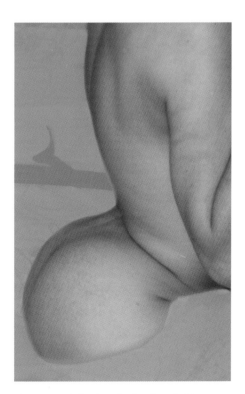

Figure 3.8. This boy had a dorsal rhizotomy with laminaplasty 4 years before this photograph. He did well for several years; however, during his adolescent growth period the lordosis increased rapidly. Over a period of 4 months, he went from having a severe cosmetic lordosis that was not painful to an increase of 30° in his lordosis accompanied by such severe pain that his sitting was limited to several hours a day. This is rather typical of the lordosis associated with rhizotomy.

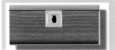

Case 3.2   Kaitlyn and Hannah

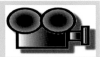

Kaitlyn and Hannah are both 4-year-old girls with diplegia who had been walking independently for 18 months; however, they are unstable and had trouble stopping and standing without holding on or falling to the floor. The mother of Kaitlyn elected to have a dorsal rhizotomy, while the mother of Hannah elected to continue physical therapy for 1 more year and then have femoral derotation and gastrocnemius lengthening. For Kaitlyn, 1 year after the dorsal rhizotomy, she also had femoral derotation, hamstring, and gastrocnemius lengthenings. As these two girls continue to mature both have done well, although Kaitlyn has had to work to overcome weakness that tended to limit her endurance for long-distance ambulation. As close as we could compare, these girls are very similar as 4-year-olds; however, Hannah, who had only orthopaedic surgery, may have had slightly less spasticity. This is a major problem in choosing the candidates for dorsal rhizotomy. Based on our experience, the child who does very well with a dorsal rhizotomy also does very well with only musculoskeletal surgery.

In summary, dorsal rhizotomy had a large burst of enthusiastic support from approximately 1987 through 1993. During this time, several thousand children had dorsal rhizotomies, and as individuals caring for these children develop more experience over time, and with the publication of two studies[36, 37] showing marginal functional benefit, the enthusiasm has decreased rapidly. The current general opinion is that there is no significant role for dorsal rhizotomy in children with quadriplegia because the complication rate is too high and the risk of functional loss is too great. Also, in the quadriplegic pattern children, unless almost all the posterior rootlets are cut, much of the spasticity will return. We had to implant baclofen pumps in three children with quadriplegic pattern CP who previously had dorsal rhizotomies and had very significant return of their spasticity 5 to 10 years afterward. In the young child, aged 3 to 8 years, who is a very high functioning diplegic ambulator with no significant muscle contractures or bony deformity, a dorsal rhizotomy can still be considered a reasonable option. However, based on a nonrandomized study[50] of ambulatory ability, these same children probably will do as well and maybe better with only orthopaedic surgery. It has been our experience that as children grow and develop, gait patterns of those who had orthopaedic surgery are somewhat different than those who had rhizotomy; however, there is no major functional improvement with the rhizotomy. The children with rhizotomy have a gait pattern in which weakness predominates, and the children with orthopaedic surgery have stiffness as the predominating factor (Case 3.2) As yet, there is no real equal comparison with the baclofen pump; however, the advantage in the few cases we have is that the pump can be adjusted to get more or less spasticity based on the clinical assessment of the child's need. With the data currently available, and the improved development of the intrathecal pump, it seems likely that rhizotomy will again become less accepted as a treatment option for spasticity in children with CP.

Electrical Stimulation

Electrical stimulation of the central nervous system to decrease spasticity has a long history both in the brain[62–64] and in the spinal cord.[65, 66] In spite of the very positive comments in these reports, the unpredictability, high complication rate, and minimal response have prevented this form of treatment from ever gaining wide acceptance. We have managed three children who had spinal cord stimulators implanted for spasticity control, and none of them has had any recognized benefit after the first several months. The use of implanted central nervous system stimulators for children with CP has enough experience in the community to safely say that it has no role, except in a very well-controlled research environment.

Myelotomy

Myelotomy, which involves cutting the spinal cord longitudinally either in the sagittal or coronal planes, was advocated extensively in the 1970s and 1980s.[67–69] However, because of the unpredictable results and high complication rate, myelotomy has been abandoned completely and has no role in the management of children with CP.

Peripheral Nervous System

Another way to decrease spasticity is by intervention at the level of the peripheral nerves. The only options involve lesioning of the nerve, either chemically or by physical transection. This lesioning mainly involves addressing the motor nerves instead of the sensory nerves, which are addressed by a rhizotomy. Chemical lesioning is almost always at least partially reversible. The chemical agents range from short-acting to long-acting local anesthetics, alcohol, and phenol. The use of local anesthetics to block nerve transmission was usually advocated as a way of doing diagnostic tests to see if a child would benefit from a surgical lengthening procedure.[70, 71] This concept makes little sense today because the blockade of nerves does not affect the contracture, which usually is the major problem to be surgically addressed. With today's modern diagnostic gait laboratories, this type of diagnostic evaluation has little use. In the 1970s, the use of alcohol was also advocated as a diagnostic and therapeutic way to reduce spasticity. Alcohol injections generally provide a decrease in tone for 1 to 3 months.[72–74] Phenol is an even more caustic agent and will destroy the nerve, so the spasticity will stay reduced for 18 to 24 months[75]; however, it is a very painful injection usually done under general anesthesia.[76] Both alcohol and phenol were very popular in the 1970s and into the early 1980s. Because of the toxic nature of these drugs and because the injections were painful, general anesthesia was required. With the availability of botulinum, there is only a rare role for their use to manage spasticity today. The use generally is in cases of botulinum immunity in which there are no other reasonable options (Case 3.3).

Direct surgical ablation of the motor nerve also has a long history as a means of reducing spasticity. Sectioning of the obturator nerve to decrease adductor spasticity at the hip is the most common indication.[77–79] In general, this procedure should be done only in nonambulatory children, and then only the anterior branch of the obturator nerve should be sectioned. Anterior branch obturator neurectomy is typically done in adolescents with severe adductor spasticity, or in younger children with severe hip dysplasia in whom an attempt is being made to reduce the hip and allow the dysplasia to recover without doing hip reconstruction. Occasionally there may be a child in whom neurectomy is a reasonable option in the upper extremity,[80] where the flexor muscles can be denervated by dissecting out the motor branches of the ulnar nerve. Also, there is a recent report of doing gastrocnemius neurectomy to control ankle equinus[81]; however, this is not a good idea from a mechanical perspective, as the muscle would lose strength. Overall, for the control of spasticity, peripheral neurectomy has a minimal role in the management of spasticity in the child with CP.

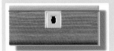

Case 3.3   Joe

At age 4 years, Joe developed a mild bleed from a brain arteriovenous malformation. This condition was surgically treated, and following the procedure he was left with mild left hemiplegia. This appeared to be a typical spastic hemiplegia until he entered puberty at age 14 years. A significant dystonic movement disorder developed in his left upper extremity, in which the elbow would flex along with strong wrist and finger flexion. An attempted treatment with trihexiphenidyl was unsuccessful. The biceps, forearm flexors, and finger flexors were then injected with botulinum toxin, which provided excellent relief, allowing the limb to remain in good position. Repeat injections were performed every 4 to 6 months over the next 2 years with gradually diminishing effect. At this time, the dystonia was so severe that finger flexion was causing skin breakdown in the palm, which was very painful. Motor point injection alcohol of the biceps and finger flexors provided only 3 months of relief. The same motor nerves, as well as the motor branches of the radial nerve, were then injected with phenol. This injection caused a severe neuritic pain syndrome for 6 weeks because the phenol also affected the sensory nerves. This injection provided almost 12 months of improvement in the dystonic movement. However, elements of the dystonia returned. The shoulder tended to go into extension and abduction, which was very annoying, because as he walked in school the arm would suddenly fly into extension and abduction, hitting walls or other people (Figure C3.3.1.). This was extremely annoying and frustrating to him. Because of the severe pain from the previous phenol injection, he refused it and other phenol injections, actually requesting amputation of the limb. It was recommended that Joe go for an evaluation for possible central lesioning to decease the dystonia; however, he refused this because he blamed his first brain surgery for all his current problems. With few other options left, he had a surgical denervation of the upper extremity, cutting the suprascapular nerve, motor branches to the triceps, and deltoid muscles. At the forearm, the motor branches to the finger and wrist flexors and extensors were cut. Because it was difficult to cut all motor nerves without cutting sensory nerves, some isolated motor function remained and got stronger over the next year following the denervation. At this time, the tendons on several finger flexors, the wrist extensor, and the biceps were released.

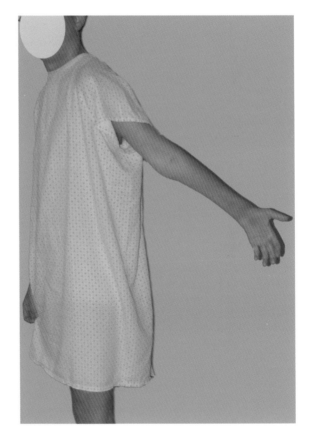

Figure C3.3.1

Neuromotor Junction and the Muscle

Decreasing tone at the muscle level by oral medication can be done with dantrolene sodium. The principal effect of dantrolene is an alteration of the calcium release from the sarcoplasmic reticulum. In addition to decreasing tone, dantrolene also decreases muscle strength.[18] This drug has been found to cause an acute decrease in spasticity similar to diazepam.[82] Dantrolene has significant complications: in addition to weakness, it can cause irreversible hepatitis in some children, chronic fatigue and dizziness, diarrhea, and increased seizures.[83] The drug has also been found to cause variable functional gains and a rapid accommodation effect.[84] With this record of poor functional gain and high complication rate, it is rarely used in children with CP today.

Local Injections: Botulinum Toxin (Botox)

Botulinum toxin (Botox) is a neurotoxin that is extracted from *Clostridium botulinum*, an anaerobic bacteria that typically causes food poisoning. Botox was initially used to treat strabismus in 1973.[85] It was approved for use to treat blepharospasm in 1987, and since that time, has been approved to treat cervical and oral dystonia in adults. In spite of these being its only approved uses, there are 297 references cited concerning the use of botulinum toxin as a treatment drug. The uses of this drug include spasticity, dystonia, cystitis, essential hyperhidrosis, facial wrinkles, facial asymmetry, debarking dogs, bruxism, stuttering, headaches, back spasms, bladder spasms, achalasia, anal spasms, constipation, vaginismus, tongue protrusion, and nystagmus. There are very few drugs on the market today with such widespread use.[85] Botox is serotype A, and is currently the only available therapeutic toxin of the seven available serotypes, although there is research on types B, C, and E.[85] The botulinum toxin binds irreversibly to the neuromotor junction, preventing the junction from functioning. With the permanent blockade, the peripheral nerve sprouts a new fiber and forms a new neuromotor junction. This process requires approximately 3 to 4 months. After new neuromotor junctions are formed, normal motor function returns (Figure 3.9). The toxin is a large protein molecule approximately 150 kilodaltons (kDa) in size.[86] Botox is frozen to preserve the drug and its function and requires reconstitution with saline at the time it is thawed. Because it is a large molecule, the

Figure 3.9. Botulinum toxin affects the neuromotor junction by irreversibly binding to the synaptic receptors to which the synaptosomal vesicles bind. This prevents the synaptosomal vesicles from releasing the acetylcholine into the neuromotor junction; therefore, activation of this neuromotor junction is no longer possible.

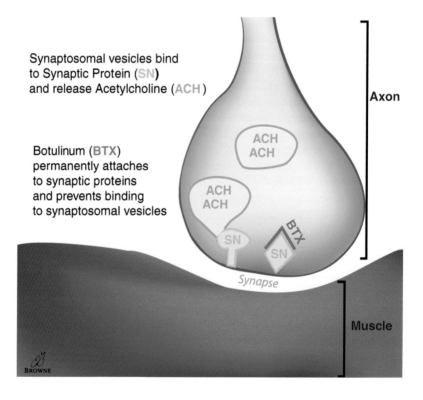

solution should not be vigorously shaken or injected rapidly through a small-bore needle or the turbulence created could potentially denature some of the protein.[87] When Botox is injected into the muscle, it causes a decreasing gradient of denervation approximately 3 cm in radius from the injection site.[88] Therefore, Botox injected into the muscle will cause temporary denervation followed by reinnervation, which takes approximately 3 to 4 months. Significant weakness occurs with a decrease in spasticity. The effect of this decrease in active spasticity is clear; however, this drug has no effect on the fixed contracture that may also be present.

The role of Botox for children with CP is continuing to evolve; however, its main use is to control spasticity. Others have promoted Botox as a pain control drug to use postoperatively to decrease postoperative muscle spasms,[89] a concept that does make some sense, although we have no experience using Botox in this way. The major use of Botox to treat children with CP is to decrease localized spasticity in a situation where some functional gain is expected. The typical situation is a 3- to 4-year-old child with a very spastic gastrocnemius who has problems wearing an orthosis. The Botox injection allows much more comfortable brace wear. Botox can be used in the cervical paraspinal muscles for severe hyperextension, opisthotonic posturing, upper extremity contractures with severe spasticity, or in hamstrings or adductors with significant spasticity. Botox injection to the adductors is not recommended as a treatment of spastic hips, except in a closely controlled clinical research trial, because there is a well-documented treatment that yields excellent results and deviation from these guidelines may increase the risk that more children will need hip reconstructions. A dose of 5 to 10 units per kilogram of weight is typically used and can be divided between two or three sites. The dose should be diluted with 1 to 2 ml saline per 100 units of Botox and injected with a small (25- to 27-gauge) needle into the neuromotor junction-rich zone of the target muscle. This zone is generally at the junction of the proximal and middle one-third of the muscle. The injections are usually done in a fan-shape fashion to help diffusion and only local topical anesthetic is used, such as Emula cream (Figure 3.10). Care should be taken not to inject the drug intravascularly; however, this has never been reported as a significant problem. Parents should expect the maximum effect to become present in 48 to 72 hours. It is possible to reinject other muscles in 4 weeks, by which time all the drug will be tissue fixed or degraded. There are almost no significant side effects except for mild pain at the injection site, similar to a vaccination. Some clinicians are using much higher doses without apparent side effects; however, the FDA approval is for only 5 units/kg of weight per day, and it is not approved for use in children at the time of this writing.

Botox is a short-acting drug by the nature of the way the neuromotor junction recovers. This character of the drug is good if the result of an injection is not considered beneficial; however, it is usually a drawback because the injection does provide a positive effect, which is subsequently lost. Repeat injections after 3 to 6 months are possible, but an immunity to the toxin develops in many children.[90] In our experience, most children have about 50% less benefit with each subsequent injection, and all children whom we have treated with more than four or five injections have developed complete immunity. This immunity is very frustrating for the child and family because the drug initially provided a very positive beneficial effect (see Case 3.3).

The typical effect of botulinum toxin is to decrease spasticity and strength in the injected muscle, with the tone and strength recovering in the subsequent 3 to 6 months. Some families report a much longer beneficial side effect; however, most studies looking at objective findings see little change

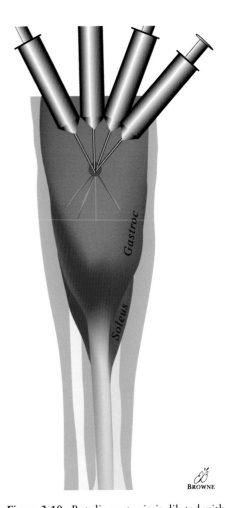

Figure 3.10. Botulinum toxin is diluted with 1 to 2 ml saline and injected into the neuromotor junction-rich zone of the muscle to be blocked. This neuromotor-rich zone is usually in the proximal one-third and two-thirds junction area. The botulinum is injected in a fan-shaped pattern with an understanding that it diffuses over approximately 3 cm from the injection site. For the gastrocnemius, separate medial and lateral injections may be made.

after this initial positive effect.[91] There may be longer-lasting functional gains in some children,[92] which may suggest that there is a reorganization that occurs such that the patient may settle around a slightly different chaotic attractor. This kind of temporary change may also allow physical therapy to have a positive effect on the individual's motor control system to shift the dynamic function. Also, many clinicians believe that Botox should be used in conjunction with other modalities, such as therapy, bracing, or casting.[93] Because of its temporary nature, this concept has good merit as a way of trying to gain more long-term functional improvement. However, if considerable effort with multiple modalities only pushes a child slightly away from a very stable chaotic attractor, the long-term prognosis is poor because the child will settle back to where she was when the efforts started. It is unclear at this time how often Botox can benefit a child by truly moving the dynamic motor control to a substantially new attractor area. Another major problem with botulinum toxin is that it is extremely expensive. As more companies develop other serotypes, perhaps competition will cause the price to drop.

Local Injection: Alcohol and Phenol

Injections into the neuromotor junction region with alcohol and phenol were also popular for a time, especially in the 1970s.[2, 75, 76, 94] Alcohol and phenol have the same problems when they are injected into the neuromotor junction as when they are used for neurolysis. In addition, if large volumes of the drugs are injected into muscles, intramuscular fibrosis can develop. The use of alcohol and phenol for neuromotor junction injections is rarely indicated for the treatment of spasticity in children today.

Direct Surgical Treatment of the Musculotendinous Unit

A very common and old treatment of spastic muscles is lengthening of the tendon, thereby releasing the contracture. In reality, the contracture is due to a muscle that has not grown sufficiently to its anatomically required length. The classic wisdom often repeated is that muscle tendon lengthening does not directly treat spasticity but only addresses the secondary effects of decreased muscle growth.[2, 7] This understanding of the effects of muscle tendon lengthening is only partly true because the hyperreflexic component of spasticity depends on the specific length and tension where the muscle is being stimulated.[1] Thus, the muscle is much more sensitive to initiate a hyperreflexive contraction when the most sensitive region of the length-tension curve is under tension. For an example, with the gastrocnemius having its most sensitive length-tension curve set at 20° plantar flexion, hyperreflexia demonstrated clinically as clonus will be easily initiated in 20° of plantar flexion. By lengthening the tendon and allowing this most sensitive aspect of the muscle length to rest at 10° of dorsiflexion, there will be significant decrease in the spasticity or the ability to initiate clonus when the ankle is at 20° of plantar flexion. By this method, lengthening the tendon has direct functional effects on the spasticity by moving the sensitive region to an area where it is less likely to be initiated during an activity such as gait. Also, lengthening the muscle will give it the ability to generate active plantar flexion moment at the place in the joint range where it is needed, instead of in significant plantar flexion in which children get little additional mechanical advantage from the contraction. This complex effect of muscle length is discussed further in the section on gait. Adjusting muscle length through the use of tendon lengthening is one of the primary options for treating the major secondary muscular effects of spasticity and also has some direct impact on the spastic response of the local muscles.

Orthotics

There has been much discussion in different venues of tone-reducing orthotics, specifically the use of various orthotic designs, such as elevated toe
plates, peroneal arch, calcaneal bar, and ankle articulations. All reported
studies that objectively evaluated these claims have not found any benefit beyond the mechanical constraint these orthoses provide.[95–97] Based on these
published data, there is no direct evidence of an impact on tone by the use
of orthotics. There may be some benefit to decreasing sensory input and
thereby decreasing muscle tone in some children. Also, based on subjective
experience reported by many clinicians, there are a significant number of
children, especially those with quadriplegic pattern involvement, whose
motor control system shifts to a different chaotic attractor. For example, by
keeping the ankle at neutral in an ankle-foot orthosis (AFO), a child has less
extensor posturing and sits better, and has better arm control. This change
in motor control is hard to directly relate to a reduction in spasticity; however, this change does occur. The orthotics have the opposite effect in some
children. Often, these children are driven to push into more plantar flexion
and hyperextension. These children get a sensory stimulus from the orthotic
that drives them toward more of the extensor posturing attractor.

Special tone-reducing casts with molded-in pressure point areas in the soles
and extended toe plates have been advocated as a technique for reducing
spasticity.[97, 98] Only small case studies have been reported that suggest a
benefit with this technique.[99] However, it seems that the positive effects of
wearing casts are directly related to the length of time they are worn.[100] It
is well known that cast wear causes muscle atrophy and weakness, which is
the likely effect seen and labeled as decreased spasticity in these children. In
our experience, the benefit of casting usually is approximately one to two times
the length of the cast wear time; therefore, if a child is in casts for 4 weeks,
the benefits will last 4 to 8 weeks. Parents tire quickly of placing the child in
casts and then having the effects quickly lost. Casting is very disruptive to
the child's lifestyle because they cannot bathe, dressing is difficult, and the
application of the cast is very time consuming. For these reasons, we do not
find the use of tone-reducing casts of much benefit in children with spastic
CP. The ankle orthotics, when they are fitting well, provide similar gains as
the use of tone-reducing casts. There are many benefits of these orthotics
over casts, including that the orthotic can be removed for bathing, the ankle
range of motion can be maintained, and there is less muscle atrophy.

The use of serial casting continues to make good therapeutic sense in very
spastic children in the acute recovery phase from closed head injury or any
other circumstance where the spasticity is resolving. The use of casts in these
children can provide a bridging effect until the spasticity resolves and they
are easier to maintain in orthotics. The primary mechanism for decreasing
spasticity by immobilization is probably immobilization atrophy of the
muscles and perhaps some stretching of connective tissue. There are no con-
vincing data available that suggest that it is possible, through immobilization
techniques, to make spastic muscles grow longer.

Therapy

The use of physical therapy techniques, such as active and passive range of
motion, are well-accepted treatment modalities in children with spasticity.
There is no objective evidence that a specific therapy can impact the degree
of spasticity permanently, although there are activities, such as horseback
riding, that patients, parents, and therapists almost uniformly report to

decrease spasticity temporarily. This same effect has been reported to us by individuals while riding in boats or doing other rhythmic activities. The effects on spasticity by these activities are hard to explain, but we believe they occur and probably are mediated through complex cerebral cortex sensory perception and motor control program generator interactions. From dynamic motor theory, this may also result from pushing the individual toward a different chaotic attractor that is not very stable, and as soon as the perturbation has subsided, the stronger attractor comes back into force and the individual's motor control system settles back to where it was before the activity. This explanation best describes what patients report; however, it is not very helpful in conceptually understanding what is happening from an anatomic perspective.

Passive stretching is a widely-accepted modality for maintaining range of motion; however, objective documentation of the exact benefit is lacking. We have seen many children in patterning therapy programs where they were receiving passive range-of-motion exercises 18 to 20 hours a day. These children do have less spasticity and better range of motion compared with similar children who get very little passive range-of-motion stretching. However, it is unclear how much passive range of motion is required to get a significant benefit, because it is neither practical nor healthy for children's overall development to be doing 12 to 18 hours per day of passive stretching.

The use of vibrators, usually at 100 to 120 hertz, also has been shown to decrease muscle tone, and they are often used by individuals who feel stiff. Some patients with CP report that the use of a vibrator makes their muscles feel less tight.[6] This feeling is a temporary phenomenon and may be related to similar benefits that others report from deep muscle massage.

A Global Approach to Managing Spasticity

There are many options available to treat spasticity. In developing an algorithm, clinicians first have to remember and educate families that spasticity is not CP, and by removing spasticity, the CP will not be cured. Also, the spasticity is an exaggeration of a normal phenomenon, muscle tone, which is an extremely important aspect in normal motor function. Therefore, the goal is never to remove all muscle tone, but to adjust the tone so it provides maximum functional benefit to the individual.

The first function of an evaluation for spasticity treatment is to tally the negative and positive aspects of the spasticity. Based on the specific problems the spasticity is causing, the clinician can choose from the available treatment options. First, the clinician needs to determine whether these problems are due to a global increase in spasticity or to increased spasticity in a local region, such as one joint or one limb. For example, the increased tone in the gastrocnemius of a hemiplegic child has very different implications compared with a child who has severe total body involvement and has problems being seated in a wheelchair.

For local problems that involve two to four specific muscles, the focus should initially be on local treatment. Examples of such localized spasticity are spastic wrist flexors and elbow flexors, equinus foot position, and spastic hamstring muscles causing knee flexion contractures. After identifying the problem as local, the clinician has to decide if it is supple spasticity only with full underlying joint range of motion, mainly a fixed muscle contracture due to a short muscle, or a combination of both supple spasticity and fixed contracture. If the problem is dynamic spasticity with no underlying contracture, then the primary treatment options are botulinum toxin injection and an orthotic. If the problem is a fixed contracture, the only option is surgical lengthening of the tendon. If the problem is mixed spasticity and fixed contracture, the options can be combined by starting with a trial of Botox and orthotics. To gain an adequate result when the Botox fails, a muscle lengthening should subsequently be done. By far the most common situation is children who fall into the mixed group with dynamic spasticity and contracture; however, there are also children who clearly fall into one or the other groups.

Children whose functional problems related to spasticity involve more than four muscle groups should be considered as the globally involved group. These children should be divided based on whether the problems are mainly caused by sleeping difficulties at night or daytime functional problems. The group of children with primarily nighttime sleeping problems is small, and it is never very clear whether these sleep problems are related to spasticity or whether they are a primary sleep disorder. This group, whose primary problem is nighttime sleeping, should be treated with a trial of oral antispasticity drugs, which occasionally work. Usually, diazepam is our first treatment preference, and we have several patients in our practice for whom this works well. Intrathecal baclofen also improves sleep and can be used if the oral trial fails. For children with daytime functional problems caused by global spasticity, the specific functional problems need to be identified. These functional problems may include difficulty with dressing, seating, and toileting or gait problems. This group should be further divided into those children with multiple functional problems and those with a single problem.

For children with multiple functional problems due to global spasticity, there usually are significantly more problems than functional benefits of the global spasticity. However, it is always important to consider what the functional benefits of the spasticity are for the individual child. If these benefits can be preserved, or are much less beneficial than the problems being caused by the spasticity, the main treatment option is the intrathecal baclofen pump.

For children with single functional problems, such as gait or problems with seating, attention should be focused on specific local treatments. For example, for children who have seating problems, a careful assessment of the seating system can often correct the problem by adjusting and providing a well-fitting seating system. For children whose primary problem is gait, a very careful assessment, usually requiring a full instrumented gait analysis, should be completed to fully understand the interactions of the spasticity, contractions, and skeletal malalignments, which all may be components of their gait impairment. For most children who are independent ambulators and have global increase in spasticity, the primary treatment is correcting the specific individual components of the disability, such as correcting bony malalignments, lengthening contracted muscles, and transferring muscles that are functioning in the wrong phase of gait. The use of intrathecal baclofen may be an option, although there is very little worldwide experience with its use in this population. For children who are ambulatory with diplegia, dorsal rhizotomy can be considered between the ages of 3 and 8 years in those individuals with no bony deformities or muscle contractures and only dynamic spasticity.

Children with global spasticity who are having significant upper extremity problems should usually be considered for surgical reconstruction. For children with global spasticity who have specific problems related to functional tasks of daily living, such as self-dressing or toileting, the first treatment should be an intensive evaluation by an experienced physical or occupational therapist. In summary, by combining all the options and careful assessment, children with CP can usually be treated in a way that makes the spasticity become a benefit and not a major component of their impairment.

Hypotonia

Hypotonia is defined as lower than normal muscle tone. Hypotonia occurs less frequently than spasticity in children with CP and, although it is still relatively common, it has not attracted the attention that hypertonia has. Hypotonia is most common in children with congenital CP, with lesions such as lissencephaly. Families usually perceive and describe the problem as the child being weak, which most children with hypotonia are. Also, there is a common confusion between hypotonia and hyperlaxity or hypermobility of joints. Each of these is a separate problem, but they are often interrelated. For example, a child with Down syndrome has hypotonia, meaning a decreased stiffness in the muscle, but also has connective tissue laxity. Together, these conditions allow for joint hypermobility. In children with hypotonia due to CP, it is usually associated with severe quadriplegic pattern involvement and mental retardation. These children have so little motor control that the system fails to even make an attempt to provide stability. Some children have hyperreflexia as a spastic feature but have low tone as a passive element. This group will be called the local mixed tone pattern. Also, there are children with definite increased tone and spasticity in the lower extremities but significant hypotonia with their trunk and head control. This group will be called the anatomic mixed tone pattern. The anatomic mixed tone pattern is very common during middle childhood, especially in nonambulatory children. Many of these children were initially hypotonic infants, which are much more common than hypertonic infants.[6] Most of these hypotonic infants develop spasticity slowly, usually starting distally and progressing proximally.[101, 102] This proximal migration of increased tone often helps the children to sit better as they get older.

The Effects of Hypotonia

Just as secondary effects of spasticity are noted, there are secondary effects of hypotonia. Muscles are the primary structures that are affected. The muscles tend to be weak, meaning they do not generate a high active force compared with a normal child, and they tend to be excessively long or do not have a good definite end feel during an examination as a normal muscle would. These hypotonic muscles are very thin and gracile when examined. Some children with severe hypotonia have a muscle that appears white during surgery. There are no data to define what these changes reflect at the histologic level. Other common changes in the limbs in hypotonic children are long gracile bones with osteopenia and osteoporosis. Joint hypermobility is often associated. There is no recognized measurement of hypotonia except the modified Ashworth scale, which assigns a single scale group to separate hypotonia from normal tone (Table 3.1).

Functional Problems and Treatment

The main functional problem is poor trunk and head control. The joint laxity and poor strength also leads to a high rate of joint dislocations at the hip and feet with the development of scoliosis. Because of the osteopenia, gracile bones, and osteoporosis, recurrent fractures become a problem in a few children.

Almost all the literature with respect to hypotonia and CP is concerned with diagnosing other common diseases.[101, 102] As opposed to spasticity, the treatment options for hypotonia are very limited because hypotonia is a situation where there is not enough tone. In almost all situations of life, it is harder to treat something that is not there than to remove something of which there is too much. This fact is well demonstrated by all the options that are available to decrease muscle tone in children with spasticity, whereas there is not one option available to increase muscle tone in hypotonic children. Stabilizing hyperlaxed joints is limited to either surgery or external orthotics. The main problem of poor sitting is addressed with well-designed seating to provide a stable, upright posture. Foot and ankle orthotics are used to stabilize the ankle and feet for standing in standers. These children often require supine standers because of poor head control. When the joint instabilities become severe, stabilization by fusion, such as posterior spinal fusion for scoliosis and foot fusion for planovalgus collapse, is commonly performed.

Movement Disorders

Movement disorders are primary problems related to the ability of children to develop and control motor movement as a pattern. The specific description of these deformities is somewhat confusing and varies among authors of different texts. Although there is a large body of scientific work evaluating the function and pathologies of the brain that lead to movement disorders, the complexities are so great that there is still no easy clear explanation of how motor control is managed in the brain.[3] The pathology of these movement disorders has been localized to the basal ganglion and the communication process between the cerebral cortex and the basal ganglion. The primary lesion in most movement disorders is in the basal ganglion, as demonstrated by the development of posttraumatic dystonia.[103] Also, some movement disorders, such as ballismus, have been localized to occur primarily in the subthalamic nucleus. It is beyond the scope of this text to review all the biochemical and anatomic bases of movement disorders that are currently understood. Understanding the specific pathology in individual children may provide important treatment options, such as medication or surgery. However, in many children, it is impossible to specifically localize the pathology, or if it can be localized, it does not help in directly treating these children.

It is extremely important for the clinician treating these children to understand the difference between movement disorders and disorders of tone, meaning primarily spasticity. The treatments for these disorders are often diametrically opposed, especially the options that the orthopaedist would consider. A helpful approach for the orthopaedic clinician who deals with these children is to approach them through the conceptualization of dynamic control theory. In this approach, their function will tend to be drawn toward a chaotic attractor, which is called the movement disorder. Many of these patterns are not clearly separate from each other, and they may be best visualized as different strength attractors. The three movement patterns that can be used to categorize most children with CP are dystonia, athetosis, and chorea or ballismus.

Dystonia

Dystonia is a movement disorder that has a torsional component with strong muscle contractions with major recurrent movement patterns. An example of such a pattern is strong shoulder external rotation extension and abduction combined with elbow extension, then alternating with the opposite extreme of elbow flexion, shoulder internal rotation, adduction, and flexion. Dystonia may occur in a single limb, in a single joint, or as a whole-body disorder. These movements cannot be volitionally controlled, although there is a sensory feedback element that sometimes allows them to be stopped or reversed. For example, a specific pressure point or body position may stop the forceful elbow and shoulder external rotation contraction. Sometimes, moving a finger passively will break up the forceful dystonic wrist flexion. There is no good anatomic understanding of how these sensory inputs function.[3] The attraction to individual patterns is weak, which means various perturbations can push the system out of the pattern; however, the system is very unstable, being drawn to either another attractor or back to the same attractor again. These attractor positions in individual patients become very well recognized and can be described easily by the patients themselves as the positions to which their limbs seem to want to go.

As noted earlier, both dystonia and spasticity can be present in the same limb, although in our experience, this is not a common occurrence in localized limb dystonia. The presence of both is much more common in generalized dystonia. It is especially difficult to separate generalized dystonia from generalized spasticity, especially when it presents as extensor posturing with opisthotonic patterning. The difference exists because opisthotonic patterning originates primarily from brainstem defects as opposed to dystonia, which originates primarily from basal ganglion lesions. Also, the children with opisthotonic patterning are often in this hyperextended position all the time, including during sleep. Children with dystonia tend to be in a more relaxed and normal position during sleep. The secondary effects of dystonia and spasticity are also very different.

Secondary Effects of Dystonia

It cannot be overemphasized how important it is for the orthopaedist to identify isolated limb dystonia from spasticity because on the initial evaluation, for example, the limb may present in fixed wrist and elbow flexed position, which has an appearance exactly like a hemiplegic, spastic limb. This same position occasionally occurs with the foot in equinovarus or planovalgus, having the same initial appearance whether the child is spastic or dystonic. The major difference between spasticity and dystonia is determined by a good physical examination and patient history. On physical examination, it often becomes clear in the limb with dystonia that there is no fixed contracture and the muscle appears to be hypertrophic, like a child who has been a weight lifter. During the examination, the child's muscles will often release and have a temporary appearance of normal tone. When the muscle releases, the joint will have a full range of motion with no contracture present. This appearance is very different compared with a child with a spastic limb in whom the contracted deformity is stiff in all conditions and the muscle often has a short, thin appearance on physical examination. A child with a severe equinovarus positioning of the foot from spasticity will always have some level of muscle contracture present. The important question to ask in the history taking is if the foot or hand ever goes in any other position except the one that it is in now. If the problem is dystonia, the parents and the child often will say very readily that sometimes instead of the wrist being in a flexed position, it is stuck back with the fingers flexed but the wrist extended. The history of how the child positions when relaxed, the appearance of the muscles, and the sense of the child's underlying tone when relaxed are the important parameters to use in separating spasticity from dystonia. This distinction is especially true for a quadriplegic child, where the child with pure dystonia will often have very large well-formed muscles and no underlying contractures. A child with significant hyperextension posturing spasticity often has significant contractures, sometimes of the extensor muscles of the neck and often of hip extensors and quadriceps of the knee.

Objective measurement of degrees of dystonia is an extremely difficult problem. There has been an attempt made to measure dystonia by the development of the Barry Albright Dystonia (BAD) scale, which focuses on generalized dystonia and mainly measures the stiffness of the child.[104] This scale is not much different from the Ashworth scale applied to the trunk, and as such really has no ability to separate dystonia from spasticity. This scale cannot be applied to isolated limb dystonias.

Treatment of Central Nervous System: Medications

The primary treatment of both generalized and localized dystonia is oral medication management. The available drug options are many and the rationale for use of a specific drug is not well defined. The available options include levodopa; anticholinergics such as trihexyphenidyl hydrochloride and diphenhydramine; and the benzodiazepins, baclofen, carbamazepine, and a large variety of dopamine receptor-blocking drugs. None of these drugs has a highly selective effect on dystonia, and the positive and negative effects of each drug have to be balanced, preferably by a clinician with experience in their use (Case 3.4).

Intrathecal baclofen has been reported to be beneficial to treat generalized dystonia; however, this is a group of children that includes extensor posturing and it is unclear whether the dystonia or the spasticity responded to the baclofen.[22] In another study where there was a major attempt to separate the dystonia from the spasticity, the effects on the dystonic patterns were less reliable, especially with localized limb dystonia.[105] It has been our experience, in two children with localized limb dystonia, that the response is not very reliable (Case 3.5).

Treatment Options: Central Nervous System Surgery

Many reports going back 30 to 40 years describe destructive surgical procedures of the central nervous system, mainly pallidotomy, to treat dystonia. The results of these procedures have been unpredictable, with a tendency for the dystonia to return.[106] Using better stereotactic localization and improved localization, there is a renewed interest in lesioning procedures to treat dystonia.[107, 108] So far, however, these are single cases or very small series, and the usefulness of basal ganglion lesioning remains unclear.

Treatment Options: Peripheral

Treatment at the level of the muscle has to be approached very carefully. Dystonia is a contraindication to muscle lengthenings or transfers. Dystonia is a very unstable motor control system, and a worse opposite deformity will invariably occur if muscle lengthenings or muscle transfers are performed. The peripheral treatment should be reversible and temporary or stabilizing in almost all cases. In the reversible category, the primary treatment is botulinum toxin injections into the main offending muscles. These injections are extremely effective because the muscle weakness also somehow decreases the initiation of the dystonia and decreases the attractor strength. The major problem with using Botox in children with CP is that dystonia is permanent and will require treatment injections every 4 to 6 months. Every child we have treated for dystonia has become immune to the Botox and it has lost all effect. Therefore, the treatment starts with impressive and wonderful

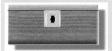   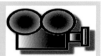

Case 3.4   Sarah

Sarah, a 7-year-old girl, was referred after having seen many other physicians. Her mother complained that she could not run or walk well. Sarah tended to get her feet tangled up and tripped over herself, according to her mother. Sarah herself was getting very frustrated and did not want to play with friends or go to school. The physical examination was completely normal, but observation of her gait demonstrated great variability with torsional elements and hyper hip and knee flexion. Kinematics showed erratic variability with extremes that indicated different patterns, not a variation from a single mean (Figure C3.4.1). With the diagnosis of torsional dystonia, she was started on trihexyphenidyl, and after 1 month, almost all the symptoms resolved.

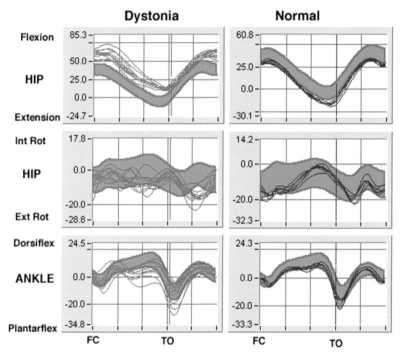

Figure C3.4.1

results and ends in approximately 2 years when it no longer provides benefit. Based on published papers, this immunity does not happen when smaller muscles are treated, such as eyelid treatment for blepharospasm.[3] For very persistent and severe dystonia in children who are resistant to Botox, phenol injections are a reasonable option. However, development of hypersensitivity and sensory pain from the use of phenol blocks of nerves that contain sensory elements is a major problem. It is very difficult to block only the motor nerves and avoid all sensory nerves, especially in the upper extremities (see Case 3.3).

Peripheral Surgical Treatment

The primary treatment of symptomatic dystonic foot deformities is to stabilize the foot with a fusion and excise the tendons of the deforming muscles.

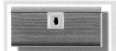

Case 3.5   Paul

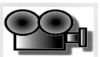

Paul, a 15-year-old boy, was referred to the orthopaedic clinic by a psychiatrist who had been treating him because of depression and a conversion reaction with a very peculiar gait. Because of Paul's persistent complaint of feeling that his knee was giving away, there was a concern that he had some mechanical knee instability. This walking pattern had been slowly and intermittently getting worse since middle childhood when he started living with an aunt. She had no history of his early childhood. Paul stated that the problem was somewhat variable but seemed worse when he wanted to walk fast or run, and got worse when he was anxious. He expressed great frustration with the problem, especially with the left leg, which did not support him. On observation of his gait, he had a consistent instability of the left leg with hyperflexion and some torsional control problem. His physical examination was completely normal with no joint contractures, no instabilities, and no increase in muscle tone. His muscle strength was excellent with manual muscle testing. On kinematic evaluation, he showed several patterns of motion with great variability that was clearly not around a bell-shaped distribution. A diagnosis of dystonia was made and he had trials of trihexyphenidyl, ankle orthotics, and botulinum toxin, all without significant benefit. Over this 2-year period, he continued to get slightly worse. After a positive trial of intrathecal baclofen, he had an intrathecal baclofen pump implanted that improved his gait pattern to some degree, but he complained of being weak when the drug dose was high enough to really suppress the movement.

This means, if there is a varus deformity with the tibialis posterior and peroneal muscles, these muscles should be excised and a triple arthrodesis performed. This approach is reliable and provides for a stable functional foot. Often, the child will need to use an orthosis because of poor control of the ankle plantar flexors and dorsiflexors. If these flexors are involved in the dystonic motor control deformity, they too may need to be excised; however, we prefer to leave them alone in the initial procedure to see if they will settle down after the foot is stabilized. The upper extremity is more difficult, but in severe cases the limb may need to be denervated and allowed to be flaccid. Also, doing fusions of the wrist and occasionally of the shoulder may be reasonable options. We had one adolescent who requested amputation of the upper limb, but a limb that is flaccid with sensation is a better cosmetic solution. Dealing with dystonia at the knee and hip is especially difficult, because it is not functional to denervate the muscles or fuse the joints. We did a rectus transfer on an adolescent whose knee stiffness was thought to be spastic but afterward was found to be dystonic. For 9 months after the rectus transfer, she held the knee in flexion when she tried to stand. Persistent physical therapy and orthotic use converted this patterning back to extension at about the time we were contemplating reversing the rectus transfer.

A Global Approach to Management of Dystonia

Treating dystonia in children can be very frustrating. Because dystonia is a relatively rare occurrence, treatment should be a combined effort of the individual who has experience with neurologic drugs and the clinician who has experience with peripheral motor management options. The initial management in most children should be to explore the possibilities of oral drugs because some children respond to very low doses and do well. If the oral medications fail, the whole body involvement group should be separated from the focal single anatomic area group (see Case 3.4).

For the whole body involvement group, a careful assessment should determine if these children really have dystonia or if their problems are due to spasticity and fixed contractures. If the problem is due to fixed contractures, releasing the contractures, usually hip flexor and knee extension contractures, and allowing them to get in a better sitting position may solve the problem. If the dystonia is the major aspect of the problem, the options to consider are intrathecal baclofen pump or a pallidotomy. At this time, the intrathecal baclofen pump is favored as the first approach if there is a positive response to a trial dose. If the intrathecal baclofen does not work, another reasonable option to consider is pallidotomy.

For children with localized dystonia who have failed oral medication treatment, a careful assessment of the area and level of maximal functional impairment is required. The first-line approach is an evaluation with the use of orthotics to stabilize the deformity. Orthotics are especially likely to work if the dystonia is affecting the foot. If this simple mechanical approach fails, the next line is to use Botox in the offending muscle; however, the family and child need to be warned that this is a temporary measure. After the Botox fails, an intrathecal baclofen trial is considered, or if the problem is localized to the foot, a fusion stabilization procedure is considered. If the baclofen trial is successful, a pump is implanted (see Case 3.5). If the pump is not successful, additional peripheral blockade using phenol may be an option. At this point, pallidotomy can also be considered as an option. If the pallidotomy is not an option, then further denervation and stabilization are the only remaining options.

Athetosis

Athetosis is a movement disorder presenting as large movements of proximal joints. Athetosis tends to be worse in the upper extremity with external rotation and abduction movements of the shoulder, often with extension and fanning of the fingers. The movement is induced by voluntary effort, although sometimes this effort is as remote as trying to speak. A variable amount of voluntary control is often improved in the context of more complex movements, such as a movement associated with walking. Athetosis is also a major component of the hyperkinetic pattern, which is the term used by some neurologists. Traditionally, athetosis has been associated with neonatal kernicturus and hyperbilirubinemia.[109] This direct relationship has become less clear as the treatment of kernicturus and hyperbilirubinemia has improved.[110] There has been a significant decrease in the number of children with predominantly athetosis in the past 30 years.[111] The pathologic etiology classically involves kernicturus in the palladium; however, investigations into cases with unclear etiology have found lesions also involving various parts of the basal ganglion. Children with isolated athetosis tend to have no intellectual deficits, but often have motor speech problems that make communication difficult. The natural history of athetosis is an infant who initially is hypotonic, then between 12 and 24 months of age, starts to have increased movement with an underlying hypotonia. As these children get to be 2 to 4 years old, the hypotonia resolves and many develop some level of increased tone that helps to modulate their movement. Typically, by age 5 years the full expression of the movement disorder is present.

Sensory Motor Effects of Atethosis

In individuals with athetosis only, there are almost no secondary effects in childhood. There may be some increased mobility of finger extension, especially at the metacarpal phalangeal joint. The muscles tend to be hypertrophic, although less so than with dystonia where the maximum contraction is held for a longer period of time. In athetosis, there is a large amount of motion but the muscle is not held in maximum contraction for an increased amount of time. The difference between athetosis and dystonia for the muscles is similar to the difference between a weight-lifting athlete and a long-distance runner. Dystonia is similar to weight lifting and athetosis is similar to running. Children with athetosis have a very high energy need,[112] as opposed to children with quadriplegic spasticity where the energy need is considerably less than normal. Athetosis usually involves significant problems of trunk control, with trunk hypotonia often significantly limiting a child's ability to gain sitting stability or to walk. Facial movements are usually part of the athetoid pattern, and are often associated with increased drooling. This movement disorder also appears to affect the vocal cords, causing a major motor speech impairment.

Treatment

The use of diazepam as an oral medication will decrease athetoid movement, but only at very high doses. Except for acute situations, such as following surgery, diazepam has little use because of the severe sedative effects at the dosage that controls the movement. There are no other medications that have gained widespread use. Baclofen is contraindicated because it will reduce the tone, which often makes the athetoid movements worse because the spasticity acts like a shock absorber to dampen the movements. Botox has little or no usefulness because of the whole-body nature of the athetoid involvement. There is rarely a single problem caused by one or two muscles.

There is a long history of central nervous system surgery, mainly ablative procedures[43, 113] or implanted electrical stimulation[114]; however, none of these has demonstrated any consistent benefit in individuals with athetosis. Currently, there is no role for central nervous system surgery for athetosis.

Musculoskeletal surgery is limited to stabilizing joints where they might provide functional benefit. Fusion of the subtalar joint and spinal fusion for scoliosis are the most commonly indicated operative procedures. However, most children with athetosis only will need no musculoskeletal surgery. Many children have a mix of spasticity and athetosis, so they develop the secondary problems of muscle contractures from the spastic component. As the patient is evaluated to determine if the contracted muscle should be lengthened, caution should be exercised when trying to determine how much spasticity is dampening unwanted athetosis.

A common combination is a hamstring contracture with or without a knee flexion contracture, which makes it difficult for a young adult or adolescent to stand. Often, the standing is an important function for the adult-sized individual because it will allow one attendant to provide for their needs as opposed to needing two attendants to do a dependent patient lift transfer. In this situation, lengthening the hamstrings and knee capsule may provide a substantial functional benefit; however, the postoperative management may be very difficult, as the athetosis tends to get worse with pain. Although this can be a very difficult time for the patient, family, and medical team, it often provides excellent functional gain in the end. A major advantage is that the patient usually has excellent understanding of the goals and will be very willing to work hard to achieve the goals.

Undertaking a major surgical reconstruction in a child with severe athetosis and underlying spasticity requires a very experienced postoperative management team. Often, there is an element of great hesitation with families

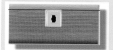 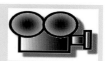

Case 3.6   Nicholas

Nicholas, a 16-year-old male with severe knee flexion contractures and torsional malalignment of the left hip with planovalgus feet, was having increased difficulty in walking. He had normal cognitive function and was academically at the top of his high school class. It was recommended that he have a left femoral osteotomy, bilateral knee capsulotomies with hamstring lengthenings, and arthrodesis for planovalgus feet. After extensive discussion, he and his family agreed to proceed, although with a lot of hesitation. Postoperatively, he had severe spasms requiring very high doses of diazepam and morphine. On the left side, he also developed a sciatic nerve palsy. After 1 week, the pain and spasms subsided and he started a long rehabilitation period requiring slow extension stretching of the left knee, as tolerated by the sciatic palsy. After 1 year of rehabilitation, he was standing and walking much more upright and he was very glad he had gone through the procedure. There were many times following the surgery where both Nicholas and his family felt like he would never recover from the surgery and the related complications. However, the sensory and motor defects of the sciatic palsy completely resolved, and the final expected outcome was similar to the expectations going into the procedure.

and young adults or adolescents to undertake any major surgical changes. This hesitation in families and patients often develops because of their own experience with the unpredictableness of athetosis. They are hesitant to undertake a treatment that they fear will leave them even worse than they are currently. Many of these families and patients have also had experience with physicians who did not appreciate the unpredictable nature of athetosis and were not willing to listen to their experience with this condition (Case 3.6).

Because of the excellent cognitive function in most individuals with athetosis, their input into rehabilitation often significantly enhances the rehabilitation period because they will know what works and what does not work. This great insight by these patients in understanding of their own body can lead to a dynamic in which therapists feel the patients are not willing to listen or want to try something new. On the other hand, these patients may feel that the therapists are not listening and only want to follow a fixed therapeutic plan. This is the situation in which both the therapists and the patients have to listen to each other, and both have to be open to try different techniques to arrive at a maximum rehabilitation potential of each individual.

Another major musculoskeletal problem of athetosis is degenerative joint disease changes in the cervical spine from the increased cervical spinal mobility. We have never seen these changes as a problem in a child or an adolescent; however, they have been well reported to occur in middle age, although the exact incidence is unclear. There are many small series reporting myelopathy with this degenerative joint disease process as the cervical spine develops instability and subluxation.[115-119] If there is any decreased motor function or change in motor function in an individual with athetosis, a full workup of the cervical spine including radiographs and MRI scans is required. The degenerative joint disease and the cervical spine instability usually require cervical spine fusion and decompression.

We have seen several children with athetosis who developed lumbar spondylolisthesis in childhood, and the only fusion for spondylolisthesis that we have done was in an adolescent with athetosis (Case 3.7). There is

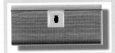

Case 3.7   Zackery

Zackery, a 12-year-old boy, presented with a complaint of back pain, especially after walking long distance. A gait analysis showed very high variability in step length and most kinematic parameters (Figure C3.7.1). He had no fixed contractures on physical examination. A radiograph of his spine demonstrated L5 spondylolysis with grade one spondylolisthesis (Figure C3.7.2). An attempt at conservative treatment with a lumbar flexion jacket for 6 months demonstrated no significant decrease in the pain; therefore, it was recommended to have a posterolateral arthrodesis from L4 to the sacrum. After this healed, all his back pain resolved.

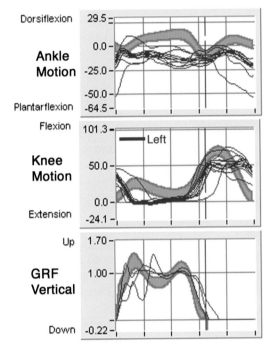

Figure C3.7.1

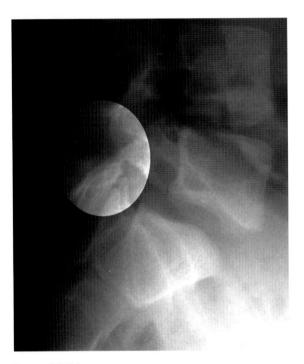

Figure C3.7.2

no specific information on the incidence of spondylolysis, or the incidence with which it progresses to an unstable spondylolisthesis.

Treatment: Therapy

The main treatment for a child with athetosis is excellent therapy by an experienced therapist. This treatment focuses on educating the family and working with the child to help them find what works and what does not work. Good seating is required to maximize upper extremity function; however, the family and therapist also have to allow the child to explore with bare feet and use her head as a motor control device. Because athetosis is usually worse in the upper extremity, there is a small group of children who have good control of their lower extremities and can do fine motor skills with their feet. Skills such as drawing, writing, and playing musical instruments are occasionally mastered. Unless the child is given options to explore these skills, they will not be recognized. The most common skill a child with athetosis can learn is to use a joystick to drive a wheelchair. Because the function of these children is often apparent by the time they are 4 to 5 years old and they are very intelligent, they are the only candidates with CP for whom an early power wheelchair fitting is a reasonable option. The power wheelchair does require the family to have transportation to carry it and an adapted home. Also, many children benefit from the use of weights on the wrists when they are trying to do specific tasks with the upper extremity, or the use of ankle weights when they are working on walking. Weighted vests can also help some children during seated activities. These weights may provide dampening of the movement similar to the presence of spasticity, or there may be a more complicated control interaction. The weights do seem to move these children to a different and more stable chaotic attractor in the motor control abilities area. Each child is quite variable, requiring an experienced and patient therapist to try many options and ascertain which combination is working best for the individual child. Some parents become excellent at defining the specific circumstances in which their child can best function.

In summary, the treatment of athetosis primarily revolves around experienced therapists who can help these children access the most useful functional motor abilities and to allow them to express their generally high cognitive function. These children often benefit greatly from the use of augmentative speech devices, and as such need to have access to excellent assistive communication services. Musculoskeletal procedures are useful only to stabilize joints, and in rare circumstances, to treat the underlying spasticity when it causes more functional problems than benefits. There is rarely any role for medication in the treatment of athetosis.

Chorea and Ballismus

Chorea is a movement disorder defined by jerky, rhythmic, small-range movements. These movements are more predominant distally in the limb; however, they are present as proximal movements of the head and trunk as rhythmic, jerky motion as well. Ballismus is large movement based at the proximal joints, primarily the shoulder and elbow or hip and knee. These large movements are unpredictable, jerky, and often have a violent character to them. Some neurologists believe that chorea and ballismus are two ends of the same movement spectrum, and from the musculoskeletal treatment perspective, this concept works well. These movement patterns are the most rare of the movement disorders in children with CP. When these movement disorders are seen to be developing, especially if significant chorea develops, the diagnosis of CP should be questioned. If significant chorea or ballismus movements start to develop in children with CP, additional workup frequently defines a more specific diagnosis, often one with a degenerative process. These movement disorders may get slowly worse if there are no mechanisms for controlling them.

The primary pathology for chorea and ballismus occurs in the basal ganglion; therefore, many drug options similar to the treatment of dystonia are considered as the first line of treatment. There have also been positive reports of ablative surgery on the internal capsule.[107, 108] There are no specific treatments for the musculoskeletal affects of ballismus and chorea in children with CP.

Summary of Motor Control Treatments

It is often very difficult to separate out exact treatment recommendations between the movement disorders, especially because there is not a clear pathoanatomic basis of one movement disorder compared with another. These disorders are somewhat overlapping in their presentation, and probably reflect movement patterns best understood as chaotic attractors in dynamic motor control without a clear anatomic separation. An analogy of these patterns might be the difference between a wind and rain storm compared with a thunderstorm or a tornado. Each of these storms is a definite recognized pattern, all occur in the same geographic region, and the cause of each is similar and not completely understood. This same analogy applies between the movement disorders of dystonia, athetosis, chorea, and ballismus. These movement patterns are fairly different and recognizable although a pathoanatomic understanding of the exact differences is not clear. However, because the patterns can be recognized, specific treatment algorithms for each can be defined. From the musculoskeletal perspective, dystonia is a nonvolitional movement pattern that is difficult to treat because of the persistent nature of the symptoms and the strength of the muscle forces. Athetosis is more predictable and is often under some volitional control that can be accessed through physical therapy intervention. There is very little musculoskeletal treatment that is beneficial for chorea and ballismus.

Disorders of Balance

Ataxia is a term used to describe poor balance in children with CP. Some children with CP seem to have an isolated ataxia, usually related to congenital cerebellar malformations.[110] Often, these are normally developing infants until 12 months of age, when it is noticed that they are not progressing with their normal motor skills development. These children have delayed independent sitting and delayed walking, often not until 2 or 3 years of age. The problem with their balance is most clear in the development of independent walking, but as the children start doing fine motor skills, they demonstrate clumsiness in writing and other fine motor skills. Ataxia often affects speech as well.

Typically, the normal development of balance reaches its maximum in middle childhood and remains stable during the adolescent growth spurt; however, these children appear to be losing balance ability. This apparent loss of balance ability is due to the rapid height gain that occurs during the adolescent growth spurt. The poor balance is a demonstration of the balancing system having trouble controlling a taller structure that is mechanically harder to control than a shorter structure. This phenomenon is also seen in completely normal children and is usually called the adolescent clumsy stage of development. After a year at the end of maximum growth, the balancing system will again gain control and these children will typically have the same function they had at 8 to 10 years of age before the adolescent growth spurt started.

Although there are children with CP whose only problem is ataxia, it is much more common to have a mixed pattern of spasticity and ataxia, or hypotonia and ataxia. Many children with athetosis probably also have ataxia, but it is very difficult to separate out ataxia in the presence of significant athetosis. Having good balance requires that the individual have a stable physical base of support and a good sensory feedback system that can interpret where the body is in space and how its position should be corrected. The lack of a stable base of support is demonstrated by an individual's experience of walking on slippery ice where the physical base of support is poor. An example of decreased balance occurs when an individual is under the influence of alcohol, in which sensory feedback and interpretation are dulled.

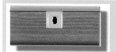

Case 3.8   Kerstin

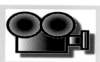

Kerstin, a girl who had a normal birth history and mild mental retardation, started walking independently at 4 years of age. She had made very little progress in the control of her gait, often having periods when she seemed to have more problems with her balance around periods of rapid growth. However, by the time she reached full maturity, her gait stabilized by being a little slower and less variable. On physical examination she had normal reflexes, muscle strength, and motor control. This is the typical pattern of primary ataxia. The main treatment is to try to teach her to know her own limitations and to use assistive devices, such as crutches or canes, which she resists because she does not feel she needs them.

In the musculoskeletal treatment plan of children with ataxia, it is important to evaluate the components of balance, such as their base of support or their sensory feedback, that are contributing to most of their functional problems (Case 3.8).

Measurement of balance in children is difficult. Most of the balance studies in adults and children involve an assessment of postural stability by measuring the impact of different sensory systems, such as eyesight, the inner ear vestibular system, and joint sensory position feedback.[120] These types of measurements have not become commonplace in clinical evaluations of children. The gross motor function measure (GMFM) has become a common clinical evaluation tool for children with CP. Although this test does not specifically evaluate and measure ataxia, it has a significant component, especially in domain 4, where tasks such as single-leg stands are evaluated. These tasks require separating out balance from motor control problems based on subjective evaluation of these children. Also, on gait analysis, temporal spatial characteristics such as step length and cadence tend to have high variability in children with significant ataxia. Children with only spasticity but good balance have less variability than normal children, and those with predominantly ataxia will have much higher variability.

This variability is also true of trunk motion and the ability to walk in a straight line. Understanding balance deficits during walking is difficult because momentum can make unstable children look much more stable than they really are. An example is a child who seems to walk very well while walking; however, every time she tries to stop, she has to grab the wall or fall to the floor. This is the analogy of riding a bicycle where the rider is very stable due to the momentum of motion. However, if the rider stops the motion and tries to sit on the bicycle, she becomes very unstable. A child who can walk well only at a certain speed may be an excellent walker; however, developing good functional walking skills requires that an individual be able to stop without falling over.

Treatment of Ataxia

Therapy to help children with ataxia improve their walking should focus on two areas. First, they must learn how to fall safely and develop protective responses when falling. They should be taught to recognize when they are falling, direct the fall away from hazards, and fall forward with their arms out in front to protect themselves. Until these children develop a good protective response to falling, they should be wearing protective helmets and have supervision when walking. There are some children who cannot learn this protective response, and they will have a tendency to fall like a cut tree; this is especially dangerous if the individual has a tendency to fall backward, which places them at high risk of head injury. These children will have to be kept in wheelchairs except when they are under the direct supervision of another individual. The second area of treatment focus for children with ataxia should be directed at exercises that stimulate balancing. These exercises include single-leg stance activities, walking a narrow board, roller skating, and other activities that stimulate the balancing system. These exercises have to be carefully structured to the individual child's abilities, with the goal of maximizing each child's ability safely and effectively.

Walking effectively as an adult requires an individual to be able to alter gait, speed, and especially to slow down speed to reserve energy as she tires. This may mean using an assistive device, such as forearm crutches. For safety and social propriety, it is important that an individual can stop walking and stand in one place. Children who cannot learn to stop and stand in one place will have to switch to the use of an assistive device, usually forearm crutches, in middle childhood or adolescence. This step may seem like a regression to parents; however, it is moving the child forward to a more stable gait pattern that is socially acceptable and functional into adulthood. It is appropriate for 3-year-old children to run and then fall when they get to where they are going and want to stop; however, this method in a 13-year-old would be both unsafe for the child and socially unacceptable. Finding the appropriate device requires some trial and error. There are rare children who can use single-point canes. Three- or four-point canes are a poor choice because they slow the child too much and are generally very inefficient. Either forearm crutches or a walker are typically the best assistive devices for an individual child. Some children's ataxia is so severe that it requires the use of a wheelchair for safe and functional mobility.

Surgery for the Child with Ataxia

The sensory perception and processing of balance cannot be altered in any predictable known way with surgery; however, the mechanical stability can be altered. Mechanical stability means that children have a stable base of support upon which to stand. Children with severe equinus at the ankle, such that they can only stand on their toes, will be unstable even if their balance is otherwise normal. Other examples of mechanical instability are severe planovalgus or equinovarus feet, severe fixed scoliosis, or severe contractures of the hip and knee. In general, the spine, hip, and knee contractures need to be very severe before they substantially affect balance. Fixed ankle equinus is the most common situation that is seen in early and middle childhood. Many of these children walk very well on their toes when they are moving with sufficient speed; however, they have no stable ability to stand in one place; this means that the children have to hold onto a wall, keep moving around in a circle, or fall to the floor when they want to stop. When these same children are made more stable by lengthening the gastrocnemius muscle to allow their feet to become plantigrade, their walking velocity slows, but they can now stop and stand in one place. This trade-off of stability and stance versus the speed of walking needs to be explained to parents to avoid their disappointment in the slower walking. This kind of fast toe walking is not a reasonable long-term option for older children for the safety reasons already explained. The safety and social inappropriateness of this gait pattern have to be carefully explained to parents for them to understand the trade-off in stability for speed provided by gastrocnemius lengthening.

Orthotics

For young children with dynamic plantar flexion causing them to toe walk, correcting the plantar flexion with the use of orthotics provides the same improvements in stability as was described for surgical lengthening of tendons. By removing flexibility of the ankle, and especially by decreasing plantar flexion and toe walking, these children will be in a more stable position to focus on controlling large joints, such as the hip, knee, and trunk. Therefore, these children will gain better experience in upright stance required for stable walking. The use of orthotics is the primary stabilizing structure that is provided to young children, usually beginning at approximately 18 to 24 months of age and then gradually decreasing instability as they get older. The orthotics also have the advantage that they can provide children a period of stability when standing with their feet flat, as well as allowing them to have time when they are walking up on their toes. This toe walking allows them to experience the stability of momentum, which stimulates the young developing nervous system. These orthotics work especially well until these children are 5 to 7 years of age.

Summary of Treatment: Ataxia

Children with ataxia need a planned approach of treatment combining a therapy environment in which the balance, sensory, and integration systems are stressed so they can learn to maximize balancing function. These children also need to have their mechanical base of support stabilized to provide a stable base upon which they can gain confidence and learn to use their motor control skills. Mechanical stability is gained through the use of orthotics and assistive devices in young children, and as they get to middle childhood, selective muscle lengthenings can be utilized to improve their mechanical stability and stance. The treatment plan should always consider how safe these children are to avoid falls, which might cause them significant injury. Children with significant ataxia are at significant risk for falls that may cause permanent additional head injuries, and because of this risk, some children with ataxia need to be kept in wheelchairs or use protective helmets based on their ability to learn protective maneuvers and the severity of their ataxia.

Spasticity Evaluation

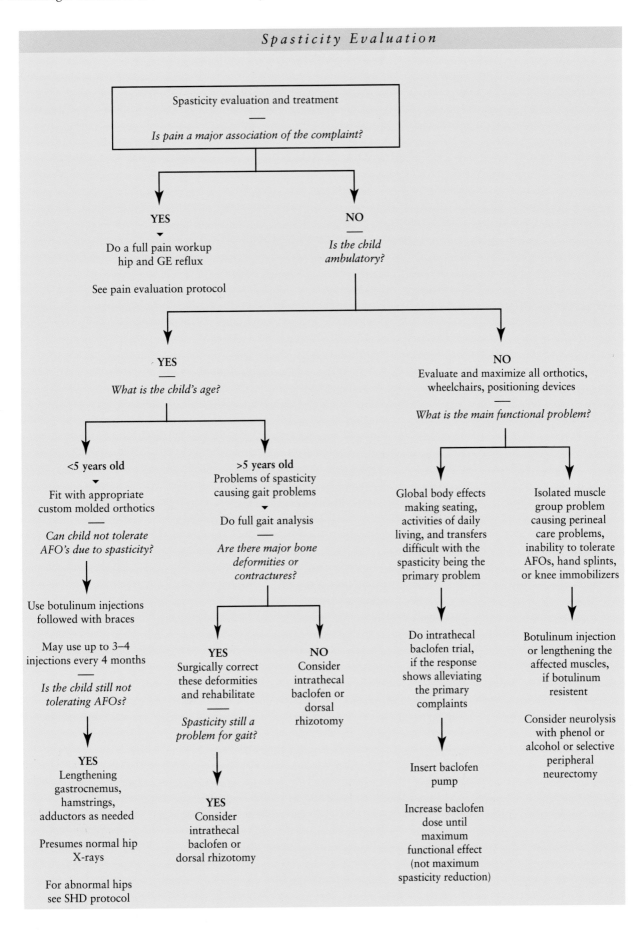

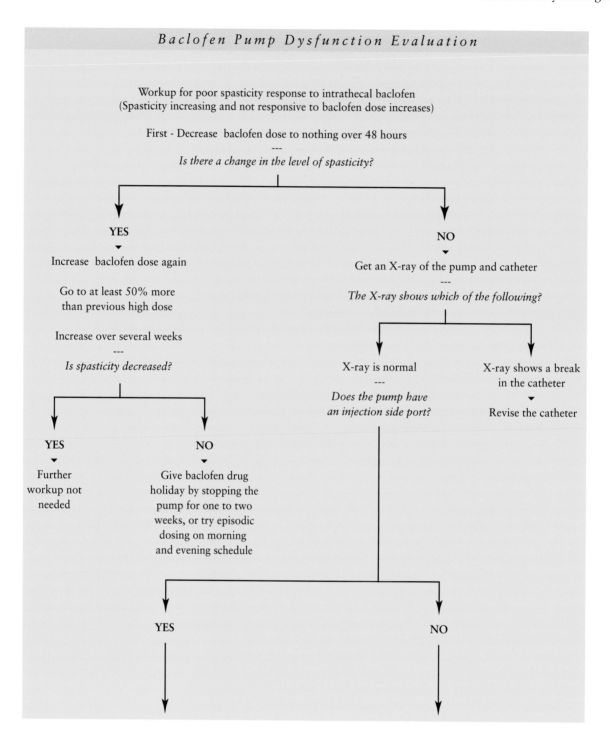

Baclofen Pump Dysfunction Evaluation

Workup for poor spasticity response to intrathecal baclofen
(Spasticity increasing and not responsive to baclofen dose increases)

First - Decrease baclofen dose to nothing over 48 hours

Is there a change in the level of spasticity?

YES

Increase baclofen dose again

Go to at least 50% more
than previous high dose

Increase over several weeks

Is spasticity decreased?

YES

Further
workup not
needed

NO

Give baclofen drug
holiday by stopping the
pump for one to two
weeks, or try episodic
dosing on morning
and evening schedule

NO

Get an X-ray of the pump and catheter

The X-ray shows which of the following?

X-ray is normal
---
*Does the pump have
an injection side port?*

X-ray shows a break
in the catheter

Revise the catheter

YES

NO

Baclofen Pump Dysfunction Evaluation

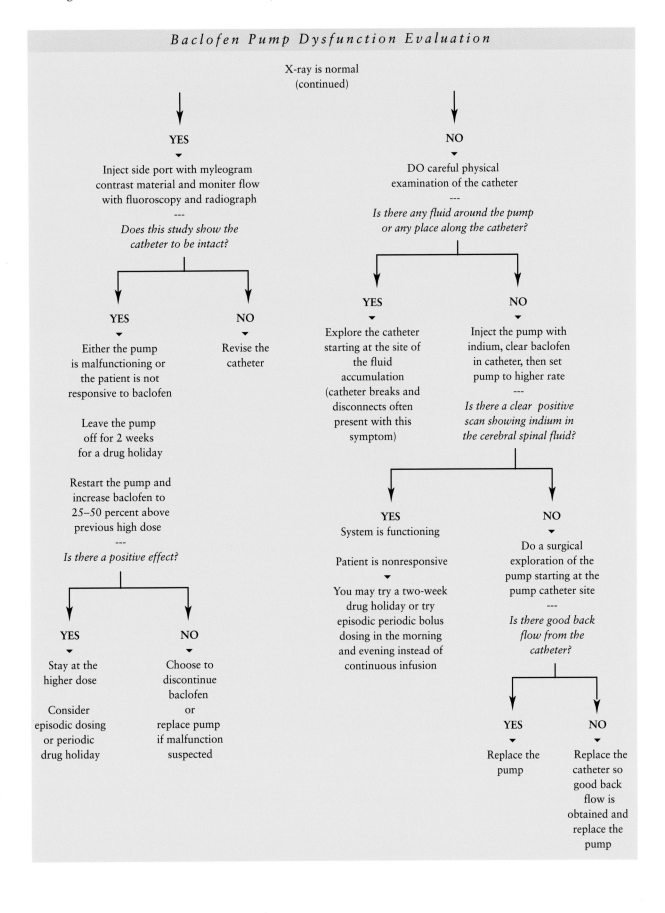

X-ray is normal
(continued)

YES

Inject side port with myleogram
contrast material and moniter flow
with fluoroscopy and radiograph
---
*Does this study show the
catheter to be intact?*

YES

Either the pump
is malfunctioning or
the patient is not
responsive to baclofen

Leave the pump
off for 2 weeks
for a drug holiday

Restart the pump and
increase baclofen to
25–50 percent above
previous high dose

Is there a positive effect?

YES

Stay at the
higher dose

Consider
episodic dosing
or periodic
drug holiday

NO

Choose to
discontinue
baclofen
or
replace pump
if malfunction
suspected

NO

Revise the
catheter

NO

DO careful physical
examination of the catheter
---
*Is there any fluid around the pump
or any place along the catheter?*

YES

Explore the catheter
starting at the site of
the fluid
accumulation
(catheter breaks and
disconnects often
present with this
symptom)

NO

Inject the pump with
indium, clear baclofen
in catheter, then set
pump to higher rate
---
*Is there a clear positive
scan showing indium in
the cerebral spinal fluid?*

YES
System is functioning

Patient is nonresponsive

You may try a two-week
drug holiday or try
episodic periodic bolus
dosing in the morning
and evening instead of
continuous infusion

NO

Do a surgical
exploration of the
pump starting at the
pump catheter site
---
*Is there good back
flow from the
catheter?*

YES

Replace the
pump

NO

Replace the
catheter so
good back
flow is
obtained and
replace the
pump

References

1. Connolly KHF. Neurophysiology and Neuropsychology of Motor Development. London: Mac Keith Press, 1997.
2. Gage J. Gait Analysis in Cerebral Palsy. London: Mac Keith Press, 1991.
3. Fahn S, Marsden CD, DeLong MR. Dystonia 3: Advances in Neurology. Philadelphia: Lippincott-Raven, 1998.
4. Nie J, DA Linkens. Fuzzy-Neural Control: Principles, Algorithms, and Applications. New York: Prentice Hall, 1995.
5. Gleick J. Chaos: Making a New Science. New York: Penguin Books, 1987.
6. Walsh G. Muscles, Masses, and Motion: The Physiology of Normality, Hypertonicity, Spasticity, and Rigidity. London: Mac Keith Press, 1992.
7. Sussman ME. The Diplegic Child: Evaluation and Management. Chicago: American Academy of Orthopaedic Surgeons, 1992.
8. Engsberg JR, Ross SA, Olree KS, Park TS. Ankle spasticity and strength in children with spastic diplegic cerebral palsy. Dev Med Child Neurol 2000;42:42–7.
9. Ashworth B. Preliminary trial of carisoprodol in multiple sclerosis. Practitioner 1964;192:540–2.
10. Sehgal N, McGuire JR. Beyond Ashworth. Electrophysiologic quantification of spasticity. Phys Med Rehabil Clin N Am 1998;9:949–79, ix.
11. Lin JP, Brown JK, Walsh EG. The maturation of motor dexterity: or why Johnny can't go any faster. Dev Med Child Neurol 1996;38:244–54.
12. Dietz V, Berger W. Cerebral palsy and muscle transformation. Dev Med Child Neurol 1995;37:180–4.
13. Ziv I, Blackburn N, Rang M, Koreska J. Muscle growth in normal and spastic mice. Dev Med Child Neurol 1984;26:94–9.
14. Castle ME, Reyman TA, Schneider M. Pathology of spastic muscle in cerebral palsy. Clin Orthop 1979:223–32.
15. Engle AG, Franzini-Armstrong C. Myology. New York: McGraw-Hill, 1994:1936.
16. Miller F, Slomczykowski M, Cope R, Lipton GE. Computer modeling of the pathomechanics of spastic hip dislocation in children. J Pediatr Orthop 1999;19:486–92.
17. Nance PW, Bugaresti J, Shellenberger K, Sheremata W, Martinez-Arizala A. Efficacy and safety of tizanidine in the treatment of spasticity in patients with spinal cord injury. North American Tizanidine Study Group. Neurology 1994;44:S44–51; discussion S51–2.
18. Gracies J, Nance P, Elovic E, McGuire J, Simpson DM. Traditional pharmacological treatments for spasticity. Part II: General and regional treaments. Muscle Nerve 1997;Suppl 6:S92–S120.
19. Erickson DL, Blacklock JB, Michaelson M, Sperling KB, Lo JN. Control of spasticity by implantable continuous flow morphine pump. Neurosurgery 1985;16:215–7.
20. Zierski J, Muller H, Dralle D, Wurdinger T. Implanted pump systems for treatment of spasticity. Acta Neurochir Suppl 1988;43:94–9.
21. Albright AL, Cervi A, Singletary J. Intrathecal baclofen for spasticity in cerebral palsy [see comments]. JAMA 1991;265:1418–22.
22. Albright AL, Barry MJ, Fasick P, Barron W, Shultz B. Continuous intrathecal baclofen infusion for symptomatic generalized dystonia. Neurosurgery 1996;38:934–8; discussion 938–9.
23. Albright AL. Baclofen in the treatment of cerebral palsy. J Child Neurol 1996;11:77–83.

24. Almeida GL, Campbell SK, Girolami GL, Penn RD, Corcos DM. Multidimensional assessment of motor function in a child with cerebral palsy following intrathecal administration of baclofen. Phys Ther 1997; 77:751–64.

25. Armstrong RW, Steinbok P, Cochrane DD, Kube SD, Fife SE, Farrell K. Intrathecally administered baclofen for treatment of children with spasticity of cerebral origin. J Neurosurg 1997;87:409–14.

26. Albright AL. Intrathecal baclofen in cerebral palsy movement disorders. J Child Neurol 1996;11(suppl 1):S29–35.

27. Gerszten PC, Albright AL, Barry MJ. Effect on ambulation of continuous intrathecal baclofen infusion. Pediatr Neurosurg 1997;27:40–4.

28. Wiens HD. Spasticity in children with cerebral palsy: a retrospective review of the effects of intrathecal baclofen. Issues Compr Pediatr Nurs 1998; 21:49–61.

29. Kita M, Goodkin DE. Drugs used to treat spasticity. Drugs 2000;59: 487–95.

30. Bennett MI, Tai YM, Symonds JM. Staphylococcal meningitis following Synchromed intrathecal pump implant: a case report. Pain 1994;56: 243–4.

31. Sweet CS, Wenger HC, Gross DM. Central antihypertensive properties of muscimol and related gamma-aminobutyric acid agonists and the interaction of muscimol with baroreceptor reflexes. Can J Physiol Pharmacol 1979;57:600–5.

32. Rode G, Mertens P, Beneton C, Schmitt M, Boisson D. Regression of vasomotor disorders under intrathecal baclofen in a case of spastic paraplegia. Spinal Cord 1999;37:370–2.

33. Agmo A, Paredes R. GABAergic drugs and sexual behaviour in the male rat. Eur J Pharmacol 1985;112:371–8.

34. Leipheimer RE, Sachs BD. GABAergic regulation of penile reflexes and copulation in rats. Physiol Behav 1988;42:351–7.

35. Denys P, Mane M, Azouvi P, Chartier-Kastler E, Thiebaut JB, Bussel B. Side effects of chronic intrathecal baclofen on erection and ejaculation in patients with spinal cord lesions. Arch Phys Med Rehabil 1998;79:494–6.

36. Steinbok P, Reiner AM, Beauchamp R, Armstrong RW, Cochrane DD, Kestle J. A randomized clinical trial to compare selective posterior rhizotomy plus physiotherapy with physiotherapy alone in children with spastic diplegic cerebral palsy [published erratum appears in Dev Med Child Neurol 1997;39(11): inside back cover] [see comments]. Dev Med Child Neurol 1997;39:178–84.

37. McLaughlin JF, Bjornson KF, Astley SJ, et al. Selective dorsal rhizotomy: efficacy and safety in an investigator-masked randomized clinical trial [see comments]. Dev Med Child Neurol 1998;40:220–32.

38. Cohen AR, Webster HC. How selective is selective posterior rhizotomy? Surg Neurol 1991;35:267–72.

39. Logigian EL, Wolinsky JS, Soriano SG, Madsen JR, Scott RM. H reflex studies in cerebral palsy patients undergoing partial dorsal rhizotomy [see comments]. Muscle Nerve 1994;17:539–49.

40. Sacco DJ, Tylkowski CM, Warf BC. Nonselective partial dorsal rhizotomy: a clinical experience with 1-year follow-up. Pediatr Neurosurg 2000;32:114–8.

41. Peacock WJ, Arens LJ, Berman B. Cerebral palsy spasticity. Selective posterior rhizotomy. Pediatr Neurosci 1987;13:61–6.

42. Fasano VA, Broggi G, Barolat-Romana G, Sguazzi A. Surgical treatment of spasticity in cerebral palsy. Childs Brain 1978;4:289–305.

43. Heimburger RF, Slominski A, Griswold P. Cervical posterior rhizotomy for reducing spasticity in cerebral palsy. J Neurosurg 1973;39:30–4.

44. Benedetti A, Colombo F. Spinal surgery for spasticity (46 cases). Neurochirurgia (Stuttg) 1981;24:195–8.

45. Benedetti A, Colombo F, Alexandre A, Pellegri A. Posterior rhizotomies for spasticity in children affected by cerebral palsy. J Neurosurg Sci 1982;26:179–84.

46. Gul SM, Steinbok P, McLeod K. Long-term outcome after selective posterior rhizotomy in children with spastic cerebral palsy. Pediatr Neurosurg 1999;31:84–95.

47. Subramanian N, Vaughan CL, Peter JC, Arens LJ. Gait before and 10 years after rhizotomy in children with cerebral palsy spasticity. J Neurosurg 1998;88:1014–9.

48. Giuliani CA. Dorsal rhizotomy for children with cerebral palsy: support for concepts of motor control. Phys Ther 1991;71:248–59.

49. Steinbok P, Daneshvar H, Evans D, Kestle JR. Cost analysis of continuous intrathecal baclofen versus selective functional posterior rhizotomy in the treatment of spastic quadriplegia associated with cerebral palsy. Pediatr Neurosurg 1995;22:255–64.

50. Marty GR, Dias LS, Gaebler-Spira D. Selective posterior rhizotomy and soft-tissue procedures for the treatment of cerebral diplegia. J Bone Joint Surg [Am] 1995;77:713–8.

51. Carroll KL, Moore KR, Stevens PM. Orthopedic procedures after rhizotomy. J Pediatr Orthop 1998;18:69–74.

52. Crawford K, Karol LA, Herring JA. Severe lumbar lordosis after dorsal rhizotomy. J Pediatr Orthop 1996;16:336–9.

53. Mooney JF III, Millis MB. Spinal deformity after selective dorsal rhizotomy in patients with cerebral palsy. Clin Orthop 1999:48–52.

54. Peter JC, Hoffman EB, Arens LJ, Peacock WJ. Incidence of spinal deformity in children after multiple level laminectomy for selective posterior rhizotomy. Childs Nerv Syst 1990;6:30–2.

55. Peter JC, Hoffman EB, Arens LJ. Spondylolysis and spondylolisthesis after five-level lumbosacral laminectomy for selective posterior rhizotomy in cerebral palsy. Childs Nerv Syst 1993;9:285–7; discussion 287–8.

56. Greene WB, Dietz FR, Goldberg MJ, Gross RH, Miller F, Sussman MD. Rapid progression of hip subluxation in cerebral palsy after selective posterior rhizotomy. J Pediatr Orthop 1991;11:494–7.

57. Heim RC, Park TS, Vogler GP, Kaufman BA, Noetzel MJ, Ortman MR. Changes in hip migration after selective dorsal rhizotomy for spastic quadriplegia in cerebral palsy. J Neurosurg 1995;82:567–71.

58. Steinbok P, Schrag C. Complications after selective posterior rhizotomy for spasticity in children with cerebral palsy. Pediatr Neurosurg 1998;28:300–13.

59. Cobb MA, Boop FA. Replacement laminoplasty in selective dorsal rhizotomy: possible protection against the development of musculoskeletal pain. Pediatr Neurosurg 1994;21:237–42.

60. Payne LZ, DeLuca PA. Heterotopic ossification after rhizotomy and femoral osteotomy. J Pediatr Orthop 1993;13:733–8.

61. Abbott R. Complications with selective posterior rhizotomy. Pediatr Neurosurg 1992;18:43–7.

62. Cooper IS, Upton AR, Rappaport ZH, Amin I. Correlation of clinical and physiological effects of cerebellar stimulation. Acta Neurochir Suppl 1980;30:339–44.

63. Davis R, Schulman J, Delehanty A. Cerebellar stimulation for cerebral palsy—double blind study. Acta Neurochir Suppl 1987;39:126–8.

64. Schulman JH, Davis R, Nanes M. Cerebellar stimulation for spastic cerebral palsy: preliminary report; on-going double blind study. Pacing Clin Electrophysiol 1987;10:226–31.

65. Barolat G. Experience with 509 plate electrodes implanted epidurally from C1 to L1. Stereotact Funct Neurosurg 1993;61:60–79.

66. Hugenholtz H, Humphreys P, McIntyre WM, Spasoff RA, Steel K. Cervical spinal cord stimulation for spasticity in cerebral palsy. Neurosurgery 1988;22:707–14.

67. Cusick JF, Larson SJ, Sances A. The effect of T-myelotomy on spasticity. Surg Neurol 1976;6:289c92.

68. Ivan LP, Wiley JJ. Myelotomy in the management of spasticity. Clin Orthop 1975:52–6.

69. Padovani R, Tognetti F, Pozzati E, Servadei F, Laghi D, Gaist G. The treatment of spasticity by means of dorsal longitudinal myelotomy and lozenge-shaped griseotomy. Spine 1982;7:103–9.

70. Carpenter EB. Role of nerve blocks in the foot and ankle in cerebral palsy: therapeutic and diagnostic. Foot Ankle 1983;4:164–6.

71. Gracies JM, Elovic E, McGuire J, Simpson DM. Traditional pharmacological treatments for spasticity. Part I: Local treatments. Muscle Nerve Suppl 1997;6:S61–91.

72. Carpenter EB, Seitz DG. Intramuscular alcohol as an aid in management of spastic cerebral palsy. Dev Med Child Neurol 1980;22:497–501.

73. Hariga J. Treatment of spasticity by alcohol injection. Dev Med Child Neurol 1970;12:825.

74. Tardieu G, Tardieu C, Hariga J, Gagnard L. Treatment of spasticity in injection of dilute alcohol at the motor point or by epidural route. Clinical extension of an experiment on the decerebrate cat. Dev Med Child Neurol 1968;10:555–68.

75. Easton JK, Ozel T, Halpern D. Intramuscular neurolysis for spasticity in children. Arch Phys Med Rehabil 1979;60:155–8.

76. Griffith ER, Melampy CN. General anesthesia use in phenol intramuscular neurolysis in young children with spasticity. Arch Phys Med Rehabil 1977;58:154–7.

77. Matsuo T, Tada S, Hajime T. Insufficiency of the hip adductor after anterior obturator neurectomy in 42 children with cerebral palsy. J Pediatr Orthop 1986;6:686–92.

78. Root L, Spero CR. Hip adductor transfer compared with adductor tenotomy in cerebral palsy. J Bone Joint Surg [Am] 1981;63:767–72.

79. Sharma S, Mishra KS, Dutta A, Kulkarni SK, Nair MN. Intrapelvic obturator neurectomy in cerebral palsy. Indian J Pediatr 1989;56:259–65.

80. Keenan MA, Todderud EP, Henderson R, Botte M. Management of intrinsic spasticity in the hand with phenol injection or neurectomy of the motor branch of the ulnar nerve. J Hand Surg [Am] 1987;12:734–9.

81. Doute DA, Sponseller PD, Tolo VT, Atkins E, Silberstein CE. Soleus neurectomy for dynamic ankle equinus in children with cerebral palsy. Am J Orthop 1997;26:613–6.

82. Nogen AG. Medical treatment for spasticity in children with cerebral palsy. Childs Brain 1976;2:304–8.

83. Pinder RM, Brogden RN, Speight TM, Avery GS. Dantrolene sodium: a review of its pharmacological properties and therapeutic efficacy in spasticity. Drugs 1977;13:3–23.

84. Joynt RL, Leonard JA Jr. Dantrolene sodium suspension in treatment of spastic cerebral palsy. Dev Med Child Neurol 1980;22:755–67.

85. Jankovic J, Brin MF. Botulinum toxin: historical perspective and potential new indications. Muscle Nerve Suppl 1997;6:S129–45.

86. Brin MF. Botulinum toxin: chemistry, pharmacology, toxicity, and immunology. Muscle Nerve Suppl 1997;6:S146–68.

87. Brin MF. Dosing, administration, and a treatment algorithm for use of botulinum toxin A for adult-onset spasticity. Spasticity Study Group. Muscle Nerve Suppl 1997;6:S208–20.

88. Borodic GE, Ferrante R, Pearce LB, Smith K. Histologic assessment of dose-related diffusion and muscle fiber response after therapeutic botulinum A toxin injections. Mov Disord 1994;9:31–9.

89. Barwood S, Baillieu C, Boyd R, et al. Analgesic effects of botulinum toxin A: a randomized, placebo-controlled clinical trial. Dev Med Child Neurol 2000;42:116–21.

90. Greene PE, Fahn S. Use of botulinum toxin type F injections to treat torticollis in patients with immunity to botulinum toxin type A. Mov Disord 1993;8:479–83.

91. Koman LA, Mooney JF III, Smith B, Goodman A, Mulvaney T. Management of cerebral palsy with botulinum-A toxin: preliminary investigation. J Pediatr Orthop 1993;13:489–95.

92. Fehlings D, Rang M, Glazier J, Steele C. An evaluation of botulinum-A toxin injections to improve upper extremity function in children with hemiplegic cerebral palsy [see comments]. J Pediatr 2000;137:331–7.

93. Graham HK, Aoki KR, Autti-Ramo I, et al. Recommendations for the use of botulinum toxin type A in the management of cerebral palsy. Gait Posture 2000;11:67–79.

94. Tarczynska M, Karski T, Abobaker S. [Hip dislocation in children with cerebral palsy—the result of illness or treatment error]. Ann Univ Mariae Curie Sklodowska [Med] 1997;52:95–102.

95. Crenshaw S, Herzog R, Castagno P, et al. The efficacy of tone-reducing features in orthotics on the gait of children with spastic diplegic cerebral palsy. J Pediatr Orthop 2000;20:210–6.

96. Radtka SA, Skinner SR, Dixon DM, Johanson ME. A comparison of gait with solid, dynamic, and no ankle-foot orthoses in children with spastic cerebral palsy [see comments] [published erratum appears in Phys Ther 1998;78(2):222–4]. Phys Ther 1997;77:395–409.

97. Ricks NR, Eilert RE. Effects of inhibitory casts and orthoses on bony alignment of foot and ankle during weight-bearing in children with spasticity. Dev Med Child Neurol 1993;35:11–6.

98. Bertoti DB. Effect of short leg casting on ambulation in children with cerebral palsy. Phys Ther 1986;66:1522–9.

99. Cruickshank DA, O'Neill DL. Upper extremity inhibitive casting in a boy with spastic quadriplegia. Am J Occup Ther 1990;44:552–5.

100. Otis JC, Root L, Kroll MA. Measurement of plantar flexor spasticity during treatment with tone-reducing casts. J Pediatr Orthop 1985;5:682–6.

101. Lesny IA. Follow-up study of hypotonic forms of cerebral palsy. Brain Dev 1979;1:87–90.

102. Nelson KB, Ellenberg JH. Neonatal signs as predictors of cerebral palsy. Pediatrics 1979;64:225–32.

103. Thajeb P. The syndrome of delayed posthemiplegic hemidystonia, hemiatrophy, and partial seizure: clinical, neuroimaging, and motor-evoked potential studies. Clin Neurol Neurosurg 1996;98:207–12.

104. Barry MJ, VanSwearingen JM, Albright AL. Reliability and responsiveness of the Barry-Albright Dystonia Scale. Dev Med Child Neurol 1999;41:404–11.

105. Ford B, Greene P, Louis ED, et al. Use of intrathecal baclofen in the treatment of patients with dystonia. Arch Neurol 1996;53:1241–6.

106. Gros C, Frerebeau P, Perez-Dominguez E, Bazin M, Privat JM. Long term results of stereotaxic surgery for infantile dystonia and dyskinesia. Neurochirurgia (Stuttg) 1976;19:171–8.

107. Lin JJ, Lin GY, Shih C, Lin SZ, Chang DC, Lee CC. Benefit of bilateral pallidotomy in the treatment of generalized dystonia. Case report. J Neurosurg 1999;90:974–6.

108. Vitek JL, Chockkan V, Zhang JY, et al. Neuronal activity in the basal ganglia in patients with generalized dystonia and hemiballismus. Ann Neurol 1999;46:22–35.

109. Kyllerman M. Reduced optimality in pre- and perinatal conditions in dyskinetic cerebral palsy—distribution and comparison to controls. Neuropediatrics 1983;14:29–36.

110. Acardi J. Diseases of the Nervous System in Childhood. Oxford, England: Mac Keith Press, 1992:1408.

111. O'Reilly DE, Walentynowicz JE. Etiological factors in cerebral palsy: an historical review. Dev Med Child Neurol 1981;23:633–42.

112. Johnson RK, Goran MI, Ferrara MS, Poehlman ET. Athetosis increases resting metabolic rate in adults with cerebral palsy. J Am Diet Assoc 1996;96:145–8.

113. Fraioli B, Nucci F, Baldassarre L. Bilateral cervical posterior rhizotomy: effects on dystonia and athetosis, on respiration and other autonomic functions. Appl Neurophysiol 1977;40:26–40.

114. Davis R, Barolat-Romana G, Engle H. Chronic cerebellar stimulation for cerebral palsy—five-year study. Acta Neurochir Suppl 1980;30: 317–32.

115. Ebara S, Harada T, Yamazaki Y, et al. Unstable cervical spine in athetoid cerebral palsy [published erratum appears in Spine 1990; 15(1):59]. Spine 1989;14:1154–9.

116. Fuji T, Yonenobu K, Fujiwara K, et al. Cervical radiculopathy or myelopathy secondary to athetoid cerebral palsy. J Bone Joint Surg [Am] 1987;69:815–21.

117. Kidron D, Steiner I, Melamed E. Late-onset progressive radiculo-myelopathy in patients with cervical athetoid-dystonic cerebral palsy. Eur Neurol 1987;27:164–6.

118. Nishihara N, Tanabe G, Nakahara S, Imai T, Murakawa H. Surgical treatment of cervical spondylotic myelopathy complicating athetoid cerebral palsy. J Bone Joint Surg [Br] 1984;66:504–8.

119. Wang PY, Chen RC. Cervical spondylotic radiculomyelopathy caused by athetoid-dystonic cerebral palsy—clinical evaluation of 2 cases. Taiwan I Hsueh Hui Tsa Chih 1985;84:986–94.

120. Watanuki K, Takahashi M, Ikeda T. Perception of surrounding space controls posture, gaze, and sensation during Coriolis stimulation. Aviat Space Environ Med 2000;71:381–7.

Therapy, Education, and Other Treatment Modalities

Almost all children with cerebral palsy (CP) will receive therapy and go to school. Most of the therapy has to be ordered by physicians as part of the medical treatment of the CP. Because education is a universal experience in the lives of these children, it behooves the physicians treating the motor impairments to have some understanding of the educational system. These children often receive therapy as early as in the neonatal intensive care nursery. This early therapy is provided in a medically-based construct. As the children get older, especially over age 3 years, the main intervention shifts to the educational system, and much of this therapy also shifts into the education milieu. As these children enter grade school, except for periods of acute medical treatment, education is predominant with therapy occurring within this context. During the children's growth and development, the therapists provide the best bridge between the education and medical systems. The final physical and emotional function and independence of these children depends on intervention by both the medical and educational systems; therefore, the bridging effect provided by the therapists is an important aspect. In addition to the standard therapy treatment in education, there are many treatment modalities that are promoted as beneficial for CP treatment. Some of these modalities may start as an alternative medicine approach, such as hippotherapy, but then develop acceptance within traditional medicine. Others, such as hyperbaric oxygen therapy, develop a reputation of possible benefit but, upon careful investigation, their validity is discredited. The physician who treats the motor impairments of children with CP should understand the techniques, goals, and expected outcomes of therapies they order while also understanding the educational context in which these children function.

Therapy

In this discussion, the term therapy applies to physical, occupational, or speech therapy, all disciplines trained in the milieu of the medical system, although these individuals often work in the educational system. These disciplines overlap significantly; however, each has a very defined area of expertise. Physical therapy focuses on gross motor function, such as walking, running, jumping, and joint range of motion. There is some overlap with occupational therapy, where the main focus is on fine motor skills, specifically upper extremity function and activities of daily living such as dressing, toileting, and bathing. This overlap between physical and occupational therapy occurs in the areas of seating and infant stimulation programs where both therapists perform the same function. Speech therapists focus on oral motor activities such as speech, chewing, and swallowing. A subspecialist speech therapist will do augmentative communication evaluations. Speech and occupational therapy overlap in the area of teaching feeding skills to caretakers and self-feeding therapy for patients. The specific areas of practice of each of the therapy disciplines vary slightly among geographic regions and facilities. A major focus of all therapy is to maximize the individual's independence. The goal of this discussion on the therapy disciplines is not to promote a full review of each discipline, but to provide only the information that a physician who treats children concurrently with the therapist should possess. Also, most of this discussion is directed at the musculoskeletal motor impairments because that is the focus of this text; however, it must be remembered that speech and communication are usually rated as more important by individuals with disabilities.

Physical Therapy

Applying physical therapy to children with CP is common and has a large body of published data. Since 1990, there have been approximately 300 citations in the National Library of Medicine reporting the use of physical therapy in children with CP. Most of these papers report physical therapy being used in conjunction with other treatments, such as surgical hip reconstructions or lower extremity reconstructions for gait improvement, or following dorsal rhizotomy and Botox injections. Many of these reports are case series without controls to evaluate the index procedure, and most make no objective attempt to evaluate the impact of the therapy program separately from other modalities. The number of reports attempting to evaluate the impact of specific therapy programs is increasing; however, many contain few patients and no control groups.[1] The role of physical therapists, and the therapy they provide to these children, is very complex. Many reports presume that physical therapy is like medication in that it can be evaluated by having a control group with no treatment. This research approach has some merit if no effect is found, such as the evaluation of therapy in infant stimulation programs.[2] However, when a positive effect is found, the intimate, personal interaction that physical therapy requires with the children and parents makes it very difficult to sort out what effect the specific therapeutic regimen or a specific treatment had on the outcome. Recognizing these complex interactions has led to recommending more complex and global evaluations using multivariate analysis in research protocols.[3] This trend in therapy research should be incorporated into the evaluation of all CP impairments because it has the potential to impart a better understanding of the effect of each modality in the treatment routine. For example, a treatment protocol where physical therapy modalities along with casting and Botox are used to treat gait abnormality in young children cannot be reasonably evaluated by any other means. Recognizing the complex interaction of physical therapy in its own right will lead to improved research techniques for other treatments as well.

The long history of physical therapy has been predominated by different theories of development and specific protocols to impact childhood development.[4] Most of these therapy protocols were designed with a theoretical understanding that distal lower-level functions will influence higher-level cortical functions to develop. In this theory the spinal cord-mediated activities, such as single synapse reflexes and spasticity, have to be corrected first before the more primitive higher reflexes can be addressed. These primitive reflexes then have to be corrected before high-functioning cortical motor activities, such as walking, can develop properly. This hierarchical theory of neurologic development has some base in animal studies. For example, the need for the eye to function properly before the optical cortex will organize and function appropriately is well documented.[5] All the major therapy protocols developed and used in modern medicine before the 1990s were based on this hierarchical theory of development.[4] These protocols are still widely used in pediatric physical therapy today, and are described briefly here because parents often ask for explanations of the relative importance of one therapy technique over another. The scope of this text, however, makes it impossible to give a full discription of these techniques. In the 1990s, the theory of neurologic development was slowly changing to a more complex, circular theory in which subsystems are recognized to interact. In this theory, the psychologic state and behavior of children are also recognized as being important in their motor function. Complex interactions exist between lower reflexes and cortical motor movement patterns, in which the interactions and impacts are both from the higher function to the lower function and vice versa.[6] This change in motor development theory has required physical therapists to incorporate multiple facets of the therapy experience and has led to the therapist becoming more a teacher or coach and less a technician who applies a treatment to a child. However, this change in approach is not universally adapted, because neurologic pediatric physical therapy is a small subspecialty of the much larger physical therapy discipline. In general, physical therapists tend to have clinical aptitudes that are similar to those of orthopaedic surgeons. Clinicians with a treatment approach like to identify a specific problem, then apply a cure to make the problem go away. This approach was feasible in the early therapy protocols based on the hierarchical development theory; however, it often frustrated the child, the family, and the therapist. Developing a concept where the child, family, physician, and therapist are one team whose goal is to make the child as independent as he or she can be when growing up is a much more functional approach. With this approach, an experienced therapist is the ideal head coach of the team, because this is the individual who knows the child best from a medical perspective and has the best relationship with the child, family, educators, and physicians. Unfortunately, because of frequent changes in therapists, this role of head coach often falls to the family. For some families, this works well, but for others, it does not.

The therapist who takes on the role of coach of a child's motor impairment management team has to develop a good relationship with the family and child. In general, this relationship does not work well if the parent or child does not like the therapist. Also, the therapist has to have some understanding of behavior management techniques to get the most cooperation from a child. Being aware of medical and other family issues is also important. The physical therapist should understand how to access social services and medical help in the community that may be needed by the family. One of the problems of this expanded role of pediatric therapists is that many therapists do not believe they have the training needed to take on this role. Most physical therapy training programs are at the master's degree level; however, the amount of training in pediatrics is minimal in many programs where there is a much greater allure to sports medicine and other adult rehabilitation directions. This experience mirrors what happens in orthopaedic training. Currently, there are a few well-developed specialty training programs for pediatric therapists, and none as well organized as the fellowship programs in pediatric orthopaedics. The trend to standardize this pediatric training is moving ahead and should train therapists who are much better equipped to take on the role in which they are currently expected to function.

Major Therapy Protocols

All modern major therapy protocols were developed from a hierarchical understanding of neurologic motor development. Many of these protocols have high regional concentrations of use, often in the area in which the system was initially developed and popularized. The same theories of therapy are widely used among both occupational and physical therapy.

Neurodevelopmental Treatment Approach (NDT): Bobath Technique

The NDT treatment approach was developed in England in the 1940s and 1950s by Dr. and Mrs. Bobath based on their understanding of neurologic development and experience gained in treating children.[7] Because of the well-developed concepts, clear rational approach, and the missionary zeal of its developer, the NDT approach has become the most widely used uniform approach of therapy worldwide. Based on the hierarchical concept of understanding development, this approach focused first on correcting abnormal tone through the use of range-of-motion exercises, encouraging normal motor patterns, and positioning. Second, abnormal primitive reflexes are addressed through the use of extinction by repeated stimulation.[7] Then, the third goal is to work on automatic reactions, such as placing a hand out in front when a fall is anticipated as in the parachute response. Another example is neck flexion as the child is falling backward to prevent the head from hitting. Altering sensory input by careful handling and positioning is also an important aspect to achieving the first three goals.[4] This aspect includes handling the child in patterns of normal movement and avoiding abnormal posturing. By having the child experience only normal movements, the brain will gradually remember the normal movements and forget the abnormal postures used by the immature brain. The requirement of very early treatment, under the theory that the more immature the brain is, the more it can be influenced to develop normally, is also stressed in NDT therapy. Another important aspect of this treatment is the insistence that the parents learn, and at all times apply, these correct handling techniques. In the earlier years of the technique, there was great focus on idealized movements, such as the perfect way to come to a sitting position from lying; however, focus has more recently been on functional patterns that work for the child.

The outcome of research has largely failed to show the benefits proposed by the founders of NDT techniques. Compared with other therapy techniques, or no therapy, there are few significant specific functional gains from the NDT approach.[8–11] There is one study suggesting earlier therapy is better, as predicted by NDT therapy[12]; however, more recent and better-controlled studies show no impact of earlier therapy versus no early therapy.[2, 13] There is also no evidence that NDT therapy can impact spasticity or primitive reflexes or specifically improve higher motor functioning. Despite the marginal evidence for direct benefit, NDT still has a widespread use, with some therapists maintaining the missionary zeal of avoiding specific movements in a child, such as extensor posturing. These therapists also focus on the children having correct crawling before they can stand or walk, and having them walk correctly with a walker before they can walk independently. This kind of missionary rigidity is inappropriate, and parents can be informed that they do not need to feel guilty when things do not happen exactly as the therapist requests. Because the objective data supporting the efficacy of NDT treatment are marginal, there is very little role for enforcing these concepts rigidly, although they may be perfectly legitimate techniques to help teach children correct movement.

Sensory Motor Treatment Approach: The Rood Technique

The sensory motor treatment approach was developed by Margaret Rood in the United States during the 1950s. Ms. Rood was trained as a physical and occupational therapist. This approach uses the same hierarchical understanding of neuromotor development, and was developed in approximately the same time period, as the NDT protocols. The sensory motor technique depends heavily on tactile stimulation to facilitate movement. The overall goal of sensory motor therapy is to activate the movements at an autonomic level similar to how postural responses in normal individuals are activated. This activation requires superimposing mobility as produced by basic muscle responses onto stability, which is produced by tonic muscle responses. Sensory motor technique uses a series of eight clearly defined developmental patterns, which children are to learn in sequence. These patterns are supine withdrawal, rolling over, pivot prone, neck co-contraction, elbow weight bearing, all four weight bearing, standing, and walking. This system incorporates many concepts similar to NDT but focuses much more on tactile stimulation and more specific functional movement patterns, as outlined in the eight steps of development. This technique was not developed for use in children, but rather for rehabilitation following brain injury. The Rood technique has been widely applied to children with CP; however, there are no reports that specifically document its efficacy. Many of the parameters of sensory motor therapy have been integrated into the NDT approach as it is currently used.[4]

Sensory Integration Treatment Approach: The Ayers Technique

This treatment approach was developed in the 1970s by A.J. Ayers, who is trained as an occupational therapist. The basic goal of this therapy technique is to teach children how to integrate their sensory feedback and then produce useful and purposeful motor responses. The sensory integration approach tries to have these children access and integrate all their sensory input to use for functional gain. Activities such as catching a ball in different positions may be used as a way of stimulating and requiring integration of visual, vestibular, and joint proprioception feedback systems at the same time. This system's underlying theory is that sensory input followed by appropriate motor function will contribute to the improved development of higher cortical motor sensory function. For young children, a single system stimulation may be used. Typical stimulations include vestibular stimulation in a swing and tactile stimulation by stroking, rubbing, massaging, or swaddling. Educating the parents is recognized as an important aspect of the treatment, especially in helping parents understand these children's problems. However, most of the treatments are therapist directed or performed. This technique has also been applied to children with mental retardation and Down syndrome. There are no papers documenting its efficacy in children with CP.[4] The understanding of the importance of sensory integration, especially for children with tactile defensiveness, is usually incorporated in the modern therapy programs for children with CP.

The Vojta Technique

The Vojta technique was developed in Czechoslovakia by Dr. Vojta in the 1950s and 1960s. This approach is applied to young infants and requires an assessment of each infant by identifying four grades of central motor coordination disturbance. The goals of this approach are to prevent at-risk infants from developing CP and decrease the effect or severity of CP in those who do develop symptoms. The basic treatment is to use proprioceptive trigger points on the trunk and extremities to initiate reflex movement, which produces rolling, crawling, and other specific functions. These massages and stimulations have to be done every day by the family, and the treatment is believed to be of most benefit in the first or second year of life.[14] The efficacy of the Vojta technique has been reported as positive in uncontrolled studies,[15] even causing a dislocated hip to reduce[16]; however, in studies compared with other approaches, there is no positive effect.[4, 17] This technique continues to be widely practiced in Europe and Japan and is sometimes combined with acupuncture.[18] The Vojta approach is used much less in North and South America.

Patterning Therapy: Doman–Delacato Technique

Patterning therapy was developed by G. Doman, a physical therapist; R. Doman, M.D.; and C. Delacato, an educator. This therapy was based on the theory of recapitulation of species developed by Temple-Fay in the 1940s.[4] This theory espouses that during development, immature activities such as reflex activities start first, and that these activities will stimulate higher brain functioning activities to develop. Furthermore, doing the activity frequently will imprint it on the brain and stimulate the brain to develop the next higher function. Sensory integration and stimulation are included as well. In recapitulation theory in combination with the hierarchical development theory, children turn over first, then crawl, which stimulates walking with all four limbs. This four-limb walking then stimulates the brain to develop bipedal standing, in turn stimulating intellectual development. This protocol also includes stimulating children to make vocal sounds and specific sensory stimulation, somewhat similar to the Vojta technique. The concept of recapitulation comes from the belief that children start out moving first by crawling like a worm, then moving like a fish, followed by walking on all fours like a quadruped animal, until finally reaching the human phase of biped walking. A unique aspect of the patterning approach is a heavy focus on doing the therapy for many hours each day, 7 days a week, every week of the year. Parents are taught the techniques and are encouraged to mount a community effort to get volunteers into the home to continue the therapy for almost all these children's waking hours. This therapy requires a huge commitment by parents and often raises the parents' hopes above what is realistic to accomplish.

The patterning approach to therapy was especially popular in the 1960s and 1970s in California and in the Philadelphia area where there were specially developed centers. There is no scientific evidence that this approach yields any of the claimed benefits. We have had many patients whose parents pursued patterning therapy for a time at some level, usually less than recommended by the original approach. There is no evidence to suggest that neurologic imprinting works; however, the extensive amount of passive range of motion many of these children receive seems to prevent contracture development. Clearly, however, the benefits are not worth the cost in time and commitment for families. During the height of patterning's popularity, there were many severely disappointed parents, several ending in parental suicides. The high rate of inappropriate expectations among parents leading to severe problems led many medical societies to issue statements condemning patterning therapy.[4, 19–21] Over the past 10 years, patterning therapy has almost disappeared, even in the region of Philadelphia, which was its last stronghold. Very little of this approach can be functionally applied, except to use it as an example of the damage that can be caused by an inappropriate therapy approach.

Conductive Education: Peto Technique

Conductive education was developed in Budapest, Hungary, in the 1940s and 1950s by Andreas Peto as an educational technique for children with CP. In North America and the rest of Europe, this has come to be viewed as a physical therapy approach. The children were treated by conductors in a facility where they lived full time. The treatment was based on educational principles in which motor skills that children could just barely perform were identified, then they were assisted over and over again until the skill was learned. This approach is the same as is typically used to teach the multiplication tables. Conductive education also includes a great emphasis on instilling a sense of self-worth and a sense of accomplishment in the children. The motor skills were performed with a series of simple ladder-type devices that can be used to assist standing, stepping, walking, and even sitting activities. This approach is only applicable to individuals with some useful motor function, but not such a high level of function that they are essentially independent ambulators. Based on this indication, approximately 35% of children with CP are candidates for conductive education.[22] Studies of the efficacy of conductive education suggest that it is equal to standard therapy programs,[23] or may be slightly better at teaching motor skills.[24, 25] The elements of the program that can be incorporated into the day school setting are a useful addition, and this approach to therapy fits into the more recent trends, which are focused on educational techniques rather than preconceived theories of neurodevelopment.

Electrical Stimulation

Electrical stimulation has always been a basic modality of physical therapy practice. The physical therapy department at Guy's Hospital in London in the 1840s was called the Electrical Department.[26] Electrical stimulation in children with CP can be functional electrical stimulation (FES) with neuromuscular electrical stimulation (NMES), or transcutaneous electrical nerve stimulation (TENS). Functional electrical stimulation means the electrical stimulation is done with the goal of causing a functional muscle contraction, such as stimulating the anterior tibialis muscle directly to cause a contraction that produces dorsiflexion. The main uses of FES in children with CP are for wrist extension and ankle dorsiflexion. The muscle may also be activated by stimulating transcutaneously or via percutaneous wires. A major problem with FES in children with intact sensory systems is the level of pain caused by this stimulation. In a group of individuals with hemiplegia, including mostly adults, the pericutaneous stimulation is less painful and better tolerated than transcutaneous stimulation.[27] Most children are not greatly enthused by frequent stimulating wires being inserted into their muscles, which makes this pericutaneous technique of minimal use in children, although there have been a few positive reports from small case series.[28–31] Another study found no improvement in gait, although passive dorsiflexion improved.[32] Because of the pain caused by FES, its minimal use is primarily in adolescents because they may be able to tolerate the discomfort. There have been no studies that suggest any long-term benefit, and unless long-term benefit can be demonstrated, there is no reason to cause a significant amount of pain by doing a therapy session with electrical stimulation.

Therapeutic electric stimulation (TES) is the use of electric stimulation below a level where muscle contraction occurs. The goal of TES is to stimulate muscle hypertrophy and strength. This technique has been widely promoted by Pape et al.[33] as a means of improving gross motor function, locomotion, and balance. This electrical stimulation is applied at night and is worn during sleep hours. The level of electrical stimulation is just at or be-low the level a child can feel. No muscle activity is initiated, and the theory for how this stimulation causes muscle hypertrophy is based on the alleged increased blood flow. Daytime TES has been proposed using slightly higher stimulation at a level at which children can feel the stimulation, but where it is not uncomfortable and causes no muscle contraction. This level would be used during therapy sessions to assist in motor learning.[26] There has been little or no published literature to objectively evaluate TES except that pub-lished by the developers, and there is one study reporting that it was well tol-erated for 1 year of use.[34] This technique has a potential for benefiting some children and would be an easy project for double-blind evaluation. Our experience is that there was very minimal functional benefit in the five or six children whom we followed while using TES over a period of time. At this time, there is no good clear indication for the use of either FES or TES in children with CP.

Tone-Reducing Casts

The concept of using casts as a method to decrease tone was initially pro-posed by Sussman and Kuszic.[35] This technique consists of applying casts with toe extension and molding insole pressure points, which are supposed to decrease spasticity and cause the muscle to lengthen. This concept, vari-ously described as tone-reducing features, inhibitive casts, or serial casting, has been widely promoted in the physical therapy discipline; however, there is no objective evidence that it has any long-term benefit. Wearing casts and having frequent applications is very energy and time consuming for families. Whatever benefit these casts provide, the same can be gained from properly constructed ankle-foot arthroses (AFOs), as described in the section on or-thotics. There is little role for the use of casts in children with CP for the treatment of chronic spasticity or contractures.

Muscle Strengthening

There has been a long-held tradition that children with spasticity should not be encouraged to do muscle-strengthening exercises; however, excellent studies by Damiano et al.[36, 37] have shown clear benefits from minimal strengthening work. As few as three times a week for a 6-week period of strengthening led to improvement in crouch gait.[36] Although this was thought to be due to strengthening of the rectus femoris muscle, it was far more likely the result of the strengthening effect on the gastrocsoleus because crouch in midstance phase is not controlled by the rectus muscle. This work has, how-ever, clearly shown positive effects, which has also been our personal expe-rience. Based on this work, many therapy protocols, especially postoperative rehabilitation protocols, should include muscle strengthening as a compo-nent of the program.

Enforced-Use Therapy

Enforced-use therapy is based on the concept that potential function is not used because the functional component of the motor control is ignored through long-term disuse. This is the basis of the widespread use of eyepatch treatment of strabismus and amblyopia ("lazy eye") in childhood. There have been periodic attempts to use this concept by short-term immobiliza-tion of the good arm in children with hemiplegia, but this practice has de-veloped a reputation for only frustrating the child. The current concept of enforced-use therapy involves total immobilization with aggressive therapy directed at learning such functional tasks as eating and dressing. We are us-ing this treatment in children with hemiplegia whose involved limb shows

promise of better functional use than the family is observing during daily activities at home. The current protocol uses a long arm cast, with the elbow
flexed 70° to 80° so that the child cannot use the arm for feeding or reaching
the face. The cast is left on for 4 weeks, during which time the child receives
therapy 3 times a week. The parents also receive instructions to encouraging
the child to be independent by forcing use of the hemiplegic arm. After the
cast is removed, therapy is recommended for an additional 4 to 8 weeks.
Based on limited experience, parents are reporting significant improvements
in functional use of the limb. There does not seem to be a place for this approach in the leg, because walking by nature requires both limbs and is an
enforced-use function. This approach to enforced-use therapy in children
with cerebral palsy is new, and many questions need to be answered before
specific recommendations for routine use can be formulated. No data currently exists to determine at what age child this works best, what level of
physical disability responds best or worst, how long the benefit lasts, if there
is a role for repeating the immobilization of the unaffected arm, or how long
the arm should be immobilized. Based on current knowledge, enforced-use
therapy looks like a useful treatment intervention, and many of the questions
will likely be answered over the next several years to allow much better definition of the specific protocol and outcome expectations.

A Current Physical Therapy Approach

Current pediatric physical therapists are moving toward an intellectual construct of being a coach or teacher of a child's motor system instead of a
molder of the brain as the child develops. This modern approach more often uses the understanding of dynamic motor control to structure tasks and
change motor patterns. This new approach requires a broader view of the
child and has to include an understanding of how he or she is functioning in
the home, family, and school environment. This approach also places the
therapist in a much better position to bridge the gap between the educational
and medical systems. Another important focus required in this role as teacher
or coach is a realistic assessment of the child's ability. For example, teachers
have to routinely make realistic assessments concerning the functional ability of a child to learn specific material. Normal children have a widely variable ability to learn a level of mathematics at each age level, and teachers
have to be aware of the level of the individual child. Some children in fourth
grade may still be struggling to learn addition, while others are ready to learn
geometry, but none would be ready to do calculus. In a community population of children, many will never be able to develop enough math skills to
learn advanced calculus. Using this same analogy, the physical therapist
needs to have a good ability to understand what the possibilities are for each
individual child, while at the same time continuing to motivate the child to
improve his motor skills. Understanding the child's functional possibilities
means the therapist can avoid frustrating them with unreasonable demands
and help their parents understand reasonable functional goals for the child.

The strategy for physical therapy is very dependent on age and functional
ability.[6] The general treatment approach varies significantly over the age
spectrum. Added to the age appropriateness, the therapy plan should have
specific objective, quantifiable short-term goals. Such goals include improving how long the child can stand on one leg, learning to jump, using a walker
independently, or improving a specific amount on a global measure such
as the Gross Motor Function Measure (GMFM). These specific short-term
goals can help the therapist, child, and parents judge progress. Also, this type
of goal setting is an important part in the reimbursement of therapy services

from insurance companies. Another part of the treatment plan includes teaching the family how to handle the child, teaching the child and family an exercise program, assessing the general function of the family in the home environment, and helping the family understand the long-term expectations of the child. A difficult aspect of the therapist's treatment plan is integrating the child's other medical treatments with fragmented medical care. The time constraint, which does not give the therapist time to attend medical appointments, leaves many therapists to gather this information from parents. Obtaining medical notes from physician visits can be another mechanism for the therapist to stay informed.[6]

Specific Age Periods

Infant

There has been considerable focus on the impact of early childhood infant stimulation programs, especially for infants from newborn intensive care units who are at risk for developing CP. The treatment program at this age, which is carried out by either a physical or occupational therapist, usually includes a combination of stimulation through handling the children, sensory stimulation through positional changes, and getting the children into correct seating. Many of the techniques used in infant stimulation approaches are combinations of NDT, sensory motor, and sensory integration approaches. Therapy frequency at this age may be two or three times a week; however, care should be taken not to place too high a burden on new parents with many medical visits. We have seen one very frustrated mother who was scheduled to see 21 medical practitioners for an 18-month-old child who had been discharged from an intensive care unit (Table 4.1). This number is far too much of a burden, and the therapists are in a good position to sense this and help parents decide what is reasonable. This is especially helpful when there are frequent team-generated treatment plans saying, for example, that a child should have four physical therapy treatment sessions in a week; however, due to the therapists' schedules, he will be scheduled to see three different therapists in 1 week. This is the worst kind of fragmented care, and it is very frustrating to parents. To parents and children, therapy is an intimate relationship and there is little benefit when it is scheduled based on whoever can be found to do therapy that day. Many of these parents will become very confused after hearing slightly different assessments from each therapist, often with different words to describe the same concern. This scenario is to be avoided; it is far better to have fewer sessions with a consistent therapist. The efficacy of early childhood therapy has not been well documented objectively, with most studies showing no or marginal measurable benefit.[4, 13, 38, 39]

Early Childhood

At 18 to 24 months of age, there is usually no longer any question as to the diagnosis of CP. This period, from 1.5 to 5 years of age, is the age of primary motor learning and the time when therapy potentially has the most impact. This time continues to be crucial in the parents' coming to understand their children's disabilities as the impairments are slowly becoming more apparent. A close, consistent relationship with a single therapist is especially beneficial during this time. This is the period where setting concrete short-term goals works well because of the children's rapid maturation, and this is also when much of children's play and free exploration time is motor based if they have sufficient motor ability for self movement. There are many developing adaptive equipment needs that also have to be assessed, fitted, and ordered for the children during this phase. In early childhood, the phys-

Table 4.1. All the professionals treating a 2-year-old child who had a prolonged stay in the newborn intensive care unit.

1. Nurses evaluating the child but providing no direct care
   - Home visiting nurse
   - Special high-risk newborn program nurse
   - School nurse
2. Physical therapist
   - Home visiting therapist
   - Two school therapists
3. Occupational therapist
   - School therapist
4. Speech therapist
   - School therapist
   - Special feeding therapist
   - Home visiting therapist
5. Social workers
   - Home visiting social worker
   - Medical counseling social worker for high-risk newborns
6. Psychologist
7. Special coordinators
   - Neonatal special program coordinator
   - Early childhood program coordinator
8. Doctors
   - General pediatrician
   - Developmental pediatrician
   - Neonatologist
   - Neurologist
   - Orthopaedist
   - Neurosurgeon
   - Ophthalmologist

The mother was visiting 21 medical professionals, many at least once a week, who were often giving the mother conflicting recommendations.

ical therapist will be focusing on gross motor skills, such as walking, and the occupational therapist will focus on fine motor skills, such as writing, using scissors, and self-feeding. Adaptive seating is important in this period, especially for feeding, toileting, and floor sitting. In establishing a treatment approach, most therapists borrow from the three predominant approaches, combined with using a model of teaching a task that involves cognitive understanding and repetition. This early childhood period is also a time when concepts from dynamic motor theory can be employed, with the goal of trying to alter the system in ways that will allow a task to find a new chaotic attractor.[40] An example of this might be using an unstable support, such as a cane in walking, to see if a child will find a better movement pattern compared with the pattern used in a walker in which he can go fast, but with very uncoordinated lower extremities. Therapy frequency at this age is variable, usually between two to four sessions per week while progress is documented. Some children will develop periods of frustration, and it may be better to give them a break of several months, and then restart therapy again. Efficacy of early childhood therapy has also been difficult to prove, although an educational model has demonstrated some improvement,[41] as has an NDT approach.[42]

Middle Childhood
Middle childhood, from approximately 5 to 10 years of age, is when the focus of children's development is shifting from primary motor to cognitive

learning. Children with good cognitive function will be transitioning into school environments, where gradually more time is taken up with cognitive learning. In this period, therapy routines should be significantly reduced, especially if they start to interfere with cognitive learning. Many children at this age can have the frequency of therapy reduced to observer status, or even discontinued if gross motor skills have plateaued. This time is also when very specific treatment goals are addressed, such as learning to use crutches instead of a walker. In this approach, a period of intensive crutch training therapy would be scheduled with the end goal being teaching these children to use crutches. Another important task at this age is the transition to regular sports activities in the community. The therapist is in an excellent position to recommend an appropriate sport activity based on an individual child's functional mobility and community availability. Sport activities that are useful to consider are horseback riding, swimming, martial arts, skating, dancing, T-ball, softball, and bicycling. For children with limited cognitive ability, focus continues to be on motor learning during middle childhood. This is the age when many children with limited cognitive function and mild CP learn to walk. The same treatment approach used in early childhood can be continued into middle childhood for this group. Frequency of therapy may vary from one to three times per week. Efficacy of therapy for this age group has not been specifically reported.

Adolescence

For individuals with good cognitive function, this period from 10 to 16 years focuses on cognitive training and there is no role for ongoing maintenance therapy, except to address specific disabilities with a goal-focused therapeutic approach at a time when there is no interference with age-appropriate cognitive learning. For a few motivated individuals, this period during adolescent growth can be a time to push to new levels of independence. However, almost no situation exists where there is a justification for children in normal classrooms to be removed from, for example, spelling class every week to receive therapy. Clearly, the long-term benefit of spelling class is much greater than the benefit of therapy to the point where it would be unethical to even entertain this kind of scenario. Therefore, intellectually normal children, regardless of their physical disabilities, should not be routinely removed from academic classes to receive therapy. However, this is a time period when teaching specific tasks, using a cognitive-based approach, can be very beneficial. This teaching will be especially beneficial if they are tasks that children will integrate into their activities of daily living and continue to use. Once learned, adolescents maintain these tasks long term.[8] Another important aspect of physical therapy for adolescents is learning to be responsible for their own stretching and physical activity. During adolescence is also the time when long-term functional motor skills can be defined, so it is important to help the family and the patient to understand these and develop plans to maximize independence within the context of these limitations. Whenever possible, the therapist should be fostering independence by encouraging the individual to get involved in appropriate physical activities and sports. Adolescents with limited cognitive ability will continue to focus on motor learning, and on rare occasions, it is possible to teach children to walk independently up to age 11 or 12 years. This means children with severe mental retardation should continue to be stimulated toward motor activities as well as other stimulation. Frequency of therapy is variable and almost always in the milieu of the educational system.

Young Adults

By young adulthood, there is little role for ongoing chronic physical therapy except to address specific functional goals. Individuals with good cognitive function should be doing their own stretching and physical activity routine if physically able, just as individuals with no disability are expected to take on their own responsibility for health and well-being. For individuals with limited cognitive ability, caretakers should be instructed on routine stretching and having a program of physical activity.

Therapy Settings

Child's Home

Home-based therapy is advantageous for the therapist to evaluate the home environment and set appropriate goals based on this environment. The home is often used for infant and early childhood therapy because children are comfortable here and it is convenient for new parents. The home setting is also useful for therapy immediately after surgery, when children may be uncomfortable moving into an automobile, or because their size and decreased function in the postoperative period makes physically moving them very difficult. The difficulty with home-based therapy is the limited availability of equipment and space in which to conduct the therapy. Also, much of the therapist's time is taken up with travel, which increases the cost of the therapy. Because of the increased cost, insurance companies will usually not pay for home therapy unless there is an extenuating specific reason why home therapy is required over therapy in a facility.

Medical, Clinic, or Outpatient Hospital Department

The ideal location for most therapy is an established physical or occupational therapy department. This location is especially important in early and middle childhood where gait training is the primary focus. This location is also ideal for postoperative rehabilitation because it provides the therapist with the equipment and space needed to do the therapy. Also, children come to this location expecting to work at therapy, and it is cost effective for the therapist's time. However, it may not be cost effective for the family, especially a family in which both parents work and the only times to do the therapy are during the daytime working hours.

Inpatient Hospital Rehabilitation

Before 1990, inpatient rehabilitation programs were commonly used for individuals with CP, especially for postoperative rehabilitation. These programs have decreased greatly because of the refusal of insurance companies to pay for the care as there is no good evidence that inpatient therapy is better than outpatient therapy. Today, the role of inpatient rehabilitation therapy is limited to very specific situations where multiple disciplines are needed in a concentrated time period. Such an example might be an individual with good cognitive function who has limited ability to receive therapy during the school year because of academic learning constraints, but would benefit from intensive therapy to assist with independence gaining skills such as self-dressing, self-bathing, improved walking, and wheelchair transfers. For the individual in late childhood or adolescence, an intensive 2- to 4-week inpatient therapy program can provide significant long-term yields. For this to be successful and for insurance companies to pay, a very detailed and specific goal has to be defined before the therapy stay. Both children and

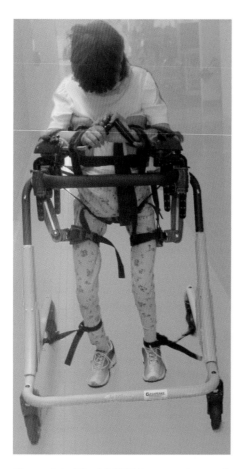

Figure 4.1. The MOVE Program is an education-based program that depends heavily on assistive devices to teach mobility. These devices demonstrate the increasing overlap of the techniques used by therapists and educators.

parents need to have a desire and commitment to make the goals and then to follow through with the goals at home after the therapy admission.

School-Based Therapy

After age 3 years, many children with CP spend most of time during the day in a school environment and therapy is often provided in school. There has been a tendency to try to segregate educational therapy from medical therapy. Educational therapy is defined as therapy that furthers children's educational goals, whereas medical therapy is directed at treating medical impairments. In some situations, these differences are clear. For example, a child who needs postoperative rehabilitation therapy clearly falls into the medically required therapy group. On the other hand, the goal of sitting in a desk chair and holding a pencil to write a school lesson is clearly a physical skill that has to be addressed in some way for effective classroom learning to occur. There are, however, many therapies that fall between these two extremes, and it seems the definition is determined most by the availability of a therapist and the attempt of school administrations to provide minimum or maximum services. The extremes range from schools that will provide increased therapy even to help with postoperative rehabilitation, to the other extreme of schools that define any specific therapy recommended from an orthopaedist as medically based therapy.

This definition of what is educational therapy rests with the educational system and not the medical system, although developmental pediatricians are seen as experts on special education and can give medical opinions for education that the school system has to consider. School-based therapy is ideal for children and families because families are not burdened with having to take children to another facility or another appointment. Most educational-based therapy is low intensity and low frequency. Often, 30 minutes once a week is the planned therapy intervention. However, educational therapy can be the focus of the educational plans for children with limited cognitive abilities. A new approach called the Mobility Opportunities Via Education (MOVE) was developed by Linda Bidade in Bakersfield, CA, as a special education teaching program, and is being adopted in some schools. Through the use of adaptive equipment, the MOVE program is able to provide significant periods of time for weight bearing, even for large adolescents and young adults (Figure 4.1). These devices include standers, walkers, and various other positioning devices that are used throughout the day, directed at a specific overall motor stimulation program. The real focus of this program is to allow the children to acquire physical skills, such as standing, that will allow them to do weightbearing transfers and to maximize an indivdual's physical function in the community. This educational therapy approach seems most appropriate for children and adolescents with severe mental retardation and limited physical abilities; however, it is very important that the therapy not interfere with cognitive educational classes, especially for individuals with good cognitive function.

Special Setting

Special environments in which physical therapy also provides a valuable service include seating clinics where physical or occupational therapists serve as primary clinicians in the role of evaluating a child's specific seating needs. The gait analysis laboratory is another environment in which the therapist usually does most of the direct patient contact testing, such as the examination and placement of markers and EMG electrodes. After the data have been compiled, the therapist is a key member of the data interpretation team.

Occupational Therapy

The theories of therapy practice for occupational therapy mirror those of physical therapy. Many of the basic therapy approaches, such as the sensory motor and sensory integrative approach, were developed by occupational therapists and are the basis of much modern occupational therapy practice. The focus of occupational and physical therapy in early childhood and in the infant period greatly overlap. As a child gains more motor function, the occupational therapist's focus shifts to functional activities of daily living and fine motor skills with the upper extremities. Upper extremity splinting to improve function or prevent contractures are also important aspects of occupational therapy practice. The efficacy of occupational therapy also mirrors that of physical therapy, in which it has been difficult to document clear objective benefits. The focus of occupational therapy is also very dependent on the age and functional ability of an individual child. The therapy plan is similar to physical therapy, in which a therapist uses a learning approach based on a specific task as the goal. The goal is planned from an understanding of a child's function, the family structure, and the physical environment in which the child lives.

Age-Specific Goals

Early Childhood

The focus shifts during early childhood from initially working on activities such as self-feeding and removing clothes, to fine motor skills such as using scissors and early writing skills.

Middle Childhood

Fine motor skills development, especially writing, self-dressing, and toilet training, if it is has not yet occurred, are the main focus. During this time, an assessment can be made of a child's ability to be a functional writer, and if it is determined that he cannot be a functional writer, an augmentative writing device should be prescribed. Typically, this would mean getting a computer and working with an effective interface with the computer to allow this to become the child's main output device. Another alternative may be the use of a dictaphone or a full-time aide who will do the writing for even more physically challenged children. The occupational therapist in the school setting often is the primary therapist working on these problems.

Adolescence

The main focus in adolescence are issues of independence. Based on individual evaluations, attempts are made for individuals to learn to do all their self-care needs, such as dressing, bathing, and cooking their own food. This is also when families start to understand what the individuals' specific, realistic, long-term goals for personal independence and self-care will be. For other children, it may be a time to focus on specific goals that are limiting their ability to be fully independent. For example, a child may be able to do all her own dressing, except putting on shoes. A specific therapy program aimed at solving this problem should be undertaken.

Young Adulthood

A major goal in young adulthood is to determine if an individual can drive a car. Many specific driving programs have been set up, often in coordination with occupational therapy programs. Also, an assessment of occupational options should be occurring, which is another area of practice where the occupational therapist usually has significant input. During this time a vocational assessment is performed for those individuals with adequate cognitive function.

Special Setting

Occupational therapists work in seating clinics and feeding clinics. Their role in these clinics is to provide clinical expertise in evaluating children and recommend appropriate adaptations. In feeding clinics, occupational therapists may also be involved in feeding therapy programs. Occupational therapists have as large a role in the school therapy setting as physical therapists.

Speech Therapy

The speech therapist's main role is to address the speech and augmentative communication needs of children. Also, feeding and swallowing malfunctions are evaluated by speech therapists. Radiographic swallowing studies are often performed by a speech therapist in coordination with a radiologist. For children with complex oral motor dysfunction, many pediatric hospitals have multidisciplinary feeding clinics in which the speech therapist is a key member. Usually, these clinics are directed by developmental pediatricians and do not have much direct interaction with the orthopaedic treatment, except when maximum oral motor function is significantly impacted by a child's seating.[43, 44] There may even be an impact on general motor function by altering oral motor function through the use of oral orthotics that enhance swallowing.[45, 46] This significant impact on general motor function has not been confirmed independent of the developer of the oral orthotic.

Therapist Assistants

There are special associate degree programs that train individuals in physical and occupational therapy. These individuals are called physical therapist assistants (PTA) or occupational therapist assistants (OTA). These assistants may carry out a treatment program as outlined under the direction of a licensed physical or occupational therapist. The level of required supervision varies from state to state; however, a PTA or OTA may not practice independent of a fully licensed therapist. The function of the therapist assistant is very similar to a physician assistant's relationship with the supervising physician. Therapy departments also use therapy aides who typically have on-the-job training to do activities only under the direct supervision of a licensed therapist.

Physical Therapist and Orthopaedist Relationship

The two main medical practitioners in the treatment of children's motor impairments are the primary therapist and the physician. This team is most commonly a physical therapist and a pediatric orthopaedist; however, it may be an occupational therapist and a physiatrist. We primarily address the orthopaedic and physical therapy relationship, but the context is similar for the other disciplines. The orthopaedist's experience is usually based on many children with whom he has had superficial contact. This experience is reflected in the orthopaedic literature of CP, in which most published papers are based on specific problems, such as hip dislocations or scoliosis, and include large numbers of patients, often 50 to 100 cases. The experience of the physical therapist is usually with of a few individual children, in much greater detail. This experience is also reflected in the physical therapy published literature, which often includes case studies or series of 3 to 10 children. Based on this experience difference, each discipline develops a different perspective. The physical therapist often feels that the orthopaedist does not understand this specific individual child, while the orthopaedist feels that the physical therapist has a narrow focus not based on a wide enough experience. These different perspectives require that the physical therapist and the orthopaedist have discussions where each is honest about the perspective from which the decisions are being made. By having open discussions, children's best interests are served because both perspectives together usually yield the best treatment plan. Often, orthopaedists are deceived by short examinations of a child who is not performing in the typical and normal way. The physical therapist has a much better perspective on how the child functions day in and day out. It is, after all, the typical daily function that the orthopaedist wants to evaluate and the basis from which decisions should be made about bracing, surgery, or seating. Alternately, the physical therapy approach of placing great weight on single case study experience does not work well in orthopaedic decision making because one bad outcome based on a surgical complication should not be used to preclude considering that surgery. Yet, it is this typical case experience approach in which a therapist will say, "I once saw a child who had this operation and he did very poorly, so we would never allow any child we are treating to have that operation." This approach would lead a surgeon to never do surgery, and is not based on scientific principles. This is the area where the therapist needs to hear from the orthopaedist what a surgical procedure is expected to do and the complication risks that are involved.

Children's medical care is greatly benefited by good, open communication between the therapist and the physician. This communication, however, is often difficult to practice in real life. The telephone seems like the ideal instrument; however, finding times when both the therapist and the orthopaedist are available to come to the telephone is often difficult. Other alternatives should be considered as well, such as the use of e-mail, letters, and, whenever possible, direct face-to-face meetings. There are occasional families who request that the physician not communicate with their child's therapist. If this therapist is, for example, a school-based therapist with whom the family has no direct contact (meaning the school hired the therapist and the family has no say in who this person is), this request may be valid at some level. We still try to convince families that it would be in their child's best interest to have communication between the therapist and physician. However, if the therapist is a primary therapist that the family is engaging to see the child, and the same family has also chosen to see us as the orthopaedist, the request that the therapist and the orthopaedist not communicate is inappropriate. If the family does not agree that the therapist and physician can communicate, they should go to either a different therapist or a different orthopaedist. Almost all families will understand the importance of this communication if it is discussed in the context of the benefits it provides to the child.

Education

The integration of children with disabilities in the educational system was variable in the United States until 1975 when Federal Law PL 94-142, entitled "The Education for All Handicapped Children Act," was passed. This law mandated free and appropriate public education for all children, including those with disabilities. This law led to the building of many schools for special education. This bill has been reauthorized in various forms and with many additions. In 1990, it was retitled "The Individuals with Disabilities Education Act" (PL 010-476). This bill and subsequent amendments, especially PL 99-457 and PL 94-142, have included infants, toddlers, and preschoolers with disabilities as part of the educational bill.

Most recently, part C of PL 105-17 has outlined the specific state-run services including early intervention that have to be provided for children from birth to age 3 years and states that children after age 3 years must be served by the school system. These acts require that the states provide appropriate education and associated services, which include occupational, physical, and speech therapy as needed for children to meet their educational goals. The school must also provide whatever adaptive equipment is needed for children to meet the educational goals set out. This law also states that these goals have to be individually defined in a structured individual education program (IEP) on a yearly basis, and that parents must be given feedback on how their children are progressing toward these goals on a frequency at least as often as other children are given report cards. The annual IEP has to include a definition of the specific special education program, the special services the child will receive, meaning therapies, and the adaptive equipment that is needed. The IEP must be explained to parents and caretakers in an annual meeting, and the parents or caretakers must agree that it is appropriate. If the parents disagree with the IEP as it is stated, they may try to negotiate. If this negotiation fails, they may appeal through an appeal structure that is defined in the special education act. The special education act also states that children's education should be in the least restrictive environment, which means that whenever possible a child should be in a normal classroom with age-matched peers. These federal education laws have greatly improved the educational opportunities for children with CP.

These laws are administered by states but interpreted and executed by local school systems; therefore, there is great variation in the quality of the educational experience individual children receive. Because of the significant subjective evaluation involved and the interpretation of the legal code, there is much more variation in the educational experience of children with disabilities than the educational experience of normal children; this is true even though there is great variation in the educational opportunities in public schools across the United States. The pediatric orthopaedist has various levels of contact with the educational system and has to understand the general milieu of special education. In addition, the orthopaedist should have a general understanding of the local special education system in which he is practicing. By nature of the special education system as it is defined in the federal code, there are many areas of frequent conflict that involve the orthopaedist directly.[47] These areas of conflict are discussed in the following paragraphs.

Separation of Education and Medical Practice

Education and medical practice are separate in our society at almost every level, and this separation has led to frequent conflicts in the area of special education. More specifically, special education law states that the educational system must pay for medical evaluations that are needed to determine children's educational goals and functions. The school system has to provide adaptive devices that are needed for children to gain an educational experience; however, the educational system does not need to purchase medical treatment required to maximize children's educational goals. The eye examination is a typical examination that the educational system is required to perform because visual acuity may be a major obstacle to a child's learning ability. If the eye examination demonstrates that the child needs eyeglasses, the school system has to pay for the glasses if the glasses are interpreted to be adaptive devices. However, if the glasses are interpreted to be medical devices, the educational system does not pay. This exact example has been litigated in several locations in various courts, and decisions have been handed down in both directions. These types of circumstances have spawned a whole legal subspecialty to help interpret and litigate areas of special education law.

What Is Medical Equipment and What Is an Adaptive Device?

The definition from the perspective of the educational system of what is educational and what is medical varies from state to state and even from school district to school district based on many reasons. Financial considerations in the educational system are often part of the reason to determine how aggressively the educational system pursues trying to shift costs to the medical payers. In general, wheelchairs, walking aids, and orthotics are considered medical equipment. Special desk seating, communication devices, writing aids, standers, and positioning devices used by children at school are considered educational devices. Devices such as standers or other adaptive equipment such as tricycles that children can also use at home may fall into either category.

Prescriptions

A major impact on the pediatric orthopaedist who manages children with CP is the need for many prescriptions, especially related to their needs in school. Although there is variability from state to state, most states require licensed therapists to provide therapeutic services only under a doctor's order. With this requirement, even therapists practicing in a school environment doing therapy to further children's education need to have a physician's prescription. If that prescription comes from an orthopaedist and is very specific for range of motion, gait training, or postoperative rehabilitation needs, with specific frequency requirements, the school administration can legitimately conclude that it is medically needed rehabilitation therapy and refuse to provide the services. The prescription that works best in the school environment is to order educationally based therapy and include specific restrictions and suggestions, such as a child's need to be in a stander every day for a certain maximum period of time.

The physician needs to understand his proper role as related to the educational system. The physician also needs to be able to clearly articulate that role to parents. A common parental concern is that the school is not providing adequate therapy to their child. In some situations this concern is true, and in others, the parents' enthusiasm for therapy and the expectations of how much benefit the therapy will provide are misunderstood. The orthopaedist should play a role in explaining to the parents that therapy is not indicated if that is his opinion, but he can also explain his role in ordering school therapy when he believes more therapy is required but the school disagrees. The parents' usual response to the physician is, "You wrote the prescription, so the school has to do what you said."

A typical example of a parent demanding therapy and the school disagreeing is a child with good cognitive ability who is an independent ambulator. In general, a child with this level of motor function probably has more long-term side effects from therapy than benefits, especially if the therapy interferes with any academic classroom work. In this situation, the parents need to be educated and the school decision needs to be reinforced with the parents. The opposite example occurs with a middle school child with severe quadriplegia, who has made no motor gains over several years, and the school IEP plans to maintain motor function with classroom activities provided by a teacher and a schoolroom teacher's aide. The educator believes that the focus of the this child's educational goals should be teaching him to use augmentative communication. The parents disagree and want everything to occur.

These are difficult subjective decisions and the orthopaedist may find himself siding with the parents; however, an aggressive response by letter or phone call will not help the parents' position because it will only give the school administration physical evidence that this need is medical rehabilitation. It is much more helpful for the orthopaedist to recognize that this is an educational decision, and offer the parents and school additional data as a way of helping the school and parents negotiate the disagreement. This negotiation will be more profitable with this approach than getting involved with a litigation.

Another major area where prescription need arises is obtaining adaptive equipment. All adaptive equipment purchased through medical reimbursement sources, such as private insurance or Medicaid, must include a medical prescription and usually a letter of medical need. Examples include orthotics, wheelchairs, and standers. If devices are purchased with educational dollars, no prescriptions are needed; these would typically include writing desks and computers used as augmentative writing devices. Many devices fall in between, such as augmentative communication, classroom standers, and floor positioning devices. The specifics of who pays for what may be negotiated at the state level between agencies, or in other states, debated at length, often to the major advantage only of the legal profession.

Physician–Educator Relationship

In almost all school environments in special education, administrators really try to provide the best services for the children in their care. A major constraint many special education systems work under is poor funding; however, cost may not legally be considered in determining what children need. The pediatric orthopaedist can be very helpful to further a child's education by providing documentation and perscriptions for the required services but at the same time must have a clear understanding of their limited role in determining the child's program. Annual visits to special schools are very beneficial to both the educator and the medical care provider. This kind of interaction helps both to understand the different environments, and it is helpful to have time for face-to-face conversation. The professionals in the educational system are very interested in staying up to date on advancing medical practice. Parents often ask for medical advice from the educational staff, just as parents ask educational questions from the medical staff. This kind of bilateral educational and communication process between the systems can only help children and families in the overall goal of allowing them to become all they can be.

Inclusive Education

The special education legislation currently requires that these children be educated in the least restrictive environment. The goal of this education is to encourage placement of these children in classrooms with their peers whenever possible.[47] This has also become a major political issue, with some parents narrowly interpreting this code to mean all children have to be in standard classrooms, with special education support provided in the classroom in the presence of normal children. The concept of this goal is valid but has limits. Because this is a very active current issue, parents frequently want to enlist the help or opinion of their orthopaedist. For many children, the correct placement is clear; for example, a child with ambulatory diplegia and good cognitive function should be in a regular classroom with their age-matched peers. Also, it is clear that a child who requires frequent nursing attention because of respiratory dysfunction and has no recognized accessible cognitive function is not served well in a standard classroom. This child also becomes a distraction to other children in the room who are trying to learn. Neither the child with the disability nor his age-matched peers gain anything from this experience. This movement toward education in the least restrictive environment has led to a great reduction in the number of special education schools that were built as a result of the 1975 legislation. Some children with severe impairments are placed in neighborhood schools and are being cared for by an on-the-job trained aide who sits with them in a classroom, with some occasional therapy services provided in the school. The therapists who provide this service often have little experience in working with children with CP.

Deciding which child is best served in a special school and which child is best served in a neighborhood school is a difficult decision for parents and children. Some of this decision depends on what services are available in the community. In general, it is much less expensive to provide services in the neighborhood school system, even for children who need a great deal of care, than providing for this care in a separate special education facility. The combination of a cheaper solution for the educational system and a politically active parent-based movement makes this concept of educating children in the least restrictive environment a very strong political and social movement. This movement has clearly benefited many children. As with most social movements, there are those children who have been hurt by the movement as well, and a basic directive of the early special education legislation was to provide for an individualized education program that best meets the individual child and family's needs. The role of the orthopaedist in this debate is marginal, but he should have an understanding of the issues involved as this often has a profound effect upon the children and their families. Case examples can help to demonstrate the impact these decisions have on some children (Cases 4.1, 4.2).

Transitional Planning and Guardianship

The special education legislation also requires the educational system to plan for transition from the school system, whose responsibility ends at age 21 years or with graduation from high school. This phase includes transition to sheltered workshops or adult day care as well as more traditional work and advanced educational opportunities, based on the abilities of each individual. Also, this transitional planning is supposed to include some education of the parents about the need to obtain guardianship for the young adult if

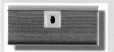

Case 4.1   Chandra

Chandra was a 12-year-old girl with combined spastic and athetoid pattern quadriplegia who had no oral speech and was totally dependent for all activities of daily living. Cognitive function was near age appropriate. Her parents felt strongly that she should be in a regular classroom with a teacher's aid and other required therapeutic support. Over several years, especially as Chandra en-

tered puberty, she became depressed and started having behavioral problems. After grade eight, her parents elected to have her move to a special education school that had an extremely high level of technical expertise. Her depression gradually lifted, her behavior stabilized, and she became a school leader over the next 5 years of her high school experience.

it is required.[47] For some environments, in facilities such as the Nemours Foundation and the Shriner's Hospital System, individuals also have to transition their medical care to adult services at this same time. This is a very stressful time for parents and young adults with CP. If the pediatric orthopaedic care has to end at age 21 years, this discussion should start several years earlier and the parents should be encouraged to see this as part of the same transition that the educational system is also working toward.

The need for guardianship must also be addressed for those individuals whose cognitive level precludes them from managing their own affairs. At age 18 years, individuals are considered adults, and from strict legal interpretations, if the individual has not been legally judged incompetent and a guardian assigned, the individual's guardianship rests with the State. This issue has special relevance for individuals who are clearly incompetent and are in need of a surgical procedure. Before age 18 years, a parent has to sign; however, after age 18 years, many parents think that it is clear that they will continue to be the guardian and to sign operative consents and other legal matters. The parents need to be informed that they have to get a court-ordered guardianship. The court will often need a statement from the physician, which

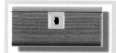

Case 4.2   Mary

A very similar case example is Mary, a girl who was in a special school until grade eight, then she transferred to a regular high school. Mary had a spastic quadriplegia and was almost totally dependent in activities of daily living; however, she was completely verbal. Her cognitive ability tested at marginal mental retardation. In her special school, she was a leader among the students because of her excellent verbal abilities. Upon transfer to the regular high school, she became depressed and developed significant behavioral problems. Some of the behavioral

problems had been apparent before entering regular high school but they became more severe. The whole high school career was a very traumatic experience for Mary and her family. It was not certain that this adolescent trauma would have been avoided in a special school environment; however, as demonstrated by these two case examples, inclusion in a regular school may create problems and does not universally benefit all students, as much of the current politictically correct discussion would suggest.

is easy in many individuals and reasonable for the orthopaedist to provide the court in clear cases of incompetency. When the situation is not clear, such as a child who can speak and seems reasonable but has some mental retardation, it is better for the court to obtain more expert opinion. In these situations, it is better to allow the psychologic and psychiatric experts make the determination. If an individual who is over 18 years has a medical problem that requires surgery, the physician's knowledge of the family and the individual with CP often means that it is all right to proceed. However, if there is a legal challenge from another family member, or there is some other liability issue, the court may find that the person who signed the consent was not a legitimate guardian, therefore putting the surgeon at risk for having done an operation without a valid consent. Also, if there is any question about the competency of the individual who is over 18 years, and the individual has not been adjudicated, the best action is to obtain the signature of both the patient who will have the surgery and the accompanying parent.

Other Treatment Modalities

There are many different treatment modalities pursued by families of children with CP. Some of these modalities are closely coordinated with or incorporated into standard therapy services. Other treatments tend to be more focused in the area of sport and athletic activities. The real advantage of the athletic activities, which are usually done in the individual's community with age-matched peers or family members, is the integration of the child into the normal community activities. Therapy services, even in a school environment, always have some sense of medical treatment and involve only the child with the disability. Some of these activities are explored in the following pages.

Hippotherapy

Providing therapy treatment using horseback riding is called hippotherapy (Figure 4.2). Hippotherapy has a long history in Europe, with one review in 1975 reporting more than 150,000 therapy sessions.[48] The vertical movements

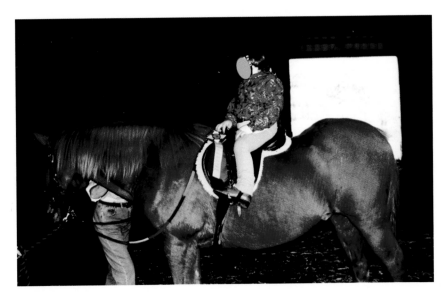

Figure 4.2. Hippotherapy is performed usually under the direction of a physical therapist using horseback riding. This therapy is usually performed in the location of a horse barn or farm, which has the additional advantage of providing the child with a different opportunity for social stimulation.

of horseback riding are thought to provide sensory stimulus, which decreases muscle tone. The shape of the horse's back also helps with stretching hip adductors and improves pelvic tilt and trunk positioning. Often, the therapist has the child riding facing forward and backward as a way of stimulating different aspects of the sensory system. Hippotherapy also provides an environment that is much more stimulating and psychologically uplifting than the sterile therapy treatment room. Published research studies have documented positive effects from horseback riding therapy. There was a decrease in spasticity immediately after the riding session.[29] There were also improvements in sleeping and bowel routines noted in the same study. Improvements in children's psychologic outlook have been reported as well.[49] A suggestion of improved ambulation skills with a more energy-efficient gait has also been reported.[50] There is enough evidence to conclude that hippotherapy is probably equal to other therapy approaches. However, the specific benefits of hippotherapy over standard therapy are not convincingly documented. Hippotherapy is a reasonable alternative to, or may be incorporated into, a standard therapy approach. A major obstacle for hippotherapy programs continues to be poor recognition of its benefit by secondary medical payors, requiring many of these programs to depend on donations or direct patient billing.

Horseback riding as an athletic endeavor is enjoyed by many children as well. We have one patient with hemiplegia who has been able to develop a national ranking in English-style riding competition. This is a very practical sport for children with CP who have enough motor skills that regular riding instructors can teach them horseback riding as a sport rather than as a therapy.

Hydrotherapy: Swimming

Therapy performed in water is called hydrotherapy. The effects of the water give children a feeling of weightlessness, which has been suggested as a way to reduce tone and allow these children to access better motor control.[6] This modality is also used for postoperative rehabilitation to allow children to start walking with reduced weight bearing. Hydrotherapy is a reasonable modality for gait training, especially in a heavy child who may be able to walk in water with relative weightlessness from the floatation effects. Also, there is a technique for using the neurodevelopmental treatment approach to teach swimming to children with CP.[51] There are no reports comparing hydrotherapy with standard therapy; however, one report suggested hydrotherapy and hippotherapy are equivalent but hippotherapy is cheaper.[49] Based on this report, hippotherapy apparently is cheaper because it is less expensive to buy a horse than build a swimming pool. Hydrotherapy is a reasonable adjunctive modality to use in planning a therapy program for a child.

Swimming as a recreational activity is excellent for individuals with CP. For many children who have a high-energy demand of walking in middle childhood, learning to swim and using this as the physical conditioning exercise is an excellent option. A major problem for individuals whose main motor ability is by wheelchair is finding an exercise technique that can be performed comfortably but still provide cardiovascular stress. Swimming is a primary option for many of these individuals. If a childhood swimming program teaches children to be comfortable in water and learn to swim, there will potentially be lifelong benefits. There are some children with diplegia who can learn to become competitive swimmers and even compete with normal age-matched peers.

Martial Arts

The martial arts are an excellent choice for some children, even those who require assistive devices for walking. The routines in martial arts are usually individualized for the speed at which a child can learn; many of the routines also stress balance reaction, stretching, and large joint range of motion. Also, there is a clear system for making progressive steps with awarding levels of achievement, which is a great motivator for many children. The training for the martial arts occurs in community locations with regular community peers, which is another major advantage. The main problem with the martial arts is the difficulty in finding instructors who are interested in teaching individuals with disabilities. Another problem of the martial arts for individuals who become very enthused about the sport is that at the higher levels of skill the motor impairments also make advancement very difficult.

Sports

Encouraging children with CP to get involved with typical age-matched sport activities is an excellent alternative to medically based therapy programs, especially for children with motor skills that allow them to enjoy the activity. Physical therapists are in an excellent position to recommend to families specific sporting activities that would likely work for their children. For ambulatory young children, the beginner soccer programs work well. For children with a need to work on balance and motor control, dance programs are an excellent option.

Acupuncture

Acupuncture with functional training has been reported to increase both children's motor function and cognitive function.[52] However, objective evidence is not strong to support the use of acupuncture. Apparently, the acupuncture meridians are closely related to the Vojta massage points, and there is a suggestion that both techniques may be stimulating the same system.[18] There may be a close relationship in these two theories of practice because there is a separate discipline of acupressure, which is alleged to have similar effects as acupuncture.[52] Because very few children enjoy injections, the routine use of acupuncture is much too stressful compared with any suggested or implied benefit to recommend its use in minor children. The use of pressure point manipulation by acupressure causes no harm if it is not uncomfortable to the children; however, there is no clear objective benefit of acupressure.

Massage and Myofascial Release Therapy

A major aspect of the Vojta technique of therapy is stimulation through a series of massage points. There has been increased use of massage by some therapists, including borrowing techniques from chiropractors. Myofascial release therapy is one such technique that has been developed emanating from chiropractor practice. Although myofascial release therapy is not usually described as massage, it is in fact a massage program with a minimal joint range of motion component. There are no English-language reports on the specific efficacy of massage compared with no therapy or other therapy modalities. Benefit has been reported for massage, reflexology, and other manipulations that are widely used in Eastern Europe and Russia.[53, 54] Based on the available evidence, massage therapy seems to cause no harm if the therapy is comfortable and the children enjoy the therapeutic experience. If the therapy is in any way uncomfortable for these children, it cannot be justified based on currently available data.

Hyperbaric Oxygen Therapy

There has been increased interest in the use of hyperbaric oxygen therapy for children with CP under the theory that more oxygen will make the brain function better. A small study suggested a possible benefit[55]; however, there have also been complications reported from this therapy.[56] Based on this minimal evidence of a positive impact, a well-designed study was conducted in Montreal. This as yet unreported study has apparently shown that there is a small benefit to the child by sitting with the parent in the hyperbaric oxygen chamber for approximately 10 hours each week. However, the addition of hyperbaric oxygen to the chamber adds no additional benefit. Based on these results, there is no role for hyperbaric oxygen therapy in children with CP.

Space Suit Therapy

Therapy with children in space suits, initially designed to counteract the weightlessness of space by being pressurized and add elastic resistance to movement, was first investigated in Russia in the early 1990s. This device has several versions but the ADELI suit has had the most reported use.[35, 57] This therapy has been popularized as a therapy treatment modality in Poland and is focused on improving sensory stimulation by providing children with the ability to stand through the resistance of the additional joint stiffness. Also, this method theoretically allows children to learn movement and standing posture and balance strategies. All the outcome studies have reported changes in vestibular and postural control activities with gains reported on short-term evaluation.[35, 57, 58] Because there are no objective functional gains reported, the measured effects are probably short term. In many patients we have examined after space suit therapy, we have not been able to determine any recognizable change. For American families with children who have CP, the opportunity to travel to Poland for 3 weeks seems to be a very positive experience. We suspect the opportunity to travel to Poland is more beneficial than the effect of the space suit. We would not recommend the use of the space suit in America because there is no evidence of functional improvement at this time.

Alternative Medicine

There are many alternative medicine techniques used to treat children with neurologic disabilities. Often, these practices arise out of local folk medicine. Many therapies used for the promotion of general health in health resort treatments are frequently promoted to those with disabilities. Such treatments as mud baths, reflexology, auriculotherapy, and various manipulations are promoted.[53, 54] There are a few alternative therapies that seem to have persisted for a significant time period and have spread beyond a small local area into wider geographic representation. Craniosacral therapy and Feldenkrais therapy, discussed next, are two examples of such techniques.

Craniosacral Therapy

Craniosacral therapy was developed from the therapy practice of treatments promoted by Dr. William Sutherland, an osteopathic physician in the early

1900s. This theory and practice was picked up in the 1970s and 1980s by Dr. John Upledger, an osteopathic physician who has heavily promoted and further developed the current practice of craniosacral therapy. The underlying therapy is based on the rhythmic pulsation and flow of the cerebrospinal fluid, which is influenced by breathing. This rhythmic movement is supposed to cause movement of the cranial joints and, in the vibration effect, movement of every joint in the body. Therefore, the craniosacral therapist can perceive this movement anywhere in the body, but it is most noticeable in the cranium and facial bones. The therapy involves palpation of the area to be adjusted to perceive the rhythmic movement. Then, using very light pressure, this rhythmic movement is altered to a better state. This change allows the individual to be more relaxed and to generally function better. There are no medical reports evaluating the efficacy of craniosacral therapy.[59, 60] Based on modern scientific understanding of anatomy, there is no theoretical reason to recommend craniosacral therapy, although a few reports of parents and children report a sensation of being relaxed and alert after therapy sessions. This effect is probably similar to typical effects reported secondary to the sensory stimulation of many massage techniques.

Feldenkrais Therapy

In the early part of the 1900s, Moshi Feldenkrais grew up in Russia and Palestine, then was educated in Paris where he received a Ph.D. in physics. During this time, he developed a relationship with Jigaro Kano, who is the developer of modern judo. From Dr. Feldenkrais' combined enthusiasm for Newtonian physics, especially with movements of mass, and the movements of judo, he devised a therapy technique that claims to increase intellect and general well-being and to improve motor function. The technique uses a therapist who gives verbal instructions on specific movements. These movements use positions and stretching specifically directed at increasing the individual's awareness, flexibility, and coordination. There are no medical reports evaluating this therapeutic approach. Based on reports of patients who have received Feldenkrais therapy, it does seem to involve many of the typical therapy positions often practiced as functional maneuvers, such as raising from the chair with a specific posture. These movements are combined with martial arts positions, which are often held for periods of time. The functional motor movements seem to be realistic as therapeutic approaches for some individual children; however, the theories and claims of benefits are totally unsubstantiated and unrealistic. There may be elements of this technique that an experienced physical therapist could use in a treatment plan. Feldenkrais treatment by an individual who is not trained in standard physical therapy is not recommended. There is a great risk of raising inappropriate expectations in families and patients, especially when the Feldenkrais technique is performed and advocated by individuals with no medical background.

References

1. Hur JJ. Review of research on therapeutic interventions for children with cerebral palsy. Acta Neurol Scand 1995;91:423–32.

2. Weindling AM, Hallam P, Gregg J, Klenka H, Rosenbloom L, Hutton JL. A randomized controlled trial of early physiotherapy for high-risk infants. Acta Paediatr 1996;85:1107–11.

3. Bartlett DJ, Palisano RJ. A multivariate model of determinants of motor change for children with cerebral palsy. Phys Ther 2000;80:598–614.

4. Harris SR, Atwater SW, Crowe TK. Accepted and controversial neuromotor therapies for infants at high risk for cerebral palsy. J Perinatol 1988;8:3–13.

5. Hubel DH, Wiesel TN. The period of susceptibility to the physiological effects of unilateral eye closure in kittens. J Physiol (Lond) 1970;206:419–36.

6. Campbell S. Pediatric Neurologic Physical Therapy. New York: Churchill Livingstone, 1991.

7. Bobath K. The Neurophysiological Basis for Treatment of Cerebral Palsy. Oxford: Spastics International Medical Publications, 1980.

8. Fetters L, Kluzik J. The effects of neurodevelopmental treatment versus practice on the reaching of children with spastic cerebral palsy. Phys Ther 1996;76:346–58.

9. Law M, Cadman D, Rosenbaum P, Walter S, Russell D, DeMatteo C. Neurodevelopmental therapy and upper-extremity inhibitive casting for children with cerebral palsy [see comments]. Dev Med Child Neurol 1991;33:379–87.

10. Law M, Russell D, Pollock N, Rosenbaum P, Walter S, King G. A comparison of intensive neurodevelopmental therapy plus casting and a regular occupational therapy program for children with cerebral palsy. Dev Med Child Neurol 1997; 39:664–70.

11. Hullin MG, Robb JE, Loudon IR. Gait patterns in children with hemiplegic spastic cerebral palsy [see comments]. J Pediatr Orthop B 1996;5:247–51.

12. Aebi U. Early treatment of cerebral movement disorders: findings among 50 school children. Helv Paediatr Acta 1976;31:319–33.

13. Rothberg AD, Goodman M, Jacklin LA, Cooper PA. Six-year follow-up of early physiotherapy intervention in very low birth weight infants. Pediatrics 1991;88: 547–52.

14. Jones RB. The Vojta method of treating cerebral palsy. Physiotherapy 1975;61: 112–3.

15. Imamura S, Sakuma K, Takahashi T. Follow-up study of children with cerebral coordination disturbance (CCD, Vojta). Brain Dev 1983;5:311–4.

16. Schutt B. Juvenile hip dislocation and the Vojta neuro-physiotherapy. Fortschr Med 1981;99:1410–2.

17. d'Avignon M, Noren L, Arman T. Early physiotherapy ad modum Vojta or Bobath in infants with suspected neuromotor disturbance. Neuropediatrics 1981; 12:232–41.

18. Stockert K. Acupuncture and Vojta therapy in infantile cerebral palsy—a comparison of the effects. Wien Med Wochenschr 1998;148:434–8.

19. Joint executive board statement. American Academy of Pediatrics and American Academy of Neurology. Doman–Delacato treatment of neurologically handicapped children. Neurology 1967;17:637.

20. Official statement. The Doman–Delacato treatment of neurologically handicapped children. Arch Phys Med Rehabil 1968;49:183–6.

21. American Academy of Pediatrics Policy statement: the Doman–Delacato treatment of neurologically handicapped children. Pediatrics 1982;70:810–2.

22. Bairstow P, Cochrane R, Rusk I. Selection of children with cerebral palsy for conductive education and the characteristics of children judged suitable and unsuitable [see comments]. Dev Med Child Neurol 1991;33:984–92.

23. Reddihough DS, King J, Coleman G, Catanese T. Efficacy of programmes based on Conductive Education for young children with cerebral palsy. Dev Med Child Neurol 1998;40:763–70.

24. Catanese AA, Coleman GJ, King JA, Reddihough DS. Evaluation of an early childhood programme based on principles of conductive education: the Yooralla project. J Paediatr Child Health 1995;31:418–22.

25. Coleman GJ, King JA, Reddihough DS. A pilot evaluation of conductive education-based intervention for children with cerebral palsy: the Tongala project. J Paediatr Child Health 1995;31:412–7.

26. Alexander MA, Molnar, GE. Pediatric Rehabilitation: Physical Medicine and Rehabilation. Philadelphia: Hanley & Belfus, 2000.

27. Chae J, Hart R. Comparison of discomfort associated with surface and percutaneous intramuscular electrical stimulation for persons with chronic hemiplegia. Am J Phys Med Rehabil 1998;77:516–22.

28. Carmick J. Managing equinus in children with cerebral palsy: electrical stimulation to strengthen the triceps surae muscle. Dev Med Child Neurol 1995;37: 965–75.

29. Exner G, Engelmann A, Lange K, Wenck B. Basic principles and effects of hippotherapy within the comprehensive treatment of paraplegic patients. Rehabilitation (Stuttg) 1994;33:39–43.

30. Scheker LR, Chesher SP, Ramirez S. Neuromuscular electrical stimulation and dynamic bracing as a treatment for upper-extremity spasticity in children with cerebral palsy. J Hand Surg [Br] 1999;24:226–32.

31. Wright PA, Granat MH. Therapeutic effects of functional electrical stimulation of the upper limb of eight children with cerebral palsy. Dev Med Child Neurol 2000;42:724–7.

32. Hazlewood ME, Brown JK, Rowe PJ, Salter PM. The use of therapeutic electrical stimulation in the treatment of hemiplegic cerebral palsy. Dev Med Child Neurol 1994;36:661–73.

33. Pape KE, Kirsch SE, Galil A, Boulton JE, White MA, Chipman M. Neuromuscular approach to the motor deficits of cerebral palsy: a pilot study. J Pediatr Orthop 1993;13:628–33.

34. Steinbok P, Reiner A, Kestle JR. Therapeutic electrical stimulation following selective posterior rhizotomy in children with spastic diplegic cerebral palsy: a randomized clinical trial. Dev Med Child Neurol 1997;39:515–20.

35. Sologubov EG, Iavorskii AB, Kobrin VI, Barer AS, Bosykh VG. Role of vestibular and visual analyzers in changes of postural activity of patients with childhood cerebral palsy in the process of treatment with space technology. Aviakosm Ekolog Med 1995;29:30–4.

36. Damiano DL, Kelly LE, Vaughn CL. Effects of quadriceps femoris muscle strengthening on crouch gait in children with spastic diplegia. Phys Ther 1995; 75:658–67; discussion 668–71.

37. Damiano DL, Abel MF, Pannunzio M, Romano JP. Interrelationships of strength and gait before and after hamstrings lengthening. J Pediatr Orthop 1999;19: 352–8.

38. Kyllerman M. Reduced optimality in pre- and perinatal conditions in dyskinetic cerebral palsy—distribution and comparison to controls. Neuropediatrics 1983; 14:29–36.

39. Palmer FB, Shapiro BK, Allen MC, et al. Infant stimulation curriculum for infants with cerebral palsy: effects on infant temperament, parent-infant interaction, and home environment. Pediatrics 1990;85:411–5.

40. Connolly KHF. Neurophysiology and Neuropsychology of Motor Development. London: Mac Keith Press, 1997.

41. Horn EM, Warren SF, Jones HA. An experimental analysis of a neurobehavioral motor intervention. Dev Med Child Neurol 1995;37:697–714.

42. Ottenbacher KJ, Biocca Z, DeCremer G, Gevelinger M, Jedlovec KB, Johnson MB. Quantitative analysis of the effectiveness of pediatric therapy. Emphasis on the neurodevelopmental treatment approach. Phys Ther 1986;66:1095–101.

43. Hulme JB, Bain B, Hardin M, McKinnon A, Waldron D. The influence of adaptive seating devices on vocalization. J Commun Disord 1989;22:137–45.

44. Hulme JB, Shaver J, Acher S, Mullette L, Eggert C. Effects of adaptive seating devices on the eating and drinking of children with multiple handicaps. Am J Occup Ther 1987;41:81–9.

45. Gisel EG, Schwartz S, Haberfellner H. The Innsbruck Sensorimotor Activator and Regulator (ISMAR): construction of an intraoral appliance to facilitate ingestive functions. ASDC J Dent Child 1999;66:180–7, 154.

46. Gisel EG, Schwartz S, Petryk A, Clarke D, Haberfellner H. "Whole Body" mobility after one year of intraoral appliance therapy in children with cerebral palsy and moderate eating impairment. Dysphagia 2000;15:226–35.

47. Effgen S. The school. In: Dormans J, Pellegrino L, eds. Caring for Children with Cerebral Palsy. Baltimore: Brooks, 1998.

48. Riesser H. Therapy with the help of a horse—attempt at a situational analysis (author's translation). Rehabilitation (Stuttg) 1975;14:145–9.

49. Barolin GS, Samborski R. The horse as an aid in therapy. Wien Med Wochenschr 1991;141:476–81.

50. McGibbon NH, Andrade CK, Widener G, Cintas HL. Effect of an equine-movement therapy program on gait, energy expenditure, and motor function in children with spastic cerebral palsy: a pilot study. Dev Med Child Neurol 1998; 40:754–62.

51. Harris SR. Neurodevelopmental treatment approach for teaching swimming to cerebral palsied children. Phys Ther 1978;58:979–83.

52. Zhou XJ, Chen T, Chen JT. 75 infantile palsy children treated with acupuncture, acupressure and functional training. Chung Kuo Chung Hsi I Chieh Ho Tsa Chih 1993;13:220–2, 197.

53. Babina LM. Health resort treatment of preschool children with cerebral palsy. Zh Nevropatol Psikhiatr Im S S Korsakova 1979;79:1359–63.

54. Mukhamedzhanov NZ, Kurbanova DU, Tashkhodzhaeva Sh I. The principles of the combined rehabilitation of patients with perinatal encephalopathy and its sequelae. Vopr Kurortol Fizioter Lech Fiz Kult 1992:24–8.

55. Montgomery D, Goldberg J, Amar M, et al. Effects of hyperbaric oxygen therapy on children with spastic diplegic cerebral palsy: a pilot project. Undersea Hyper Med 1999;26:235–42.

56. Nuthall G, Seear M, Lepawsky M, Wensley D, Skippen P, Hukin J. Hyperbaric oxygen therapy for cerebral palsy: two complications of treatment. Pediatrics 2000;106:E80.

57. Sologubov EG, Iavorskii AB, Kobrin VI. The significance of visual analyzer in controlling the standing posture in individuals with the spastic form of child cerebral paralysis while wearing "Adel" suit. Aviakosm Ekolog Med 1996;30:8–13.

58. Semenova KA. Basis for a method of dynamic proprioceptive correction in the restorative treatment of patients with residual-stage infantile cerebral palsy. Neurosci Behav Physiol 1997;27:639–43.

59. Green C, Martin CW, Bassett K, Kazanjian A. A systematic review of craniosacral therapy: biological plausibility, assessment reliability and clinical effectiveness. Complement Ther Med 1999;7:201–7.

60. Rogers JS, Witt PL, Gross MT, Hacke JD, Genova PA. Simultaneous palpation of the craniosacral rate at the head and feet: intrarater and interrater reliability and rate comparisons. Phys Ther 1998;78:1175–85.

5

Durable Medical Equipment

Durable medical equipment is the category of devices that are prescribed to ameliorate the disabilities from the motor impairments. Each of these devices, such as orthotics to assist with limb positioning or a seating system to assist with sitting, has very specific indications and contraindications. For physicians who care for children's motor impairments, many more prescriptions are written for durable medical equipment than for drugs. Because each durable medical equipment device has its own indications, contraindications, and risks, after a physician examination, a careful consideration of the risk–benefit ratio should be performed before a prescription is written. Many of these durable medical devices are very expensive, often ranging from $1,000 for an orthotic to more than $20,000 for a very sophisticated power wheelchair. It is the responsibility of the physician writing the prescription to understand the specific benefit the device is expected to provide and to know its contraindications and possible risks. It is the responsibility of both physicians and the durable medical equipment suppliers to inform patients and caretakers of the side effects and risks of the device. This process is exactly the same as used when physicians prescribe a drug, in which they are expected to understand the indications and contraindications of using specific drugs in specific patients whom they have examined. Just as physicians should not write prescriptions for drugs they are not familiar with, there is no place for them to write prescriptions for durable medical equipment that they do not understand. Therefore, when a new device becomes available, physicians have to spend time and effort to learn about the device before it can be prescribed. The regulation and oversight of durable medical devices by government agencies is slowly getting better; however, there is still considerable room for entrepreneurs to develop and market a device with little scientific background. This development is especially common in the area of orthotic design, where there is minimal objective documentation available even for well-established designs. This area requires care, consideration, and evaluation of individual patient response to gain experience with specific new device designs. Often, the advertising rhetoric has little basis in the physical facts of how patients respond. More commonly, the new device or design has a narrow application in which it does make an improvement; however, there is a tendency to generalize this improvement to all patients with cerebral palsy (CP), which does not work. The major categories of durable medical supplies that the physician who treats motor impairments must know about and be able to prescribe are orthotics, seating and mobility systems, and ambulatory aids.

Orthotics

The use of orthotic devices for children with CP has a long history, reaching its zenith just after the poliomyelitis epidemics of the 1950s. At this time, children were usually prescribed heavy, full hip-knee-ankle orthotics to control crouch and provide support. This practice came from the polio experience, which is a condition characterized by profound muscle weakness or paralysis. The very important difference between poliomyelitis and CP was not initially recognized. Although children with CP have weakness, the typical predominating problem is spasticity with decreased motor control and poor balance. These heavy braces do nothing to help children with CP move. Also, in this earlier era the use of heavy, stiff orthopedic leather shoes that were felt to provide good support to the foot was widespread; however, all these shoes did was cover up the equinus deformity so it was not visible. Invariably, the ankle was still in equinus when a radiograph was obtained with the foot in the shoe. With the advent of modern thermoplastics, lightweight, form-fitting plastic orthotics have become the norm.

Terminology

The terminology for prescribing orthotics can be confusing. The most general rule for spine and lower extremity orthotics is that the orthosis is named for the joints that are crossed by the orthotic. For example, an orthosis that covers the ankle and the foot is called an ankle-foot orthosis (AFO). Often, modifiers are added to make the name more specific. For example, the term molded may be added to AFO, which then becomes a molded ankle-foot orthosis (MAFO). The term MAFO is used to describe a plastic brace made from a mold produced from a cast of a child's extremity where the orthotic is to be fitted. Sometimes functional modifiers are added, such as ground reaction AFO (GRAFO), to describe an orthotic used to prevent knee flexion in the stance phase of gait. Upper extremity orthotics more commonly carry functional terms, such as a resting hand splint or a wrist orthotic. Many of these orthotic names are very regionally specific or in fashion because of specific marketing campaigns by orthotic manufacturers, and thus change over time.

Upper Extremity Orthotics

Upper extremity orthotics are used almost exclusively to prevent deformity or reduce contractures. The most common use of upper extremity orthotics is in children with quadriplegic pattern involvement who develop significant wrist and elbow flexion contractures. Using orthotics to stretch against these deformities may slow the development of more severe contractures; however, objective evidence to support this concept is not well documented. There is little or no harm from the use of these orthotics so long as the children are not uncomfortable and there is no skin breakdown caused by the orthotics. From a rationale perspective, the use of these orthoses during the adolescent growth period makes some sense. The orthotics may stretch the muscles and provide some stimulus for them to grow if the stretch can be maintained for many hours each day. The exact amount of time an orthotic should be worn to be beneficial is unknown, but 4 to 8 hours of brace wear a day are probably required.

Very few children get functional benefits from the use of upper extremity orthotics. Sometimes a very small thumb abduction orthosis will allow a child to hold a toy with finger grasp, which she could not do with the thumb in the palm. The benefit of upper extremity orthotic wear is not documented objectively; therefore, a child's functional use of the limb should always be the determining factor. For example, if a child has a thumb-in-palm deformity that can be corrected with a thumb abduction orthotic but she refuses to bear weight or use the hand when the orthosis is applied, the orthotic should be abandoned.

Shoulder Orthoses

There are no useful orthotics for the shoulder. Attempts at abduction bracing of the shoulder are uniformly unsuccessful. An occasional child will have an abduction external rotation contracture of the shoulder with athetoid movement or spasticity that can be controlled using a wrist band and securing the forearm to the waist belt or lap tray of the wheelchair. Some children also develop shoulder protraction, and occasionally a parent or therapist will want to try a figure-of-eight shoulder retraction orthosis; however, the strength of this protraction cannot be overcome with a figure-of-eight shoulder orthosis because of its extremely poor mechanical advantage.

Elbow Orthoses

The principal deformity at the elbow that is amenable to bracing is flexion. In children with strong spastic flexion deformity, the use of a bivalve custom-molded high-temperature plastic orthotic is required. The use of fixed dial locks allows these orthotics to be placed in different degrees of flexion depending on the tolerance of the individual and their skin. Sometimes individuals can tolerate more extension on one day and less on the next. If the spasticity is weaker or the children are less than 10 years old, a low-temperature plastic orthotic that is molded to the flexor surface of the elbow with straps around the olecranon is simpler and much cheaper to construct. Usually, these orthotics are fabricated by an occupational therapist, and they can also be easily modified with a low-temperature heat gun if more or less flexion is required. There has been a recent commercial promotion to use elastic hinges at the elbow, which have continuous passive stretch on the elbow. No objective data exist to support this concept, and the standard teaching is that spastic and elastic do not mix. This saying comes from the usual finding that a constant elastic stretch on a spastic muscle usually continues to initiate the spasticity. A fixed stretch will allow the muscle to slowly relax and stop contracting. However, this dogma is not well substantiated by objective testing. Pronation contractures are very common in the forearm of children with spasticity. There are no orthotics that can effectively control a spastic forearm pronation deformity, although trying circumferential wraps are usually not uncomfortable for the child with a mild deformity (Figure 5.1).

Hand and Wrist Orthoses

Wrist and finger flexion combined with thumb abduction and flexion are very common deformities in children with CP. Wrist extension orthoses are used mainly after surgical reconstruction to protect the tendon transfers for some additional months after cast immobilization has been discontinued. Usually, these orthotics are volar splints, which maintain the wrist in 20° to 30° of wrist extension and are worn full time (Figure 5.2). These wrist splints seldom provide a functional benefit to children and are usually poorly tolerated for long-term use. In children or adolescents with hemiplegia, there is a major cosmetic concern about the appearance of the limb. The orthotic provides no functional gain and is very apparent; therefore, it is usually cosmetically rejected. Most children with good cognitive function object to wearing a wrist orthosis for more than a short postoperative period. A dorsal wrist extension splint is sometimes better tolerated; however, there is no

Figure 5.1. Using a soft foam material with Velcro closures, a circumferential wrap can be designed to provide some supination (A) stretch along with wrist dorsiflexion and thumb abduction (B). Many children with strong pronation spasticity do not tolerate these wraps.

A

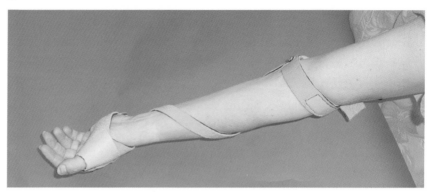

B

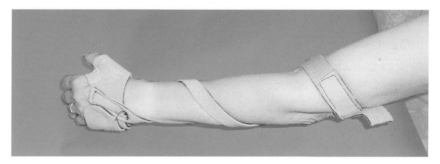

apparent improvement in function over the volar splint. The benefit of the dorsal splint is that it covers less of the palm and volar surface of the wrist and should therefore make more sensory feedback available to children during functional use. The disadvantage of the dorsal splint is that the force in the palm to extend the wrist is applied over a much smaller surface area, and if high force is required because of strong spasticity, the skin will often become irritated or develop breakdown.

Resting Splints

Resting hand splints, in which the wrist and fingers are all maximally extended to the comfort level of individual children, are good splints to help stretch the forearm muscles during the adolescent growth period. This splint may be made with a dorsal or volar forearm component (see Figure 5.2). The dorsal forearm component is easier to stabilize on the arm; however, it is often harder for caretakers to apply. The opposite is true if a volar forearm component is used. The resting hand splint can incorporate thumb abduc-

Figure 5.2. A splint that is entirely volar based can provide finger support or have the fingers free. This splint is very easy for caretakers to apply.

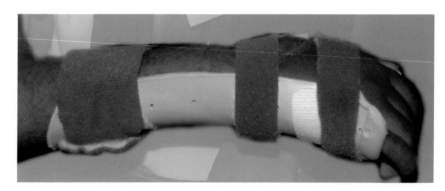

A

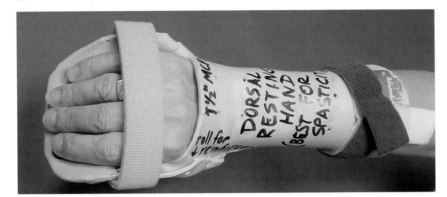

B

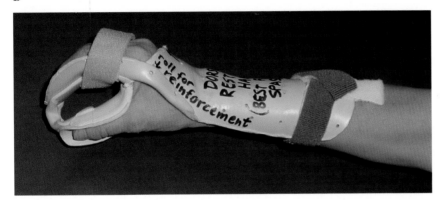

Figure 5.3. A dorsal-based resting hand splint will provide wrist dorsiflexion, finger extension, thumb abduction, and correction wrist ulnar deviation (A, B). The splint tends to be easy for caretakers to apply and is comfortable if no excessive stretch is applied at the time of construction. For postoperative support, the dorsal-based wrist extension splint is used during the day so that the child can start using active finger flexion.

tion and extension as well as finger abduction (Figure 5.3). Often, children tolerate these splints poorly immediately after initial splint construction. However, if the wear time is gradually increased, a goal of 4 to 8 hours per 24-hour period can often be achieved. This goal is ideal if children can tolerate the orthotic for this length of time; however, it is still worthwhile even if they can only tolerate the orthotic for 2 to 4 hours per day.

Thumb Splint

Thumb abduction and flexion is another common deformity. In most cases, this thumb deformity is combined with finger flexion and wrist flexion contractures, especially in children with quadriplegic pattern CP; therefore, the thumb deformity can be splinted using the global resting hand splint. For younger children with hemiplegia, thumb abduction can make finger grasp difficult. Using small, soft thumb abduction splints or low-temperature-molded abduction splints (Figure 5.4), the thumb can be positioned out of the palm in such a way that children can develop finger grasp. These splints should be limited to the absolute minimal amount of skin coverage possible because all skin coverage will reduce sensory feedback and the children will tend not to use their extremity.

Swan Neck Splints

Extensor tendon imbalance in the fingers may cause the fingers to become locked, with hyperextension of the proximal interphalangeal joint (PIP). This imbalance is most common in the long and ring fingers but occasionally occurs in the index finger. A metal or plastic figure-of-eight splint to prevent this hyperextension can be made (Figure 5.5). Usually, a plastic splint is used

A

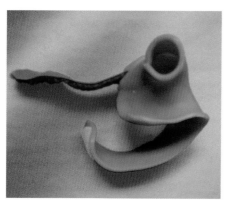

B

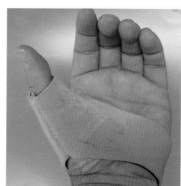

C

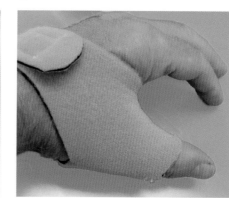

Figure 5.4. Thumb abduction splints can be constructed from a number of materials. Using low-temperature plastic, a well-molded splint can be formed (A). There are also many commercial splints available that are often more comfortable for the child (B, C). These are also available in different colors.

first and, if individuals find the splinting function beneficial, a metal splint is made, which is very cosmetically appealing because it looks like a cosmetic finger ring. In some individuals, these rings become uncomfortable because of the amount of force that the ring exerts over the very narrow area of skin. It is this narrow skin pressure that may limit the use of ring orthoses.

Spinal Orthoses

Soft Thoracolumbar Sacral Orthosis (TLSO)

Most children with CP who develop scoliosis are nonambulatory children with quadriplegic pattern involvement. The scoliosis is in no way impacted by the use of orthotics.[1] There is a role for the use of spinal orthotics to support sitting in children who are not independent sitters. The preferred orthotic is a soft thoracolumbar sacral orthosis (TLSO) with metal or plastic stays that are embedded in a soft plastic material (Figure 5.6). This soft material is well tolerated by sensitive skin and does not apply high areas of pressure. This soft TLSO works like a corset to support sitting. The orthotic may be worn over thin clothing so it is easy to apply and remove by caretakers. The TLSO is worn only at times when caretakers feel that the children have direct functional benefits. These orthotics are never worn during sleeping hours. Breathing may be restricted if the orthotic is too tight; however, the gain from upright sitting is approximately the same as the restriction from the orthotic.[2] For children with gastrostomy tube feedings, an abdominal

Figure 5.5. Finger proximal interphalangeal joint (PIP) joint hyperextension can be a difficult problem that is easy to control in some individuals with extension block splints. One type of commercially available splint is plastic-covered wire (A), and another common type is a molded figure-of-eight type plastic orthotic (B).

A

B

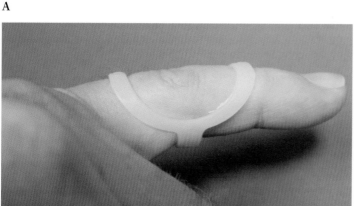
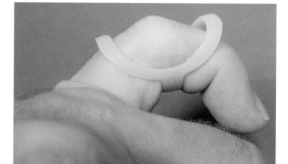

A

B

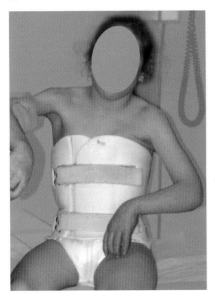

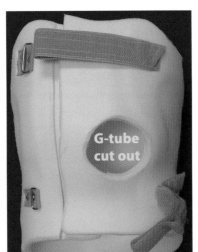

Figure 5.6. Although scoliosis in children with CP is not impacted by bracing, some children can sit much better with improved trunk support using a soft corset-type thoracolumbar sacral orthosis (TLSO). This orthosis is available in an off-the-shelf version; however, most children are more comfortable with a custom-molded orthotic (A). This orthotic is made with a soft plastic in which stiffer plastic stays are embedded to provide better support. The orthosis is only worn when it provides functional benefit, such as during sitting activities, and is never worn at night. If the child has a gastrostomy tube, the orthotic can be cut out to accommodate the tube (B).

cutout is required, which provides sufficient space and does not cause irritation. The indication for a soft TLSO is determined by the families' and caretakers' goals, with many families finding the adaptive seating working very well and thus no orthotic is needed. For families with children who sit in many different seats, the soft TLSO is especially helpful. The soft TLSO is made from a mold produced from a cast of the child's body. No attempt is made to get specific scoliosis correction, only to provide trunk alignment that maximizes children's sitting ability.

Bivalved TLSO

Usually, kyphosis is the result of truncal hypotonia and poor motor control. This deformity may slowly become fixed in some children; however, for most, it slowly resolves during adolescent growth. The initial treatment of kyphosis is by wheelchair adjustment and the use of a shoulder harness or anterior trunk restraint. However, there are children who do not tolerate the strong anterior trunk restraints or shoulder harnesses. Orthotic control of kyphosis requires the use of a high-temperature custom-molded bivalve TLSO (Figure 5.7). This orthosis must extend anteriorly to the sternal clavicular joint and inferiorly to the anterosuperior iliac spine. An abdominal cutout may be used if needed for a gastrostomy tube, but this should not be used routinely. The posterior shell needs to extend proximally only to the apex of the kyphosis. This orthotic provides three points of pressure to correct the deformity. Because kyphosis requires a very high force to correct the deformity, the orthotic will deform if it is not very strong. For this reason, the soft material construction of the scoliosis TLSO does not work for kyphosis. There are no data to suggest that the kyphotic-reducing bivalve TLSO has any impact on the progression of the kyphotic deformity; therefore, the orthotic is prescribed only for the functional benefit of allowing children to have better upright sitting posture and better head control. This orthotic should be used by children during periods of sitting when it is providing a specific functional benefit. The bivalve TLSO is never worn during sleep times. This bivalve orthosis is also constructed over a custom mold made from a cast of the child.

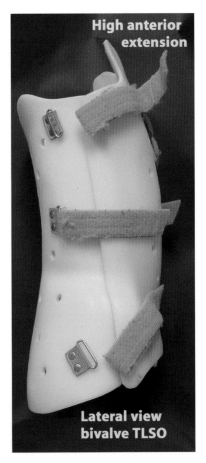

Figure 5.7. To control a kyphotic deformity, much stronger anterior support is required. The anterior aspect also needs to be high to the level of the sternal notch and low to the pubis; this requires a bivalve design in which there is an external shell of high-temperature plastic lined inside with a softer plastic.

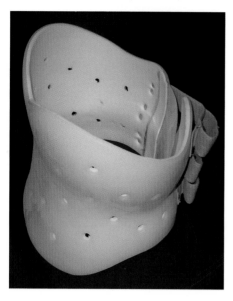

Figure 5.8. For children who develop low back pain, usually from acute spondylolysis, a lumbar flexion jacket is required. This orthotic is higher in the back to prevent lumbar extension or lordosis and is low in the front and usually front opening. Many types of this orthotic are commercially available; however, many children need to be custom molded because the appropriate fit cannot be obtained from the available models.

Lumbar Flexion Jacket

Often, low back pain is the presenting symptom of acute spondylolysis and mild spondylolisthesis. If the pain is protracted, or the spondylolisthesis is acute, the pain should be treated for 3 to 6 months with a flexion lumbosacral orthosis (LSO) (Figure 5.8). This lumbar flexion orthosis is usually made from a low-temperature plastic that wraps around the lumbar spine and abdomen, maintaining the lumbar spine in flexion. The lumbar flexion orthosis may be molded directly on a child, or made from a mold produced from a cast. There are some commercially available lumbar flexion orthoses; however, they usually do not fit children well, especially children with CP whose body dimensions do not fit typical age-matched peers. This lumbar flexion orthotic should be worn full time for 2 to 3 months except during bathing. After this, the orthotic is worn only during the day for an additional 2 to 3 months, and then children are gradually weaned from the brace. Back pain should diminish very quickly after the initiation of the orthotic. Usually, within 1 week of full-time orthotic wear, children will report a significant reduction in their level of back pain. The spondylolysis may not heal during the brace wear and often remains; however, the pain almost always disappears and does not return.

Lower Extremity Orthotics

Hip Orthoses

The use of a hip abduction orthosis is often discussed in conferences; however, there are few objective data to support this use. The use of a hip abduction orthosis before surgical lengthening of the adductor muscles causes more harm than benefit based on modeling studies and objective reports.[3] Therefore, abduction bracing of the hip should not be used to prevent hip dislocation before hip muscle lengthening surgery. Abduction bracing after muscle lengthening may improve the recovery of the hip subluxation; however, it may also increase the risk of severe abduction contractures.[4] Therefore, in the balance, abduction bracing has little use after muscle lengthening. There is no objective evidence that abduction bracing is functionally beneficial to control scissoring gait in children with poor motor control. Rather than using large hip abduction orthoses, a much simpler and easier method to control scissoring gait is to use strings from the shoes attached to rails along the lateral sides of the walker. These strings will laterally restrain the feet so they do not cross the midline. A few walkers also have thigh guides (Figure 5.9). These lateral restraints are available with commercial walkers, or can be easily made with long shoestrings tied over the lateral edge of the walker frame.

Twister Cables

Internal rotation of the hip is very common in children with CP. There has been a long history of using twister cables or similar devices that are attached to waistbands proximally and to the feet distally, often via an AFO. These externally rotating devices have no published documentation of providing any functional benefit to children, or of aiding the resolution of the internally rotated gait either in the short term or in the long term. These externally rotating devices often slow children because they increase stiffness in the extremities. In this way, the use of these devices is somewhat similar to adding increased muscle tone or spasticity, of which these children usually have too much already. Also, the externally rotating stress tends to be concentrated at the knee joint, which is the joint with the least muscle force available to resist the torsional stress that the orthotic applies. This external rotation force can potentially cause damaging stretching of the knee ligaments. Because there is no functional benefit and significant potential for harm, the use of rigid strong twister cables to counter internal rotation of the lower extremities should be abandoned.

Elastic Wraps

The use of elastic wraps has also been advocated to help control hip internal rotation. Usually, these wraps are attached to the proximal end of an AFO, wrapped around the thigh, and attached to a waistband proximally. These bands add relatively little force and almost no weight. Therefore, the negative effects of the twister cables are eliminated, and there are occasional children who seem to gain some minimal benefit from the use of these bands. These twister bands cause little harm and are reasonable to try in children who do not have strong spasticity or high fixed femoral anteversion but are mainly having internal rotation deformity of the hips secondary to poor motor control.

Knee Orthoses

Knee orthotics have a very limited use. Rarely, in children with back-kneeing that is causing knee pain or a worsening deformity, the only option may be limiting knee extension with a knee-ankle-foot orthosis (KAFO) using a free knee hinge that prevents hyperextension. Also, children with severe knee flexion contractures who have undergone posterior knee capsulotomies need to have prolonged postoperative bracing to prevent the recurrence of the flexion contractures. The best orthotic to use is a KAFO with a step-lock or dial-lock knee hinge so the knee can be gradually extended further as tolerated by the child (Figure 5.10). These orthoses cannot be used immediately

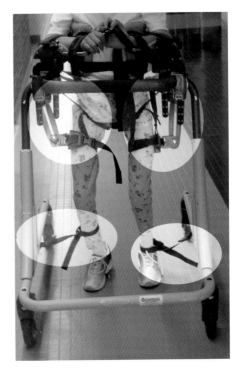

Figure 5.9. In general, hip abduction orthoses are too heavy to help children prevent scissoring. An excellent mechanism to control scissoring is to use the thigh and foot guides that are part of many gait trainers or walkers. Because almost all children who have substantial problems with scissoring require the use of a walker as an assistive device, this is a simple, effective, and easy solution.

A   B

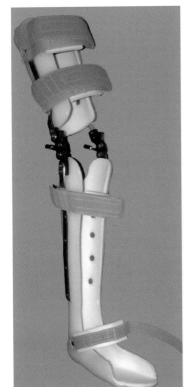   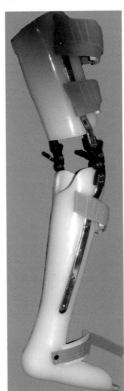

C

Figure 5.10. There are a few children with severe knee flexion contractures, especially those in whom surgical release is planned, who need progressive strong extension stretch. For these, a custom molded knee-ankle-foot orthosis (KAFO) with soft plastic lining (A) is excellent. A variable lock or step-lock knee hinge allows the child to spend time in varying degrees of extension (B). This orthotic is especially useful for a teenager in whom progressive stretching is desired (C).

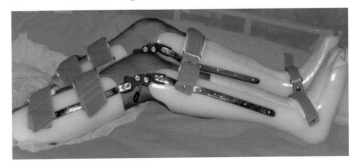

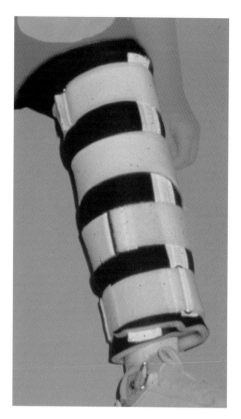

Figure 5.11. A very common need is to provide a knee extension splint for a child with CP, and most of these can be addressed with a foam wrap that includes metal stays and Velcro enclosures. These commercially available knee immobilizers are cost effective, comfortable for the child, and easy for the caretaker to apply and remove.

postoperatively until the acute swelling subsides. For the first month, bivalve casts are usually used until children can tolerate the orthotic. The KAFO should be used for 12 to 16 hours per day after posterior knee capsulotomies, with the goal of having children sleep in the orthotic with their knee fully extended. After 6 months in the KAFO, and when their knee extension has remained stable, the orthotic can be slowly weaned and then discontinued sometime between 6 and 12 months postoperatively. The most common knee orthosis is the knee immobilizer, which is usually constructed of foam material in which plastic or metal stays are embedded. The orthosis is wrapped around the limb and held closed with Velcro straps (Figure 5.11). The knee immobilizer is used as a knee extension orthotic after hamstring lengthening or for nighttime splinting for hamstring contractures.

Ankle-Foot Orthoses

Ankle equinus is the most commonly recognized joint malposition in children with CP. Orthotic control of this equinus position has a long history and is the oldest treatment of the motor impairments of CP. The availability of modern thermoplastics has greatly increased the options for orthotic management compared with the old heavy metal and heavy leather shoe devices. The plastic braces provide a much larger skin contact, so the forces from significant spasticity are distributed over a larger surface area and are better tolerated. Because of wide size and shape variation of the feet in children, most of these orthotics should be custom molded for the best fit (Figure 5.12). The use of AFOs includes many different variations, and all the published studies have confirmed the mechanical effects of these orthotics. For example, if the ankle is blocked from going into equinus by the orthosis, there is decreased ankle range of motion and decreased ankle equinus.[5–7] These same studies do not show predictable effects at joints not covered by the orthotic. Also, if the orthotic has a hinge that allows dorsiflexion, there is more dorsiflexion present than when the orthotic has a fixed ankle.[6] There are no data to suggest that one type of orthotic or different design is better than any other. The concept of pressure points in specific molds to reduce muscle tone has no objective data to support their use. There is objective evidence that these orthotics can improve children's balance ability.[8] Balance may be better with hinged AFOs than with solid AFOs.[8] Others have found no difference between hinged and solid AFOs,[6, 7] or between hinged and solid AFOs and tone-reducing designs.[9] There is improved stability in the stance phase of gait[10, 11] and improved ankle position in swing and at foot contact.[12] Also, improved stability by the use of AFOs in children who are coming to stand in the preambulatory phase has been documented.[13] Based on these limited objective data, most specific prescriptions for foot orthotics require a consideration of the skills of the available orthotist and the specific mechanical goals desired in the individual child.

Confusing Terms

The terminology used in describing specific components of AFOs is very confusing. The term dynamic is used in the literature to mean an AFO with a hinge joint at the ankle; however, it is also used to mean a solid plastic AFO made of thinner, more flexible plastic that wraps around the limb to gain stability. Tone reducing is another term that is widely used but has no specific standard meaning. To avoid confusion, the terms dynamic and tone reducing are not used further in this discussion. Hinged or articulated will be used to mean an orthosis that contains a joint at the ankle, and the term wraparound will be used to refer to the thinner plastic with a fuller circumferential mold.

A

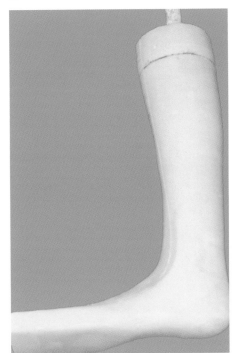

B

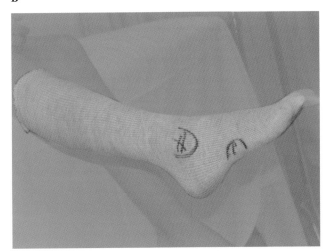

Figure 5.12. Because of the wide variation in foot size and shape in children with CP, AFOs usually should be custom molded for the best fit and tolerance. This process starts with application of a stocking on which specific bone landmarks are outlined so the mold can be later modified to prevent pressure on these areas (A,B). Next, either a premolded plantar arch mold is applied or the arch has to be molded by hand (C). Plaster is now rolled over the foot using an anterior rubber bolster to protect the skin for cast removal (D).

C

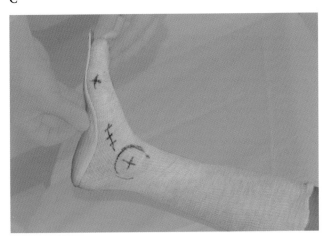

D

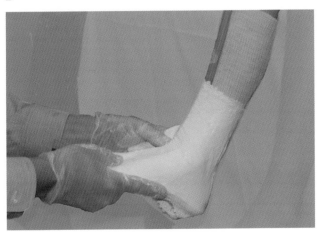

E   F   G

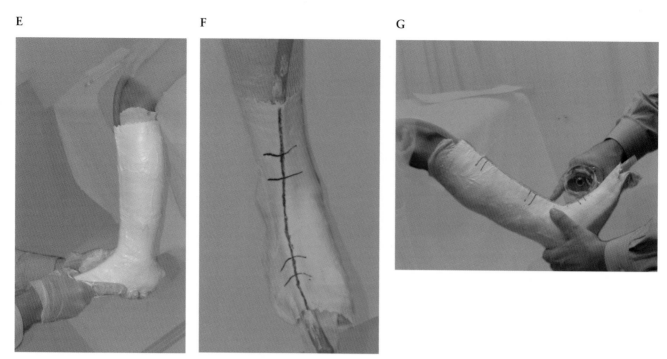

Figure 5.12 (continued). After the plaster   H
has been rolled on the whole leg, the foot is
carefully positioned and held by the orthotist
in the desired corrected position until the plaster hardens (E). The plaster is now marked
anteriorly where it will be cut; this will allow
the cast to be closed accurately for pouring
of the mold (F). The cast is now removed (G),
and the bolster is removed, splitting the cast
open (H).

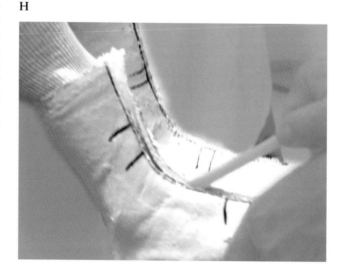

AFO

A solid AFO with an anterior calf strap and an anterior ankle strap is
the most versatile orthotic design and is the orthosis most often prescribed
for children at the preambulatory stage, usually between the ages of 18 and
24 months (Figure 5.13). This orthotic provides stability to the ankle and
foot to give a stable base of support for children to stand. This orthosis is
reasonably easy for caretakers to apply and is lightweight. As children gain
better stability and start to walk using a walker, usually between the ages
of 3 to 4 years, the ankle hinge can be added to allow dorsiflexion but limit
plantar flexion. This transition to a hinged AFO is contraindicated if children have severe planovalgus or varus foot deformity (Figure 5.14). The
hinge will allow movement through the subtalar joint rather than the ankle
joint and, as a consequence, will allow worsening of the foot deformity in
the orthosis. Also, the hinged AFO is contraindicated if the children are

I   J   K

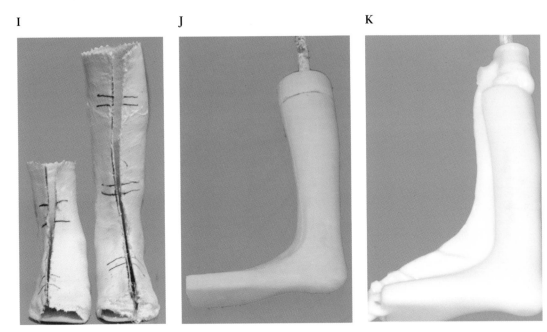

developing increased knee flexion in stance or a crouched gait pattern. Most children who have good walking ability with diplegic and hemiplegic pattern involvement benefit from the transition to a hinged AFO at approximately 3 years of age. Most children who are marginal ambulators or non-ambulators will be best served by staying in solid AFOs. Hinged AFOs are preferred for children who back-knee because of gastrocnemius contractures. By setting the plantar flexion stop at 5° of dorsiflexion, these children will be forced into knee flexion in stance if they are independent ambulators. If they use assistive devices, such as walkers or crutches, they may still back-knee by allowing the forefoot to come off the floor. If this occurs, the shoe should have a good wide stable heel; however, in spite of this, some children will persist with back-kneeing and can be controlled only with a KAFO that blocks knee hyperextension directly.

Ground Reaction AFO

Controlling crouched gait with increased knee flexion and ankle dorsiflexion in stance phase is best done using solid AFOs with wide anterior proximal calf straps until children weigh 25 kg, usually at about 8 to 10 years of age. For children who are over 25 kg, the solid ankle ground reaction AFO, which is rear entry in the calf, is recommended (Figure 5.15). The use of this orthosis requires that the ankle can be brought to neutral dorsiflexion with the knee in full extension. If this cannot be accomplished, the orthosis cannot work and these children first need gastrocnemius and hamstring lengthening before the orthosis can be used successfully. The successful use of this orthotic requires that there be very little knee flexion contracture. Because this orthosis depends on the mechanics of an effective ground reaction force, the foot-to-knee axis has to be in a relatively normal alignment, meaning less than 20° of internal or external tibial torsion. This solid ground reaction AFO does not work with severe internal or external tibial torsion or severe foot malalignments. The ground reaction AFO only works when children are standing on their feet, and as such is useful only for ambulatory children. As these children get heavier, this orthosis becomes more effective; however, it also has to become stronger. As children approach 50 to 70 kg, the orthosis

Figure 5.12 (continued). Following removal, the casts are inspected to make sure they are plantigrade and have the desired correction (I). The cast is then filled with plaster to make a positive mold, which has the relief areas increased further (J). The mold is then placed in a high-temperature oven over which a plastic cover is vacuum formed (K). The orthotic is then cut from the vacuum-formed plastic, trimmed, smoothed, and pads and straps applied.

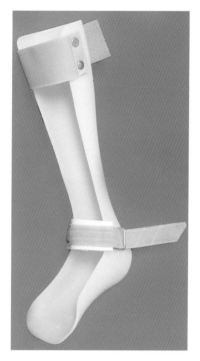

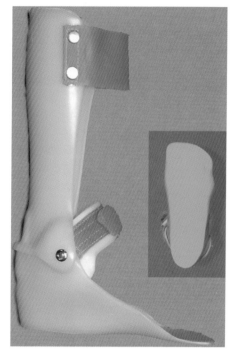

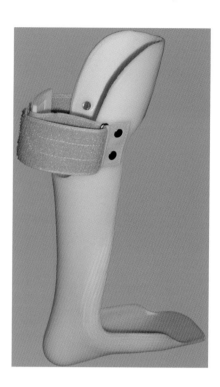

Figure 5.13 (left). The most basic AFO has a solid ankle, an anterior ankle strap, and an anterior calf strap. This is the preferred orthotic for preambulatory children and most marginal ambulators.

Figure 5.14 (middle). As children gain ambulatory ability and the main goal of the orthotic becomes preventing plantar flexion, a plantar flexion-limiting ankle hinge joint can be added. The remainder of the orthotic is similar to the solid ankle, with perhaps a flat sole or additional arch molds added. These tone-reducing features have not been shown to change gait in any measurable way.

Figure 5.15 (right). The solid ground reaction AFO is entered from the rear at the calf level. This is an anticrouching orthosis and has very specific requirements to work. The knee must be able to fully extend, the ankle has to be able to dorsiflex to neutral with an extended knee, the foot progression angle must be within 30° of neutral, and the tibial torsion must be less than 30°. This orthosis depends on the action of the ground reaction force, and as such is only effective when the child stands or walks and if the child has enough weight, usually 30 kg or more.

has to be constructed with a composite of carbon fiber or laminated copolymer to withstand the applied forces.

Articulated Ground Reaction AFO

The ground reaction AFO may be hinged to allow plantar flexion but limit dorsiflexion (Figure 5.16). This orthosis is primarily used after surgical reconstruction of the feet and muscle lengthening as a bridge to allow development of increased muscle strength in the plantar flexors, with the long-term goal of individuals being free of an orthotic. However, some individuals continue to use this articulated ground reaction orthosis long term. The orthosis can be used before surgery on rare occasions; however, a prerequisite for using articulated ground reaction AFOs is normal foot alignment. The articulated ground reaction AFO is entered posteriorly into a circumferentially molded forefoot, but with no hindfoot control. If there is any planovalgus or varus hindfoot deformity, the foot will deform even more severely into planovalgus or varus under the strong force of the ground reaction moment. Because this articulated ground reaction AFO contains no resistance to prevent deformity, the orthotic is usually not tolerated because of significant skin pressure on the forefoot when any degree of planovalgus foot deformity is present. Older children weighing more than 25 kg who meet the other criteria will usually be very comfortable with the articulated ground reaction AFO, and the orthotic will be very effective in controlling crouched gait. However, it must be emphasized that this orthosis works only when all the indications are appropriate. Another option for using the articulated ground reaction AFO that may be useful in younger children who weigh less than 20 kg is to use the standard articulated AFO and then attach a posterior restraining strap, which prevents dorsiflexion at a certain predetermined amount (Figure 5.17). Often, these restraining straps are made of a fabric material and stretch over time, so they have to be reset fairly frequently. This design never works for heavy adolescents because there is no orthotic material that is strong enough to resist the force of dorsiflexion from the ground reaction AFO.

A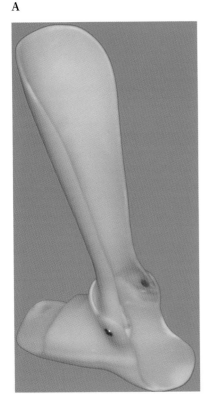

B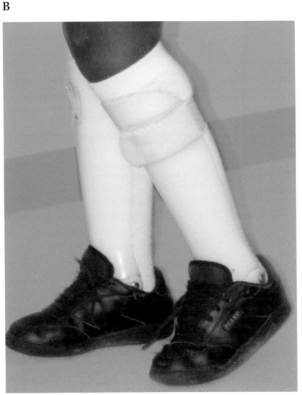

Half-Height AFO

The use of a solid AFO without an anterior calf strap is a design to control plantar flexion that will allow free dorsiflexion (Figure 5.18). If children use considerable dorsiflexion, their calves move away from the shank of the orthosis and can be very uncomfortable. Because it is uncomfortable when the calf presses against the edge of the orthotic shank, these solid ankle AFOs without anterior calf straps are usually cut low to only half the normal calf height. This design works well if children have very mild plantar flexion force and mainly need a gentle pressure reminder to prevent plantar flexion in swing phase or early stance phase. This design is contraindicated if there is strong plantar flexion spasticity or significant stance phase-back kneeing, as the orthosis does not provide adequate mechanical control of the ankle to control these deformities. Also, the half-height design can cause a high-pressure area in the posterior aspect of the calf, leading to a fracture of the subcutaneous fat and a permanent transverse line on the middle of the posterior calf (Table 5.1). Also, some children are irritated by their pant legs getting pinched between the orthotic and their skin. This half-height AFO brace design is very useful in middle childhood at a point when children almost do not need an orthosis, but still have a tendency to back-knee or to intermittently walk on their tiptoes.

Wrap-Around AFO Design

Other specific design features include the choice of the material for the orthotic. Most children's AFOs are custom molded and made of high-temperature, vacuum-formed thermoplastics. This material is available in several thicknesses, with a thickness chosen by the orthotist to meet the perceived demands based on the size of the individual child. Most commonly, this orthotic

Figure 5.16. The ground reaction concept can also be applied with the goal of increasing ankle plantar flexion while preventing crouching. This requires an orthosis that limits dorsiflexion and allows plantar flexion. The use of this rear-entry orthosis has all the requirements of the solid ankle ground reaction AFO, and in addition requires that there be no foot deformity (A). Because the rear entry does not allow any orthotic control of the hindfoot, varus or valgus foot deformities make this orthosis not useful. The most common reason to use this orthosis is following surgical reconstruction of severe crouch gait, in which the planovalgus was corrected and the goal is to gain improved plantar flexion strength with the eventual goal of the child becoming brace free (B).

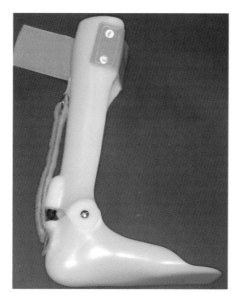

Figure 5.17. There are a group of children who are smaller, especially with some plano-valgus foot deformity, in whom some ankle motion is thought to be beneficial. One alternative is to use a standard articulated AFO and attach a posterior restraining strap to prevent hyperdorsiflexion. Although this seems like a good goal, unless the child is very light, there does not seem to be any cloth material that can be attached to the orthotic that does not rapidly stretch out.

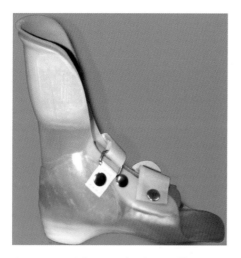

Figure 5.18. The use of a short calf segment with no anterior calf strap is an alternative to an articulated AFO. This design works well if the plantar flexion force is mild and the child just needs a little reminder to stay out of plantar flexion. If the child has strong plantar flexion, the calf segment will gradually erode a crease in the subcutaneous fat and can leave a permanent crease in the calf.

covers the posterior half of the calf and plantar aspect of the foot. The orthotic can be customized further with soft pad inserts (Figure 5.19), and it has some limited ability to be expanded by the orthotist by heating the material or being able to weld material on at the end of the toe plate or at the shank. Most of these orthotics can be made to fit for 12 to 18 months in growing children. Another design that has recently gained popularity is the use of a thinner thermoplastic plastic, which wraps circumferentially around the limb (Figure 5.20). The strength of the orthosis is gained from the circumferential wrap. This thin plastic tends to be more flexible and therefore deforms slightly when force is applied. Also, the circumferential wrap tends to apply a wider contact area to the skin, often distributing forces over a larger area of skin. The negative aspects of this thin plastic wrap-around technique is that the orthotic is difficult to apply to uncooperative children because caretakers have to use two hands to open the orthotic and to apply it to the foot. Also, it is difficult for some children to self-apply this orthotic for this same reason. Because the plastic is very thin and closely conforming, it cannot be modified for rapidly growing children and in some situations will only fit for 6 to 9 months. Because the plastic is also not very strong, it cannot be used in high-stress situations like ground reaction AFOs.

Anterior Ankle Strap

The design of the anterior strap is another variable feature, with some methods working better than others. All AFOs made for individuals with spasticity need an anterior ankle strap. For children with strong plantar flexion spasticity, the ankle strap should be fixed at the level of the axis of the anatomic ankle joint, then brought to the opposite side through a D-ring and wrapped back on a Velcro closure (Figure 5.21). This method proves to be the strongest direct force to control the plantar flexion. A figure-of-eight strapping may be used as well; however, this does not provide very strong control over the anterior ankle, although it does distribute the force over a larger area of skin. If children have varus deformity of the foot, the strap should be fastened on the inside of the lateral wall of the orthotic and brought through a medial D-ring. If the foot has a valgus deformity, the strap should be attached on the inside of the medial wall of the orthotic and a lateral D-ring should be used.

There are many variations of molds on the sole of the foot, none of which have any documented objective benefit (Figure 5.22). Some of these molds seem to make some subjective difference. Using an elevated toe plate seems to decrease the plantar flexion push in some children and helps in rollover in the forefoot in terminal stance in other children who are very functional ambulators. The only drawback of the elevated toe plate design is the difficulty of extending the orthotics to increase wear time because of growth. Also, the elevated toe plate cannot be moved once it is molded into place. Contouring for a medial longitudinal arch, a distal transverse arch, or a lateral peroneal arch is used by some orthotists. So long as these contours are not excessive, they may help to stabilize the foot in the orthotic, but they provide little other benefit that we can identify and no benefit that can be measured objectively.[6]

The distal extend of the orthotic has to be specified in the prescription. Almost all children with spastic deformities should have the orthotic extend to the tips of the toes to provide control of toe flexion. Almost all children with spasticity tend to have a toe flexor response when there is stimulation on the plantar aspect of the toes. The toes tend to always flex as if they were trying to hold or grab onto something. This is often the first area where children outgrow the orthotic and is the primary area that needs to be monitored for adequate AFO size. Children with hypotonia or predominantly

Table 5.1. Problem-based understanding of orthotics.

Anatomic problem	Proposed solution	Pros and cons of the solution
1. Flexed toes, spastic toe flexion	A. Biomechanical foot plate (BMFP) B. Standard foot plate to toe tips	Pro: BMFP - foot more stable and better rollover in third rocker Con: BMFP - not adjustable for growth, and need wider toe box in shoes
2. Forefoot abduction or adduction	A. Thin plastic wrap around B. Heavier plastic mold with distal side supports	Pro: good control, thin Con: difficult donning Pro: easy donning Con: bigger shoes needed

3. Hindfoot varus or valgus
  a. Mild deformity
    Causes mild discomfort walking
    No mechanical impact walking
  b. Moderate deformity
    Discomfort walking
    Impacting mechanical stability walking
  c. Severe deformity
    Significant discomfort
    Significant lever arm disease
	A. University of California Biomechanics Laboratory (UCBL) wraparound
	B. UCBL solid plastic
	A. Supramalleolar orthotic (SMO)–ankle-foot orthosis (AFO) wraparound
	B. SMO-AFO solid plastic
	A. Full-AFO wraparound
	B. Full-AFO solid plastic
		Wrap around: Pro: good control, thin
		           Con: difficult donning
		Solid plastic: Pro: easy donning
		           Con: bigger shoes needed
		Wrap around is more flexible and will allow collapse in the brace but may cause less skin pressure
		Solid plastic is stronger and will hold the deformity correction better because it is stronger and will not collapse, high skin pressure can occur, which may become painful

4. Ankle plantar flexion control
  a. Due to weak dorsiflexion
    Weak tibialis anterior
  b. Poor muscle control
    Poor control in both medial-lateral and dorsiflexion
  c. Spastic gastrocsoleus
    Causing toe walking
    i. Poor control severe spastic
    ii. Some control moderate spastic
	Full-height leaf spring AFO
	Half-height AFO
	Full-height solid AFO
	Full-height articulated AFO
	
	Full-height articulated AFO
	Half-height AFO
		Leaf spring: Too flexible, will break quickly
		        Too stiff will have no ankle motion
		Half height: Pro: small for cosmesis
		        Con: too much calf pressure can cause permanent skin mark
		Solid AFO: Better foot control, tighter fit, and smaller brace with solid ankle
		Articulated AFO: Dorsiflexion in 2nd and 3rd rocker with muscle stretching with articulated ankle joint

5. Ankle dorsiflexion control
  a. With need to control plantar flexion, i.e., crouch gait with equinus in swing phase
  b. Active dorsiflexion and weak Plantar flexion
    No foot deformity or torsional deformity
	A. Solid ground reaction AFO (GRAFO)
	B. Standard solid AFO with wide anterior calf strap
	Anterior articulated ground reaction—Art GRAFO
	
	Art GRAFO
		GRAFO: This can accommodate mild to moderate foot deformity but must have normal thigh-foot alignment in torsion. Child should weigh more than 30 kg and must have near full knee extension.
		AFO: Easy to don and works well for child less than 30 kg.
		This rear-entry brace requires a normally aligned foot in both varus/valgus and torsion as well as near full knee extension.

6. Too much knee flexion in stance phase	Ground reaction AFO based on ankle control as noted above	Must have passive knee extension and adequate hamstring length.
7. Knee hyperextension in stance phase (back-kneeing)	Articulated AFO set in 3°–5° of dorsiflexion for plantar flexion block	Passive dorsiflexion must be possible.

ataxia often need only a distal extend to the base of the metatarsals or the base of the toes. In these hypotonic or ataxic children, there can be a detriment to extending the orthotic because it makes rollover in late stance phase more difficult.

Foot Orthotics

Orthotics that do not control plantar flexion and dorsiflexion of the ankle are called foot orthotics. None of these orthotics has any impact on ankle plantar flexion or dorsiflexion.[6] The role of these orthotics is to control deformities of the foot, mainly planovalgus and equinovarus deformity. These orthotics are primarily used in children with hypotonia, or in middle childhood

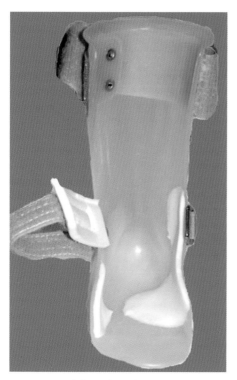

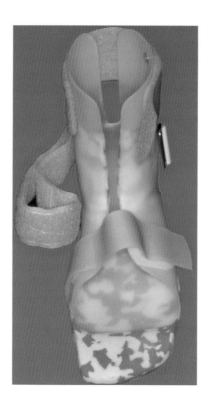

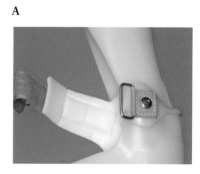

A

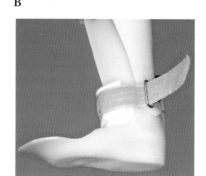

B

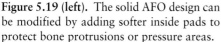

Figure 5.19 (left). The solid AFO design can be modified by adding softer inside pads to protect bone protrusions or pressure areas.

Figure 5.20 (middle). An orthotic design that uses a thinner, more flexible plastic with a circumferential wrap can be used for many of the different designs. Its major limitation is that the thin plastic is weaker and gains strength by the circumferential wrapping nature of the design. It does not work for high-stress environments, such as ground reaction AFOs, and can be difficult to put on and take off, especially for children just learning to dress themselves.

Figure 5.21 (right). AFOs made for children with spasticity need a good stable anterior ankle strap that is directed across the axis of the ankle joint. One of the best options is a padded anterior ankle strap that loops through a D-ring fixed on the side opposite the main deforming force (A). If the child has a planovalgus foot, the D-ring is lateral and if the foot is varus, the D-ring is medial; this allows using the D-ring to provide leverage to tighten the strap and allows the Velcro to hold better (B).

and adolescents with spastic foot deformities. The supramalleolar design extends above the ankle on the lateral side with the goal of controlling varus or valgus deformity (Figure 5.23). The foot orthotic can have all the same design features and options that were discussed in the section on AFOs. Usually, an anterior ankle strap is used; however, in some older children with good ankle plantar flexion control, this is not needed. Also, the heel is typically posted on the side opposite the deformity. This means a lateral squaring of the heel is added for varus deformity so the ground reaction force will tend to counteract the deformity. The opposite is done for valgus deformity, in which a post is added to the medial side of the heel. This supramalleolar foot orthotic design also works well with the wrap-around thin plastic design; however, the same problems occur as noted with the standard AFO. It is more difficult for children to don the orthotic, and heavy children tend to collapse the orthotic the same way a shoe deforms with long-term wear. There is no clear choice between the thin plastic wrap-around design and the solid plastic half-mold design. Input from the families and children should be considered as well as the preference of the orthotists. Most children who need control of planovalgus or varus, but have good plantar flexion and dorsiflexion control of the ankle, should be fitted with a supramalleolar orthotic (SMO).

There are a few children, mainly those with hypotonia and ataxia, who have moderate planovalgus that is easily controlled but who can be fitted with an inframalleolar orthotic (Figure 5.24). This orthotic contains a good heel mold, a medial longitudinal arch mold, a heel post, and typically stops at the metatarsal heads proximally. These orthotics can be set into shoes, have no anterior ankle straps, and are very easy to don because they do not need to be removed from the shoe. Applying this orthotic is no more difficult than putting on children's shoes. The use of this orthosis in spastic foot deformities is limited because of its limited ability to provide corrective force. Another name that is used for this inframalleolar orthotic in some locations is a "University of California Biomechanics Laboratory" (UCBL) orthotic.

A

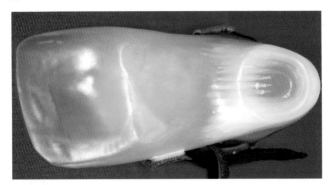

B

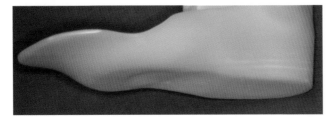

C

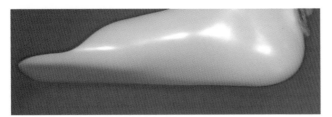

Figure 5.22. The degree of contouring and molding of the plantar surface of the orthotic inspires a lot of discussion and strong feelings; however, objective data currently do not suggest that it makes much difference. The tone-reducing features are varied; however, they tend to include some combination of transverse metatarsal arch, medial arch, peroneal arch, and transverse calcaneal arch (A,B). When comparing the relatively flat sole often used (C) with the highly contoured sole, there is minimal functional difference. The same benefit can also be obtained by adding pads to the inside of the orthotic using a soft plastic (D). These pressure areas can also be molded directly into the orthotic. Some also like to square off the heel on the outside to give better control of the orthotic in the shoe (E). This feature makes application of the shoes harder than leaving the heel rounded, and less contouring on the toe plate allows easier extension of the orthotic as the child grows. Another technique used is to flatten the sole externally with a rubber material; however, this increases the height of the orthotic and makes shoe fitting more difficult (F).

D

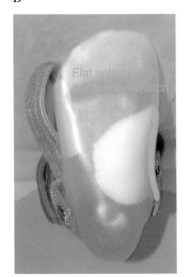

E

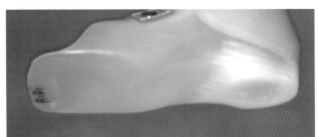

F

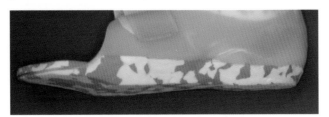

A   B

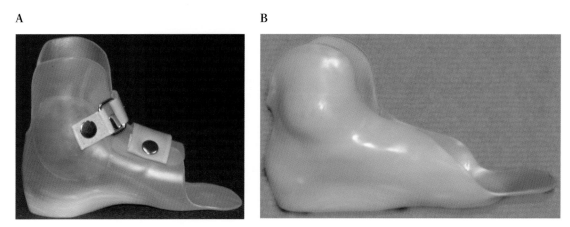

Figure 5.23. In-shoe foot orthotics are used primarily to control planovalgus or varus foot deformities. These can be constructed with the wrap-around design (A) or with the solid plastic, which sits in the shoe (B). Both of these are supramalleolar type and provide support for the foot.

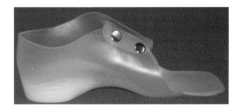

Figure 5.24. For feet that need only mild support, an in-shoe arch support can be constructed, again either with the wrap-around thin plastic, or the heavier, no-deforming material; these are commonly called inframalleolar orthotics or "University of California Biomechanics Laboratory" (USBL) orthotics.

The use of shoe inlay arch supports have little role in the management of foot deformities in children with CP. The force of the collapsing foot is so high that the shoe and inlay orthotic make no impact. Orthotics to control toe deformities are also of little use, although some children find the use of soft toe spacers helpful to keep the toes from overriding and getting compressed in shoes.

Seating

The single most important device for children with CP who are nonambulatory is the wheelchair. For these children, the wheelchair is an ambulatory orthotic, and as they get older and bigger, they become more and more dependent on the wheelchair for mobility. For example, a 12-month-old child can be carried when the family leaves the home; however, a typical-size 12-year-old will not be able to leave the house without a wheelchair. This evolution of importance of the wheelchair occurs slowly to parents. Initially, parents may be very resistant to the concept of a wheelchair because it forces them to acknowledge the degree of their child's disability, and having a wheelchair in public draws attention from surrounding people. This whole concept takes time for parents to come to terms with and to understand. It is important for physicians and physical therapists to have open discussions with parents of young children. By explaining this natural resistance, parents are given permission to feel hesitant about obtaining a wheelchair for their children. This discussion also allows parents to think realistically about their own fears and anxieties about being in public with a child who is clearly disabled. For children with good cognitive function, their response and that of their parents are often very different. Usually, at about 5 to 7 years of age, cognitively normal children will resist being in public in a device that looks like a baby buggy, and they would much rather be in a wheelchair, which they tend to see as a grown-up person's chair. Children's feelings have to be brought to parents' attention because the parents may still be in the phase of wanting the baby buggy stroller because it does not draw as much attention and looks less "disabled."

Considerations in Obtaining a Wheelchair

Many parents of children who have some ambulatory ability, but not sufficient functional ambulatory ability to function efficiently with community ambulation, resist obtaining a wheelchair because of their concern that their child will then want to give up walking. There is no basis for this fear any more than a normal 16-year-old will stop walking or riding a bicycle after getting a driver's license. Initially, there is great novelty in the wheelchair; however, wheelchairs have many limitations, especially in homes, and children who have any ambulatory ability soon discover this and will abandon the wheelchair for their walker, crutches, or whatever other device works for them. These same children will also discover that going long distances, such as shopping in a shopping mall, is much more comfortable in the wheelchair than with very slow, labored walking using a walker. Also, parents soon discover the advantage of speed and flexibility the wheelchair offers. Parents should be encouraged not to feel guilty about using the wheelchair for convenience of mobility instead of pushing their children in every circumstance to walk. There is a time when children need to be encouraged to do exercise ambulation and to push walking ability; however, comfort and convenience in day-to-day activities have to be given importance as well. After all, it is important for therapists and physicians to keep in mind that having children with disabilities is not the full-time focus of families. These children will need to fit into the families' other demands and activities, even when this means doing less walking than some therapists or physicians might feel is ideal. There is no evidence that the function of individuals as adults is significantly determined by how much they are pushed to walk as children. Clearly, however, work on maximizing children's walking ability should not be ignored, but rather has to be balanced with the other demands of these children and their families.

Seating Clinics and Their Role

For children with limited ambulatory ability, the need for a wheelchair often becomes obvious. However, for some families who primarily keep these children at home, this need for a wheelchair will occur much later than for active families who take them into the community for many activities. The educational system now requires education to start at age 3 years, and often the school system may say that children have to get a seating system to come to school. It is also important to inform families that the seating system in the wheelchair has other benefits besides mobility. Proper seating has demonstrated improved respiratory function,[14] improved speech ability,[15] improved oral motor function during eating and feeding,[16] and improved upper extremity function,[17, 18] as well as improved comfort in sitting for these children. As parents come to understand the importance of good seating for the child's global function and interaction, they invariably will want to pursue the most appropriate seating system. Obtaining a wheelchair for children with CP should be handled in the same way that prescriptions for foot orthotics or medications are handled. No physician would send a patient to a pharmacy with an order to get medicine for their CP; however, there are doctors who will send parents to a store "to buy a wheelchair" for children with CP. This is totally inappropriate. In the 1970s, the importance of seating was recognized for these children who are nonambulatory and seating clinics were widely established.[19] These seating clinics usually have input from a physician, physical or occupational therapist, rehabilitation engineer, and a wheelchair vendor. The seating clinic serves the function of assessing how the seating system will be used, the home situation of the family in which the wheelchair will be used, especially to make sure that the seating system and wheelchair will function in the home. Important in considering the seating system is the child's neurologic level of function and associated musculoskeletal deformities. The assessment should consider the timing of future planned medical treatments such as spine fusions or hip surgery that dramatically impact the seating system. The clinic also needs to make sure families have adequate and appropriate transportation to be able to transport the seating system. Finally, the seating clinic will make specific recommendations for the type of wheelchair based on all these multiple concerns. These seating clinics have been set up in almost all major pediatric hospitals and in some large special education schools. Because of the multidisciplinary nature of the clinics, these evaluations are expensive, but compared with the cost of a wheelchair, the evaluations are an excellent investment. The final result of an evaluation in a seating clinic is a specific prescription for a wheelchair and seating system, which the vendor is then responsible to obtain and build for the individual child. Under the cost-cutting efforts of American health care, especially by health maintenance organizations, there has been an increased resistance to pay for seating evaluations. Because of poor initial evaluations and prescriptions, children will not only receive a less-appropriate seating system, but due to the need for many adjustments, often the cost of the final product is significantly increased over what an initial appropriate system would have cost.

In the 1970s and 1980s, many children with CP who needed seating and mobility systems were in special schools, where school-based therapists experienced in seating were often available to assist in the seating and mobility design planning for these children. There has been a great push to move these children to regular neighborhood schools, and thus experienced therapists are seldom available. If the children see a therapist, it is seldom one who has any special knowledge or experience in seating. This trend further raises the importance of the assessments in hospital-based seating clinics where the experience is available even if there is some increased initial upfront cost for the evaluation. In general, the short-term goals of the healthcare payers, however, do not consider the total cost over the life of the wheelchair and the wheelchair's effectiveness.

Another trend that is occurring is direct advertising to families by wheelchair manufacturers. This advertising leads especially to adolescents demanding a specific brand or type of wheelchair. If the chair is not appropriate for an individual, the seating team and physician must be clear about this and refuse inappropriate requests. Allowing an inappropriate wheelchair is no more ethical than giving a medication prescription to a patient just because she wants it even though the physician believes it is inappropriate for her.

Prescribing a Wheelchair

To evaluate and prescribe a wheelchair and seating system, multiple factors have to be considered. Children's age is often an important deterrent, especially because most children's wheelchairs are expected to last 3 years. After the end of growth and during adulthood, wheelchairs are expected to last 5 years. These expectations come from United States federal guidelines, which the states do not have authority to change. The needs of children and families have to be considered over this 3-year period, and the system should have sufficient growth potential to accommodate this time frame. When a specific system is being designed, the base with the wheels needs to be considered first and then the seating system considered separately. However, there are some seating systems that will fit only on certain wheelbases, so there is sometimes a need to negotiate this balance. The discussion should start first with the children's level of function.[20] Children should be categorized into those with some ambulatory ability, those who do standing transfers, and those who require full dependent transfers. It is important to remember that the wheelchair needs of adolescents with spinal cord dysfunction-induced paraplegia are totally different from those of adolescents with CP. This difference is completely missed by many children, families, and even some vendors and therapists. Many of the wheelchairs that are heavily marketed directly to families are meant for the paraplegic spinal cord-injured population. These individuals have normal upper extremities, trunk balance, and trunk control. These patients do sliding transfers with no standing. Children and adolescents with CP almost never fit these parameters, because if they had normal or near-normal upper extremity control and normal trunk control, they would not use wheelchairs but walk with crutches or walkers.

Children with Some Ambulatory Ability

Childhood Needs

Children who are being considered for wheelchairs but ambulate in childhood usually ambulate with a walker; however, their ambulation is slow with high energy demands such that long-distance functional ambulation is limited. Most of these children have functional bilateral upper extremities and functional, although not completely normal, trunk and head control. Most are transported by parents in normal strollers until they are 5 to 7 years old. Typically, the first wheelchair is purchased when children are between 5 and 7 years of age and, because of functional upper extremities, this should be a wheelchair that children can push if their cognitive and behavioral function is such that they are responsible. If children are not responsible, then the chair design should be such that it can be locked or not pushed by them when they are sitting in the chair. This wheelchair should have swing-away or flip-up footrests so children can stand up out of the wheelchair. Adjustable armrests are required to allow children to help push themselves into a standing position (Figure 5.25).

Figure 5.25. A common first device many parents obtain is the stroller base wheelchair, which works well for rapid transport outside, such as shopping trips in early childhood (A). At middle childhood, if the child is safe and physically able to push a wheelchair, a standard large wheelchair should be obtained (B). If the child is unreliable but physically able to push herself, the wheelchair should be of the small wheel design to prevent the child from harming herself in the chair (C).

A

B

C

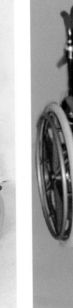

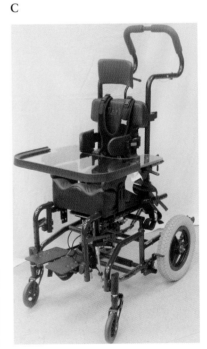

A

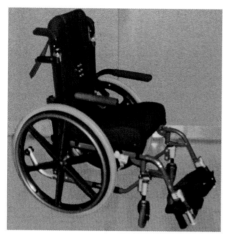

B

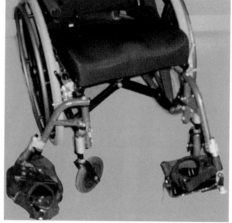

C

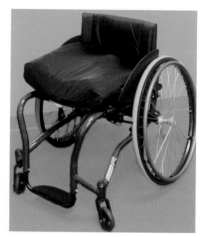

Figure 5.26. Adolescents who have some ability to ambulate, usually with the use of crutches, need a simple large wheelchair they can push (A). This chair should have swing-away footrests to make it easy for them to get out of the chair (B). Although these teenagers often are interested in a paraplegic-type design with a low back and fixed frame (C), this type of wheelchair is totally inappropriate for teenagers with CP who need a wheelchair. The teenagers with CP who need a wheelchair will always have some problems with trunk control and upper extremity control or they would be walking with crutches and would not need a wheelchair.

Typically, the seating system only needs a solid seat and solid back with a seat belt. Some children with marginal trunk control will need lateral chest support, and some may need a shoulder harness to assist with anterior trunk support. A headrest is needed only if the children are going to sit in the wheelchair during transportation in a van or on a school bus.

Adolescent Needs

A small group of children will be able to ambulate in the community until they start their adolescent growth, then their increased body weight will make walking so inefficient that it is no longer functional for long-distance community ambulation needs. Many of these adolescents will need a simple wheelchair, with a very simple solid seat and solid back, swing-away or flip-up footrests, and seat belt, in which they can propel themselves. This is also the group that will likely want the inappropriate paraplegic wheelchair (Figure 5.26). The wheelchairs should be lightweight and fold for flexibility so they can be used with different vehicles. Another group of adolescents, who are functional household ambulators but cannot functionally ambulate in the community, will also require wheelchairs. Many of these individuals have significant limitations in the function of the upper extremities. It is reasonable to consider power mobility for this group if their families have transportation available for a power wheelchair. If transportation is not available, a manual wheelchair is required. Wheelchairs for individuals who are functional household or minimal community ambulators should have crutch holders added if they use crutches. These holders allow children to carry the crutches on the wheelchair for circumstances when they need to get out of the wheelchair, such as for use of wheelchair-inaccessible bathrooms.

Children Who Are Exercise Ambulators and Transfer Standers

Childhood Needs

Children whose function is limited to exercise ambulation or standing transfers usually have their first mobility and seating system ordered at age 2 to 3 years when they enter the school system. Depending on these children's upper extremity function, a stroller base or a large wheelchair base may be ordered (see Figure 5.25). The stroller base may seat the children higher and make functional activities, such as feeding the children, easier for parents and caretakers. If children have the upper extremity functional ability, cognitive ability, and behavioral stability, the self-propelled wheelchair should be ordered. The footrests can be solid or swing-away, based on the perceived ability of these children to come to standing from the wheelchair. Power mobility should be considered when children enter middle childhood, usually at age 7 to 9 years, as the second or third wheelchair is required. The decision of power mobility is based on children's upper extremity function and general cognitive function.

The seating system for these children needs to include good chest lateral support and usually anterior trunk support. The need for a supported headrest in this group is variable, and has to be assessed on an individual basis. A lap tray should always be ordered for use when children are sitting in the chair and engaged in upper extremity activities. The lap tray is also an important assist for postural control to prevent forward slouching. Especially for young children, the work surface to do upper extremity activities is almost never at the right height unless a lap tray is routinely used. This lap tray allows children to have the ideal level and most functional work area for fine motor skills activity development (Figure 5.27). Usually, these trays are attached to adjustable armrests so they can be raised or lowered to the correct height for the individual child.

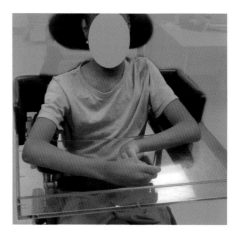

Figure 5.27. The lap tray is very important and should not be forgotten as part of the wheelchair. It is an important aspect of positioning to prevent the child from leaning forward. It is a work and feeding area for the child, and if the tray is made of clear material, it is easy to monitor the child's seating posture.

Adolescent Needs

There is a group of adolescents with fair upper extremity function who can propel themselves in the community. However, it is much more common for adolescents who require a wheelchair for all community ambulation to have so little upper extremity function that self-propelling a wheelchair is not possible. If these individuals are otherwise appropriate, a power mobility system is preferred. At this age, it is very important to have flip-up or swing-away footrests as the caretakers now depend much more on standing transfers. Usually, the seating system must continue to have a similar construction, as described earlier. Again, some of these adolescents can use crutches for short household ambulation, and in these cases, the wheelchair should be fitted with crutch holders.

Children Who Are Dependent in All Transfers

Childhood Needs

Children who are fully dependent for all their transfer needs usually require significant supportive seating by age 12 months, and the first special seating and mobility system is typically obtained between the ages of 12 and 24 months. Usually, this first chair is a tilt-in-space stroller base with solid footrests. The seating system requires full chest laterals, anterior trunk support, and a headrest to assist with head control. A lap tray should be included because the system is often used as a feeding and seating system, and is a play area for these children's play stimulations and fine motor skills development. By the second or third wheelchair, usually obtained around 5 or 6 years of age, a standard wheelchair base is ordered. A completely supported seating system is still required. Often, a tilt-in-space base is helpful to allow children to tilt back and rest. These children are seldom candidates for power mobility consideration until late childhood or early adolescence. Exceptions to this are children with athetosis who often have excellent cognitive function and demonstrate sufficient hand function. Occasionally, children with these indications may be considered for power mobility as young as 4 or 5 years of age.

Adolescent Needs

Most of these children who are fully dependent in transfers will continue to require a fully supported seating system with headrests and lap trays through adolescence. Usually, at age 10 to 12 years, a final evaluation can be made to assess the possibility of these adolescents using power mobility. This age is also when skeletal deformities are most common and problematic to deal with from a seating perspective. As children are getting heavier and having some increasing deformities, the possibility of skin breakdown also becomes most predominant. Skin breakdown is especially problematic over the prominent sacrum and ischial tuberosities for individuals who are very thin. Contoured or specially padded seating may be needed.

Specific Components of Seating and Mobility

Obtaining a seating and mobility system for children requires making decisions about many specific components of the system. Each of these systems, such as the wheelbase of the chair, comes with general design options. For example, the wheelbase may have small or large wheels, and each design tends to be available with some variations from different manufacturers. Purchasing a wheelchair is in many ways similar to purchasing a vehicle to drive on the highway where one has to choose between an automobile, a pickup truck, a station wagon, or a van. With each of these categories, each manufacturer has different small variations but one often chooses the manufacturer based on availability of service, prior experience, and options such as color and price. Most people intuitively know that they would not go to a car dealership and ask for a vehicle without first making some basic decisions about their needs for the specific vehicle. In the same way, it is inappropriate for parents to go to a wheelchair salesman and ask to buy a wheelchair for their child. The remainder of the discussion on the components of seating and mobility is directed at general design features; however, there will be no discussion on the options offered by specific manufacturers because styles and models change as rapidly as automobile styles and models. The general difference between cars and pickup trucks, however, remains constant from year to year, as do the different categories of wheelchairs.

Wheelchair Base

The wheelchair base is available in a number of options, such as a stroller base, large wheels for self-propelling, single-arm self-propelling, small wheels, and power mobility. Each of these options has specific advantages and disadvantages.

Stroller Base

This base tends to have the least medical appearance and can sometimes visually pass for a standard baby buggy or toddler stroller, which appeals to some families. The primary use of the stroller base is in young children, less than 3 years of age, as their first wheelchair. Often, this base is lightweight and easy to collapse and thus place into car trunks, which is another advantage. Large strollers can also be purchased that can handle even adult-sized individuals. Some families find these strollers very helpful as backups to the standard wheelchair, which is often very heavy and hard to transport if the primary transport vehicle is not available. These large strollers often have sling seats and small wheels, which means that they can be used only for short-distance transportation on flat pavement. These strollers work well for parents who want to use them for trips to the store or to the doctor's office, but cannot be the primary wheelchair because of poor seating support and because their use is limited to single-level flat surfaces. Most insurance companies and Medicaid payers will purchase only one wheelchair for a child, so if the company pays for a stroller, the company then will refuse to pay for the more appropriate wheelchair and seating system, which is also much more expensive. For this reason, it is better for the parents to purchase the stroller themselves if they are able and save the insurance benefit for the much more expensive system, which is what these children will be using most of the time. Because there are no strollers that can effectively be self-propelled, the stroller is seldom considered as the primary mobility system except in very young children, less than 3 years of age.

Standard Wheelchair Frame with Small Wheels

The standard wheelchair frame allows excellent flexibility in designing a seating system that meets children's needs. By using small wheels, usually 10 to 12 inches in diameter, the system still somewhat has an appearance of a stroller (see Figure 5.23C). For children with excellent arm function but cognitive and behavioral limitations that preclude self-propelling, this system prevents them from moving themselves. The major disadvantage of the small wheel is the increased resistance to rolling provided on uneven surfaces or soft ground. This resistance becomes a major concern when individuals with CP are very heavy, or when the family tries to use the chair on a surface other than completely flat pavement or a hard floor. The regular frame with small wheels is primarily indicated for early and middle childhood and for children who cannot or should not self-propel their wheelchair.

Standard Wheelchair Base with Large Wheels

A standard wheelchair frame with large wheels on the back and small wheels (casters) on the front is the most typical wheelchair used in middle childhood and adolescence. This wheelchair is the ideal setup for individuals who can propel the chair with both upper extremities. Also, it is the best setup for large patients or situations where families are often on uneven or soft surfaces. The larger the wheels, the easier the wheelchair is to roll over uneven and soft terrain. Also, it is easier to take the chair up and down stairs if the rear wheels are large. The major disadvantage of this chair setup from the parents' perspective is the chair's typical appearance of a wheelchair. For most children with CP, the front casters should also be large, meaning 4 to 5 inches in diameter (Figure 5.28). There is no role for the small 1- or 2-inch-diameter casters sold with paraplegic wheelchairs. The small casters are designed to rest the chair and to be in minimal contact with ground during

Figure 5.28. The front caster of the wheelchair is important to how easily the chair can be pushed in different environments. In general, the larger front casters (A) or the medium caster size (B) are the most functional for individuals with CP. The very small casters typical on wheelchairs for paraplegia have no role for children with CP (C). These small casters are designed mainly to rest on with the presumption that most propelling will be done with the front casters not even in contact with the floor.

A

B

C

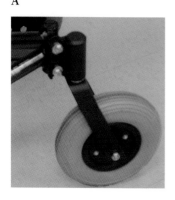
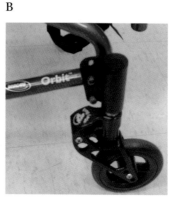
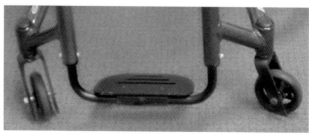

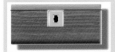 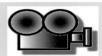

Case 5.1   Shannon

Shannon, a 15-year-old girl with spastic diplegia, was brought for the first time to the CP clinic with her mother's complaint that she is doing almost no walking except in her own home and using her wheelchair for all community mobility. Shannon had never been taught to use crutches, but as she entered puberty and had more difficulty walking, someone gave her a paraplegic type of sports wheelchair, which she liked. Now at age 15 years, she complained of increased difficulty walking and knee pain. Her primary outside activity was playing wheelchair basketball. The significant physical examination findings included knees that demonstrated increased flexion at foot contact, late knee flexion, ankle equinus, and severe internal rotation of the hip (Figure C5.1.1). Although Shannon was not in favor of surgery, her mother wanted her to have the procedures, which included femoral derotation, hamstring lengthening, rectus transfers, and gastrocnemius lengthening. During the postoperative period, she was not very motivated to work with the physical therapy program and kept complaining of pain in the hip and knees. She continued to insist she could not walk and was totally dependent on her wheelchair, in spite of an energy cost of walking and a walking speed that was mildly elevated but not in the severe range (Table C5.1.1). Shannon had an excellent technical outcome of the surgery but a complete functional outcome failure. This failure was probably because she was allowed to become wheelchair dependent in early adolescence by poor medical advice in which she was given a wheelchair instead of being taught how to use Lofstrand crutches. Her social activity revolved around wheelchair basketball, so if she started to walk, she would have to give this up. Her mother wanted her to walk, so the wheelchair use was another way to assert independence from her mother and her mother's goals. By not walking, she has become extremely deconditioned to the point where walking was uncomfortable unless she was willing to endure rigorous rehabilitation.

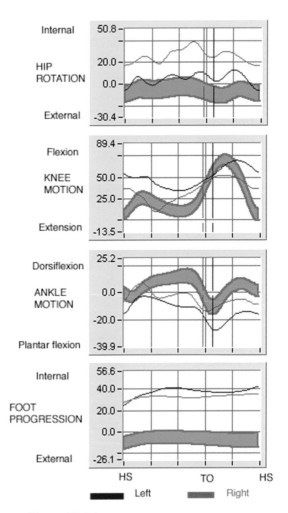

Figure C5.1.1

Table C5.1.1. Oxygen cost.

Parameter	Preoperative	Postoperative
Walking velocity (110–140 cm/s)	107	63
Oxygen cost (0.23 ml O$_2$/m/kg)	0.43	0.48
Heart rate (beats/min)	168	172
Respiratory rate (breaths/min)	47	57

mobility (see Figure 5.28). Few individuals with CP can handle a wheelchair with this dexterity or they would typically be walking and not using a wheelchair (Case 5.1). The standard wheelchair frame with large back wheels and large front casters is the ideal choice for most individuals from middle childhood to adulthood.

Standard Wheelchair with One-Arm Self-Propelling Feature

There are a few individuals with significant asymmetry in arm function such that they can propel a wheelchair with the use of only one arm. Depending on the level of cognition and motor function, individuals may be considered for either a manual self-propelling system or a power system. The standard manual self-propelling system has a double rim on the side of the functional limb, and by holding the rims together, the chair is propelled forward. Turns are made by differential turning of the rims. This system is very effective but requires a very functional and strong upper extremity with relatively good cognitive function. This chair design can be easily pushed from the back by attendants or caregivers and adds very little additional weight to the wheelchair. There are several other single-arm drive options available, using hand cranks or pumps for the single-arm drive mechanism. In many ways, these devices are easier for individuals to use and often provide better mechanical leverage; however, all these systems are very prone to breakdown, require the addition of a significant amount of extra weight to the wheelchair, and make it almost impossible for caregivers to push the wheelchair from the back. Parents almost universally come to hate these wheelchairs because of these problems. None of the currently available systems should be ordered for children with CP. The double-rim system is mechanically simple, does not get in the way of others pushing the chair, is relatively reliable, and therefore is the only reasonable choice for one-arm self-propelling.

Power Mobility

Power mobility is one of the most stimulating and freeing choices for the right children. This mobility allows children with CP, who often have not had the ability to move about under their own power, to suddenly be able to explore their environment. Developing personal freedom to move in space is a very freeing experience for these children. This mobility allows children to act like children. Although power mobility is a wonderful functional enhancement for appropriate children with CP, it is an option only for the minority of children with CP who are wheelchair dependent. The use of a power wheelchair comes with significant risks, problems, and dangers. Many children can manually learn to drive a car by the time they are 12 years old; however, our society does not allow driving on the road until children are 16 or 18 years of age because of the need for maturity in judgment and stability in behavior. Likewise, there are definite criteria that have to be present before children can be given a power wheelchair (Figure 5.29).

There are three major requirements that children have to meet before a power wheelchair should be prescribed. The first requirement is children need to have the motor ability to safely operate some switching mechanism to drive the wheelchair, have adequate eyesight, and be cognitively and behaviorally reliable to understand the dangers, such as road traffic and stairs. They must follow commands reliably, such as stopping if they are told to stop. Because power mobility is very expensive, it is never considered for short-term use during several months of postoperative rehabilitation, or for children who are expected to progress to functional ambulation over the next year or two. Children have to demonstrate that they can physically operate the power chair, which means a mechanism for switch interfacing must be found that works. There are many options for switch access, the most common being joystick use with the hand (see Figure 5.28B). Head switches, or a combination of leg and head switches, are also available and useful for children with CP. Mouth joysticks and oral sip-and-puff controls have very little use in children with CP because of uniformly poor oral motor control

A

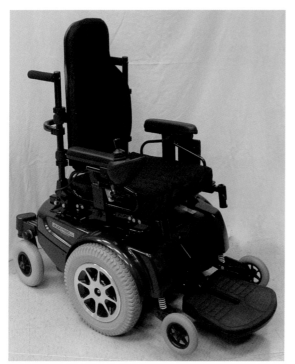

B

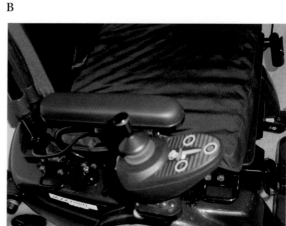

Figure 5.29. A power wheelchair provides a significant amount of independence for children with CP (A). The use of the chair, however, requires specific criteria of cognitive ability, behavioral stability, and motor function. Specifically, the child has to be able to control the chair through some controller mechanism, with a joystick being the most common arrangement (B).

in the CP population with this level of motor involvement. These systems are mainly for use in high-level spinal cord injuries. It is not mandatory that the exact control system be set up before a power mobility system is ordered; however, it is not appropriate to order a power wheelchair with the goal of seeing if a way can be found for children to access its controls. These systems are simply too expensive, and there is good expertise available to make these determinations in a general way before a power wheelchair is actually ordered for an individual child.

The second obligatory factor related to physical ability requires that children be able to see where they are going. Ordering a power wheelchair for a blind child makes as much sense as giving a driver's license to a blind person. For children with marginal eyesight, a training period should be performed so they can demonstrate that their sight is adequate to safely see where they are going.

The third and very important factor in deciding if children are candidates for power mobility is their cognitive understanding and behavioral stability. Children need to understand the concept of backing up when in a corner, to learn to avoid stairs and other drop-offs, and to understand the danger of specific areas, such as roadways. They must reliably follow directions such as stopping when told to stop. Children must have enough behavioral stability to not use the wheelchair as a weapon to injure caretakers or other children. Only when all these requirements are met is it reasonable to order a power mobility system for a child. For children with CP, this usually starts between 7 and 9 years of age. There are occasional children with athetosis who are ready as early as age 4 years. There has been discussion about fitting children as young as 2 or 3 years of age with power wheelchairs; however, this is almost never appropriate for children with CP. The considerations of early power mobility are most appropriate for children with severe arthrogryposis, osteogenesis imperfecta, or congenital limb deficiency. Almost all

A

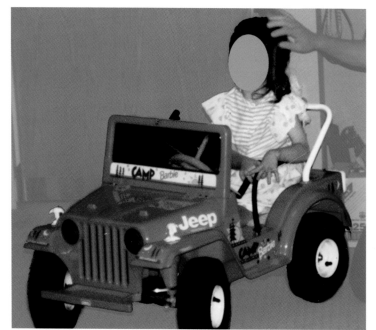

B

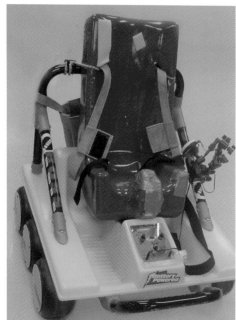

children with CP who could operate a power wheelchair this young will not need the wheelchair in a year or two as they will be walking. For young children who are marginal candidates for power mobility, other options include the purchase of battery-powered toy cars in which they can be seated with simple adaptations to see if they can drive the toys. Usually, using these toys has to be done under direct supervision of an adult for safety reasons. These toys are a cheap and simple way for children to gain early experience in operating a power mobility device (Figure 5.30). Many special schools have adapted toys in which children can also practice in a very limited, safe environment. On many occasions, ill-advised parents have obtained power wheelchairs for children as young as 3 years of age, but then found the chairs too heavy to push as transportation for the children because these power chairs cannot be pushed effectively as a manual chair. In the end, the power wheelchairs sit in the basement and parents have no seating or mobility system for their child. There is no excuse for this wasteful spending based on poor advice to parents if appropriate evaluations are performed and specific criteria are applied (Table 5.2).

Figure 5.30. Toy cars that are battery powered may be used for children who are young and marginal candidates for power mobility (A). These self-propelled toys tend to be safe and often need to be used with the supervision of an adult, which adds an extra layer of safety. Similar power bases are used in some schools to teach early mobility (B).

Table 5.2. Criteria to meet before ordering a child a power wheelchair.

1. Child cognitively understands concept of forward, backward, and turning side motions.
2. Child has demonstrated the ability to use a control switching interface, which will be used to operate the chair.
3. Visual acuity is sufficient to see surroundings where the chair will be operated.
4. Neurologic maturation is not expected to continue and allow functional independent ambulation.
5. Parents' home is accessible to power wheelchair.
6. Parents have a mechanism to transport power wheelchair.
7. If the parents are not able to transport the chair or have the chair in the home, a well-adjusted and fully adapted manual wheelchair is the first priority. Only when this is in place can a power chair be considered for school-only use, even if the child is otherwise an ideal power chair candidate.

There are some other hurdles that need to be overcome for children to effectively use a power chair. First, the family house has to be accessible, meaning no stairs are in the way of entering the house. Also, the doors need to be wide enough to accommodate the power wheelchair. If families are going to use the wheelchair when they are doing community mobility, there has to be a way to transport the chair, usually either a ramp or a wheelchair lift into a van. The school system likewise has to be accessible to children in power chairs, and wheelchair lift buses need to be available for transportation.

Choosing the Type of Power Base

After the full evaluation and the decision to move ahead with power mobility has been made, a choice has to be made about the specific type. In general, there are four options, including an add-on motor to a standard wheelchair frame, a permanent power mobility base for power mobility driving only, a deluxe power base with many other power option features, and a power scooter. The power add-on packs have the advantage of being a lightweight system that can be converted to a manual wheelchair when desired. In general, this is a system that works well if it is lightly used by individuals without heavy body weight. This add-on motor primarily brings the disadvantages of both systems together without the durability that many of the permanent power bases currently have developed. This system usually does not have enough power for heavy-duty use outside on uneven ground. This add-on power pack system is best suited for middle childhood when families are not quite prepared for power mobility. The permanent power mobility base is the best choice for most children with CP. In general, these systems are durable with good power for outdoor use. Again, a large wheel size improves the outdoor use and is an option that varies with different manufacturers. Some of these systems also have a center drive wheel, which provides for a tighter turning radius (see Figure 5.29). The deluxe power bases often offer a combination of seat elevation, power standing option, power leg rests, power recline, power tilt, and power floor sitting in addition to other features (Figure 5.31). There are only rare children for whom these options can be justified, and each child must be individually considered. Except for one manufacturer, these deluxe power bases have a poor history of durability with frequent breakdowns. These systems are expensive, typically costing over $20,000 compared with approximately $8,000 for a standard power

Figure 5.31. The deluxe power wheel base (A) allows power floor sitting (B), standing, seat raising, reclining, tilt-in-space, and foot elevation. These systems are expensive and often require a high level of maintenance.

A

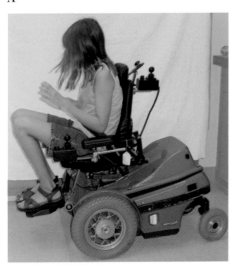

B

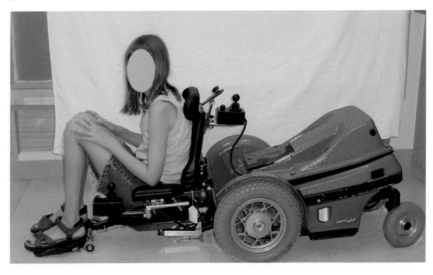

wheelchair and seating system. The fourth power option is the scooter commonly used in nursing homes by the elderly. The only role for the power scooter is in young adults or adolescents who go to large high schools or colleges and whose ambulation speed is so slow that they are not able to get to the locations needed in the allotted time. Typically these scooters do not have the option of adding adaptive seating and are generally limited to sidewalks or hard surface mobility.

Wheelchair Frames

Wheelchair frames are usually available in lightweight tubular steel, or even lighter designs in carbon fiber composite, titanium, or aluminum. There is an extra cost for these lightweight materials compared with the standard metal frame, but these lighter frames are easier to lift into car trunks and move up and down stairs. These frames are also available as fixed frames, tilt-in-space, or reclining. Most children with reasonable hip control should get a fixed frame that is strong and lightweight. The tilt-in-space frame is used for individuals with severe quadriplegic pattern involvement who need periods of time when they can be tilted back to rest. This feature adds a significant amount of weight to the chair and makes it almost impossible to collapse it and place into the trunk of a car (Figure 5.32). The reclining back is used only for specific rare deformities in children with CP, most commonly for significant fixed hip extension contractures.

Footrests

Some wheelchair frames, depending on the specific design, do not have the flexibility to add different types of footrests. Therefore, obtaining the correct footrest has to be coordinated with choosing the specific wheelchair frame. The options in footrests include swing-away, flip-up, elevating, spring-extendable, and different shoe attachments. The swing-away feature is often the easiest for children who are able to get out of the chair unaided because the release for the swing-away is the easiest to reach (Figure 5.33). The flip-up feature is the most durable and simple but requires reaching almost to the floor, a task few individuals with CP can do when sitting in a wheelchair. Either swing-away or flip-up or both are the required features of wheelchairs for individuals who come to a standing position from a sitting position in the wheelchair. This task of coming to a standing position requires that the

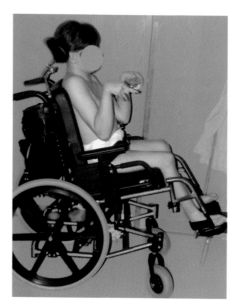

Figure 5.32. The tilt-in-space frame allows the child to lie back with loosening of the seating positioning. The tilt-in-space frame tilts both the seat and back at the same time compared with a reclining wheelchair, in which the back folds down but the seat stays in place.

Figure 5.33. It is very important to consider the needs of the child relative to their sitting knee angle. If the child has severe knee flexion contractures or hamstring contractures, the goal should be to obtain 90° foot hangers (A). However, if the child is large and the knees are relatively free, a better seating position may be obtained with 70° hangers, which are more common on larger wheelchairs because of the common interference with the front casters (B). The position of the foot plate on the hangers and the shoe tiedowns also have to be considered (C).

A

B

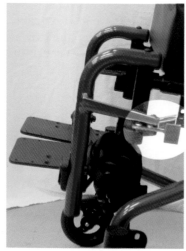

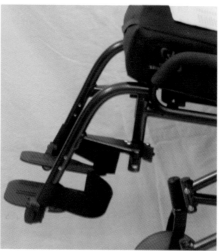

C

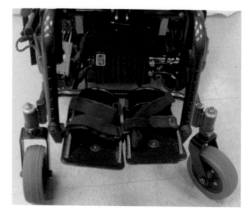

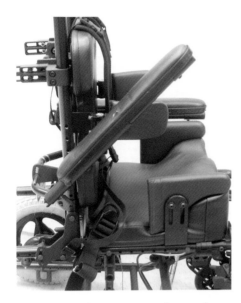

Figure 5.34. Armrests are almost always needed for children with CP because they almost universally need to use the arms to help with trunk balance. If the wheelchair is often pushed up to tables to work, study, or eat, the armrests should be flip-up in nature so they can be brought out of the way of getting under a table surface.

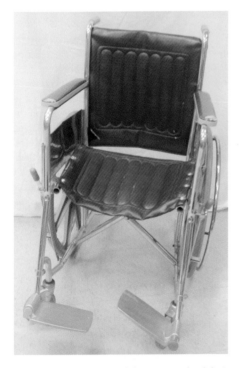

Figure 5.35. The typical drugstore wheelchair with a sling seat and sling back is always inappropriate for individuals with CP. If they need a wheelchair for long-term use, they will need more trunk support and better seating stability than this chair provides.

feet be placed in the midline under the seat for maximum ease. Elevating footrests allow the feet to be elevated, a feature that is needed only after injuries or surgery on the lower extremities for most children with CP. This feature adds weight and complexity and has a tendency to break down. Elevating footrests are rarely indicated as standard equipment on wheelchairs for children with CP. Vendors and wheelchair clinics should keep several pairs of elevating legrests available for rent during the brief postoperative period when these footrests are required. The spring-loaded, extendable feature allows footrests to lengthen when individuals push hard against the footrests. This feature has a place only rarely in adolescents who, secondary to behavior or spasticity, repeatedly push forcefully against the footrests, causing the solid tubes of the foot rests to fail frequently. If these individuals cannot voluntarily keep the feet on the footrests, which is common in many individuals with spasticity and athetosis, shoe holders and shoe tie-downs are required for the footrests (see Figure 5.33). This is an important safety feature that parents and caretakers have to be informed about, because one of the most common wheelchair-associated injuries is from feet getting struck as children are being pushed through doorways or other close quarters. We have seen multiple cases of fractured tibias, feet, and toes from feet being struck, especially on walls and door jambs, while individuals are driving power wheelchairs because they often cannot see their feet (Case 5.2).

Another aspect of footrests that has to be considered is the angle of the footrest hanger. Most hangers come in 70° and 90° options, although some frame designs can accommodate only one or the other (see Figure 5.33). Children with kyphotic posture and tight hamstrings have to be fitted with 90° hangers to inactivate the hamstring effect. Also, many individuals who have a tendency to do extensor posturing do better with full knee flexion to inactivate the extensor response, and they should also be placed in 90° footrest hangers. The advantage of the 70° hanger is that this position may be more comfortable for long-term sitting if there are no significant contractures. The 70° angle also allows a frame design with larger front casters, such that the casters do not hit the footrests. This design feature is often important for tall young adults, where it may be difficult to get enough length on the footrest hanger in the 90° position.

Armrests

The role of armrests on wheelchairs allows individuals to have a place to support the trunk with the upper extremities and provides a place from which to push up with the upper extremities when coming to stand. The armrests also provide a place to attach trays and power control switches. For individuals who are efficient in self-propelling with the upper extremity, armrests may be an obstacle and therefore are not needed. Because individuals with CP who use a wheelchair have problems with trunk balance and control, armrests are always needed (Figure 5.34). The armrests are an important aspect in getting proper positioning of the trunk balance and control; therefore, armrests should be adjustable, allowing them to be raised or lowered as needed.

Seating

The most important aspect for comfortable and maximum functional benefit of a mobility system for individuals with CP is proper seating. Almost all wheelchairs are sold with fabric-based sling seats and backs, which are inappropriate for all individuals with CP (Figure 5.35). Because of difficulty with trunk control, a solid seat and back are needed. In the 1970s, when the importance of seating was first recognized, two general approaches were

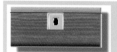

Case 5.2   Luke

Luke, a 16-year-old boy with a quadriplegia, was an excellent power wheelchair user. He did not like to keep his feet restrained in the shoe tie-downs. One day, as he was driving at his high school talking to another student, he caught his foot on the corner of the wall as he was turning into another corridor. He had severe immediate pain and heard an audible crack. He was brought to the hospital where a spiral fracture of the tibia was found (Figure C5.2.1).

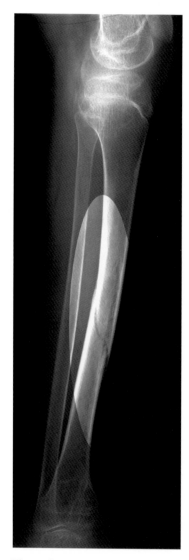

Figure C5.2.1

developed. One approach was to make form-fitting custom molds that would perfectly support individuals,[21] and the other approach was to develop modular pieces that can be assembled to provide the support needed.[22] The custom-molded form-fitting approach works well immediately after production with exactly the same clothing that children had on when molded. There are many problems with this concept. First, it is very expensive, and getting the correct mold is difficult if children are not exactly positioned correctly. It is difficult to make significant changes after the molds have been made, short of remolding the children. This system does not allow for different levels of clothing, such as clothing variation from winter to summer.

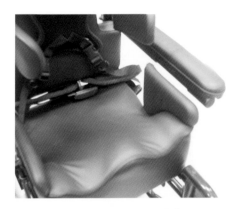

Figure 5.36. There are many different seats available as options for wheelchairs; however, most have some contouring, and many have anterior elevation to place more weight on the fleshy anterior thigh than the bony, more posterior iliac crests and sacral prominences.

In growing children, these molds only fit for 6 to 9 months and then have to be remade.[21] The main advantage is that custom molding can accommodate any type of deformity. For children and adolescents with CP, these custom-molded seating systems have far too many problems and are much too expensive to have any significant useful benefit. The other seating design approach is to use premanufactured off-the-shelf components to build a custom modular seating system. The advantage of this system is its ease of modification for the desired seating position, adjustment for growth, and level of clothing wear. Today, because of the excellent availability of commercial modular components, this is the system most suited to almost all individuals with CP. The major drawback of the modular system is a limitation in accommodating some difficult positional problems. The custom molding concept can be added to make specific custom-molded components on the rare occasions when this is needed. This is an option available in many seating clinics or from major vendors.

The Seat

The seat should have a solid base with a thin layer of soft, durable, deformable material. The main deformable materials are gel pads or closed-cell t-foams. The closed-cell t-foam is excellent to build up areas of the seat, and because it is available in different levels of stiffness, it can also be used to provide areas of pressure relief. The gel pads are excellent because they flow away from high-pressure areas. The simple flat or mildly contoured closed cell t-foam seat is best for young and light children who weigh less than 30 kg. As children get heavier and the skin pressure per square centimeter of skin surface increases, the gel pads often provide better pressure distribution. An advantage of the solid closed-cell t-foam is that it always stays in place on the seat; however, it is only comfortable for children when they are sitting in the correct position on the seat. The gel, on the other hand, tends to move and flow so the seat has to have some way to restrain the gel pad, usually by attaching it to the seat using Velcro. Over time, this gel tends to flow out of the area where it is intended to provide pressure relief; therefore, the gel pad needs to be readjusted frequently. Also, using modular contouring pads in the seat helps to keep children centered on the seat. For some individuals who have a tendency to slide to one side, a solid hip guide restraint may need to be added. This hip guide can also be extended anteriorly for children who have excessive hip abduction. In summary, the seat needs to have a solid base to provide children a stable base on which to stabilize their limited trunk control (Figure 5.36). The surface should have enough soft padding to keep the children comfortable and prevent skin breakdown. Very deformable, air-filled seats or thick, soft cushions are to be avoided because they add to trunk and pelvic instability.

Occasionally, children will develop problems with skin breakdown over the sacrum, coccyx, or ischial tuberosities. These children need a detailed pressure mapping of their seat to define the positions in which the breakdown is occurring and to also define the specific areas that need relief (Figure 5.37). After the relief has been constructed, repeat mapping should be performed to demonstrate that the pressure relief has occurred. During this pressure relief mapping, it is important to check the pressure that occurs during other positions in which children spend significant amounts of time, specifically in positions such as side lying or supine lying. Often, these pressure sores are not coming from sitting, but are coming instead from lying, and pressure mapping of only the sitting position will miss the source of the problem.

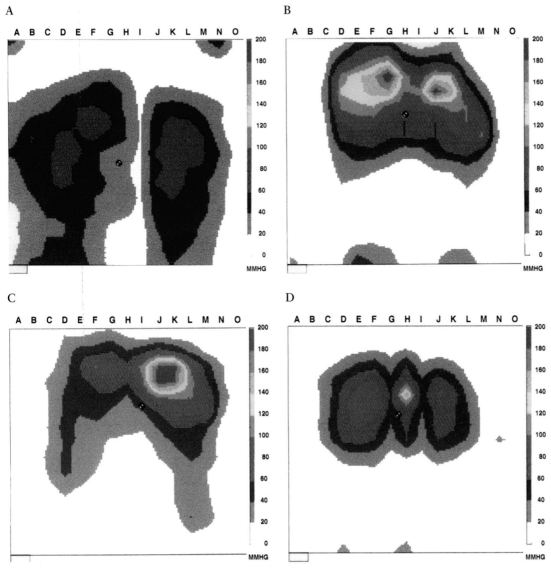

Abduction Wedges

A strong adductor response is present in some individuals with spasticity, which sometimes causes crossing of the legs while sitting. This adductor response may make it hard to keep children centered on the seat. A small modular wedge may be added directly on top of the seat in cases where this tendency for adduction is mild. For more severe cases of adduction, a larger wedge that children cannot cross over needs to be added. This larger wedge should be removable or flip down, especially if these individuals do standing transfers (Figure 5.38). Also, the wedge often makes lift transfers difficult, and even in this situation, the design of the wedge should allow for it to flip down or be removed. These wedges need to have padded and rounded edges to prevent injury to the children. The abduction wedge should not be used to keep children back in the wheelchair. This concept has to be explained to the caregivers and parents, who often want to use these wedges instead of seat belts to hold children from sliding out of the chair. If the abduction wedge is used to resist hip extension posture or to keep children from

Figure 5.37. When there are problems with seating pressure, mapping of the contact surface is required. A normal pressure contact pattern has relatively symmetric distribution between the right and left side with no areas of high pressure, and good anterior distribution on the thigh (A). Some typical abnormal patterns include high pressure over the ischial tuberosities (*red areas*) in a child with no pressure on the thighs (B). Children with pelvic obliquity will develop high pressure unilaterally over the ischium (C). Children with lumbar kyphosis have posterior pelvic tilt and high pressure over the coccyx and sacrum, leading to possible skin breakdown (D).

A

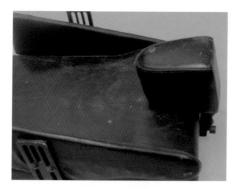

B

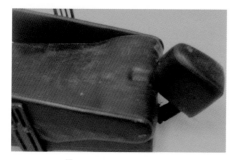

Figure 5.38. Midline hip adductor wedges may need to be added for children who have a tendency to adduct the hips while sitting (A). If the wedge needs to be large to keep the knees from crossing over, it should be mounted on a flip-down hinge to allow the child to be transferred in and out of the chair with greater ease and safety (B). These wedges are not to serve as blocks against the child sliding forward in the seat. This is the role of a seat belt.

sliding forward out of the wheelchair, it will cause significant pressure and excoriation in the perineum.

Seat Belts and Restraints

All individuals with CP must have a seat belt added to the wheelchair and used at all times. The seat belt is a basic safety measure for individuals with poor trunk control, which means that it has to be applied to all individuals with CP in a wheelchair, because if they did not have poor trunk control, they would be walking. The seat belts may be a simple design, like a standard car seat belt. The belt should be fixed so that it crosses the hip joint center laterally, pulling posteriorly and inferiorly at approximately a 45° angle. Special consideration should be given to children with strong extensor posturing responses by fitting them with double-pull seat belts. This type of belt can be closed with a standard closure in the front, and then there are two pull belts on each side, which allow it to be snugly pulled down. These belts often need frequent readjustment, as they tend to work loose and lose their ability for tightening. Children who have behavioral problems and are unreliable but have enough motor function to release the seat belt should be fitted with a release buckle that they cannot open. On rare occasions in difficult cases, the belt may be fitted so it closes in the back of the wheelchair as a way of avoiding children releasing themselves. The opposite consideration should be applied for individuals who can transfer themselves, in that the belt-release mechanism must be of a design that they can manipulate. Another option for individuals with strong hip extensor posturing is to use a solid bar instead of a seat belt. These bars, called subanterior superior iliac spine bars (SUBASIS), are attached to the seat (Figure 5.39). These padded bars apply pressure primarily downward toward the seat on the anterior thigh just distal to the hip crease. The restraining pressure from these bars has to be on the anterior thigh and not against the abdomen. When these bars are properly positioned they are very comfortable and provide excellent control of posture. The main problem with some children is that these bars are difficult to get into position, and if they are not correctly positioned the bar tends to be uncomfortable. There is also a tendency for these SUBASIS bars to not be adjusted correctly, especially by vendors with poor under-

Figure 5.39. For some children, the extensor posturing tends to be so severe that more rigid restraint is required. The subanterior superior iliac spine (SUBASIS) bar works well if it is properly adjusted. This bar presses down onto the anterior thigh and not against the abdomen. With the child relaxed, the pressure on the anterior thigh should allow insertion of a finger between the bar and thigh; however, there should be no contact with the abdomen.

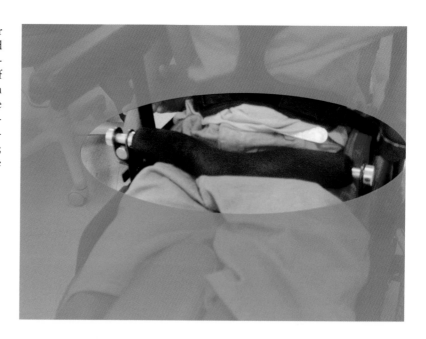

standing of their function. The correct adjustment of a SUBASIS bar is that it should be in contact with the anterior thigh when children are relaxed to the point where a finger can just be inserted between the bar and the anterior thigh. The SUBASIS bar should not be in contact with the abdomen when children are sitting relaxed.

Back

Most individuals with CP are best served by a simple flat solid back with a thin, soft padding layer as a covering. There are many modular pieces available, such as lumbar support pads and kyphosis contours, but these add no functional gain and may make individuals more uncomfortable. It is not important to have total contact against the back, so having some open area, especially in the lumbar region, causes no known problems or recognized discomfort. It is very important to keep the back high enough above the level of the shoulders, especially if there is a shoulder harness attached. There is no role for the very short, flexible backseat rests usually advertised with paraplegic-equipped wheelchairs (see Figure 5.26) because these greatly destabilize the already poor trunk control present in the CP population.

Lateral Trunk Support

Many, but not all, individuals with CP have significant instability in the trunk to the point where they require support to prevent from falling to the side. This lateral trunk support is usually fixed to a solid back. Some manufacturers sell lateral supports fixed by Velcro, and these uniformly fail over time, even in relatively small children. The lateral should be fixed solid to a solid back, but the attachment should be adjustable. For children who are very dependent on the lateral support and live in a climate of significant temperature changes, easy adjustment of the medial to lateral position of the trunk lateral is desirable. These are often called summer–winter chest lateral attachments. The disadvantage of the easy adjustment is that it requires caretakers to be attentive to the correct position of the lateral. The attachments of the lateral should also allow vertical adjustment to accommodate for growth and changing spinal deformity. The correct position of the chest lateral in most children is at the midchest level, and the width of the lateral should be approximately one third the height of the chest. The laterals should extend anteriorly far enough so that children do not move anteriorly out of the confines of the restraint. Usually, this position is approximately three fourths of the diameter of the chest wall. The lateral may be constructed with thin, soft pads or contours to the chest wall. For small children less than 30 kg, the flat laterals are simple and work well; however, as these children get heavier and apply more pressure, the contoured laterals may be more beneficial (Figure 5.40). A small group of children without scoliosis always lean to one side but have reasonable trunk and head control otherwise. These children may benefit from the use of only one chest lateral on the side they lean toward. This lateral seems to give them an area to lean against, which they may end up using primarily when they are tired.

Anterior Trunk Support

A tendency to drop into the kyphotic position when sitting is present in some individuals with poor trunk control. This tendency has to be controlled with an anterior trunk support that is available in designs of flexible fabric vests, flexible fabric straps, solid plastic straps, or solid anterior vest molds (Figure 5.41). There are no recognized functional benefits from any of these designs.[23] The function of the different designs seem to depend much more on the correct adjustment rather than the specific design. We have found that

Figure 5.40. Many children need lateral support on the chest to help them remain upright. These laterals need good stability, and it is helpful if they are articulated to swing away for transfers.

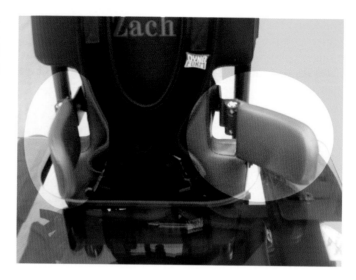

the fabric vest design works well for small children and the fabric strap design works better for older, heavier children. The most important aspect by far of the use of anterior supports is that the mechanical function of these systems is to pull the shoulders superiorly and posteriorly, which means the superior straps must be fixed above and behind the shoulders when the children are sitting upright. Many vendors, therapists, and parents see these straps as suspenders holding the wheelchair up against a child's bottom. We have, on many occasions, seen chairs fitting with the back 2 inches below the shoulders and then the vest harness tightened so it depresses the shoulder and encourages the children's spines to roll into kyphosis, exactly the opposite of the desired goal. Also, when children are growing fast, they should have the shoulder harness attachment adjusted every 6 to 9 months to maintain a proper fit. The inferior attachment of the anterior shoulder support needs to be fixed posteriorly to assist in creating a posterior vector at the

Figure 5.41. Many children need some chest restraint at some time to assist with upright sitting. There are a variety of different designs, although almost all fix over the shoulder and come in some anterior vest design (A). Distally, these vests should be fixed posterior and above the hip joint level. It is very important that the chair back be kept high superiorly so the shoulder straps do not depress the shoulders, because the goal is to pull the shoulders posteriorly, not for the straps to act as suspenders to hold the wheelchair onto the child (B).

A

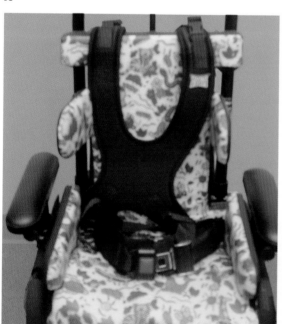

B

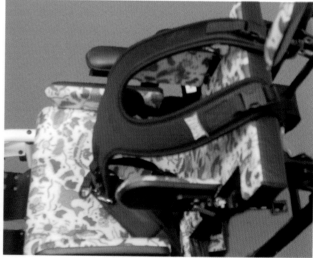

shoulder; however, this attachment point is not as crucial to good function as the proximal attachment. Another option that can occasionally be used in adolescence is a strap attached to the chest lateral crossing in front of the chest wall. These anterior chest straps only work if the force or tendency to fall into kyphosis is not very strong. These straps are especially useful in female adolescents with large breasts for whom the harness type of restraint is hard to use. The strap is placed immediately inferior to the breasts. Another very important aspect of controlling the anterior fall of the trunk is to have a lap tray and armrest placed in an elevated position. By using the upper extremity on the arm rest or lap tray, children are encouraged to sit upright. In some children, the tray may be placed as high as the nipple line, which will greatly encourage sitting upright.

Headrests

Headrests provide two functions, first, to provide support for individuals with poor head control, and second, as a safety feature when riding in a vehicle. For children who have good head control but sit in a wheelchair while riding in a van or school bus, the headrest may be needed only during vehicle transportation. This headrest can be a simple flat extension of the back that can flip down or be removed easily when not needed. For individuals who need head control, a more elaborate system may be needed. If the only head control needed is to prevent hyperextension, a simple flat or mildly contoured headrest only may be required. If a lateral support is needed, a lateral extension, usually coming inferiorly and anteriorly, is preferred. These anterior extensions should be inferior far enough to avoid causing irritation to the ears (Figure 5.42). Proper anterior trunk control is important for the best function of these head restraints. To restrain the severe anterior drop of the head, a mobile forehead strap may be used. This system only works if the forehead has a shape with some ledge or protrusion, which will allows the strap to stay in place. A forehead shape with a posterior slope does not allow this system to work. Another approach to preventing anterior drop of the head is to use cervical collars that place the support under the mandible. Some of these are attached to the chair posteriorly and some are free floating on the children. The free-floating collars, either anterior opening or posterior opening, are safer and are more comfortable for children. These free-floating collars are excellent options for use in vehicles for individuals with marginal head control.

Figure 5.42. A very important component is the headrest. There are many different systems available, and often trial and error is required to find the one that works best. Many headrest systems have modular posterior and lateral sections (A). The lateral sections can be adjusted separately, which is helpful in children with significant asymmetry (B). The lateral parts provide good side-bending control (C), whereas the posterior element prevents hyperextension.

A

B

C

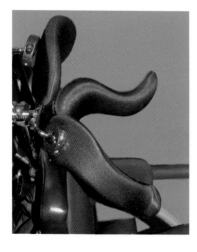
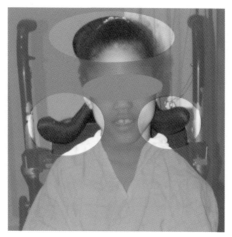
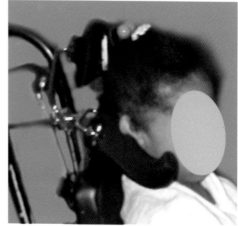

Back-to-Seat Position

The best position for the back-to-seat angle has been extensively debated, with many therapists feeling that individuals do better with the back inclined forward slightly, up to 20°, or the seat raised anteriorly 10° to 20°. All studies that have evaluated these different constructs have found that there is no consistent functional benefit from either position.[17, 24, 25] Seating position, especially the back angle, however, does affect upper extremity function.[17] In general, children with functional upper extremities should be seated straight upright to slightly inclined forward relative to the floor. Some individuals seem more comfortable with a seat that has anterior elevation of 5° to 10°, but these factors are variable and require individual evaluation. The seat-to-back angle should almost always be close to 90° or greater.

Tray

For individuals who spend most of their time in a wheelchair, the availability of a good stable lap tray is very important for sitting in an optimal upright posture and having a work surface that is always at the right height. Clear, plastic material is best because it is easy to clean, lightweight, and the child's position in the wheelchair can be monitored more easily while the tray is in place.

Attachments

It is very important for the seating clinic to do a good medical and social history to understand all the needs of caretakers and families for the use of the wheelchair. The wheelchair has to be adapted to carry all the things caretakers need when these children are taken out in the community because the caretakers cannot push a wheelchair and also carry a large bag of other things. This careful history should make sure that these things are not overlooked because commonly, when something is overlooked, it takes 6 to 12 months from the time the item is found to be missing until it is ordered, approved by the insurance company, and placed on the wheelchair. Crutch holders are often overlooked and should be added on the wheelchairs of all individuals who use crutches. Other overlooked items are augmentative communication attachment devices, feeding pump holders, and intravenous pump holders, which should be ordered when they are needed for the routine care of these children. Also, suction machines should have a place to be carried if they are required when these children leave the house. Wheelchair frames with respirator supports have to be special ordered if these children use a respirator. This kind of careful medical evaluation is part of the standard expected full seating evaluation.

Cosmetic Appearance

The major element in the choice of which automobile a person chooses to purchase is often based on cosmetic appearance. Likewise, in choosing a wheelchair, the cosmetic appearance is important to caretakers and to the individual wheelchair user. The ability to choose a color gives the user an important task in the process of selecting the system. Although function must not be compromised for the sake of cosmesis, it is important to consider the appearance of the system. Another area of cosmesis to consider is the durability of the seating system, especially the material the seating cover is made of and ease of cleaning. Because this seat is expected to last for approximately 3 years and will be used for long periods of time every day, high wear stress occurs. This high wear stress is an area where different manufacturers try to make improvements and experience gained by vendors, rehabilitation engineers, and families can help guide a selection. It is recommended to families to be very suspicious of new materials with which no one has experience, because these materials will occasionally be found to function poorly, and it is typical for manufacturers not to know this until the first group of patients has tried them.

Making the Specific Wheelchair Prescription

Most insurance companies require physicians to sign a prescription and to dictate a letter of medical necessity to document why each specific component of this wheelchair is needed. Physicians who sign these prescriptions should have examined the children and understand the appropriateness and need of each component. Although the full list is usually compiled by the seating team, it is still the physician's responsibility to know that the system meets the needs of the individuals for whom it is ordered. Physicians who sign prescriptions for patients they have not seen or order things that they cannot evaluate because of insufficient knowledge of the equipment, disease process, or specific patient can be held liable for fraud.

An example of the prescription and letter of medical necessity that we use for the evaluation team, which allows physicians to evaluate each component and the specific rationale for which it was ordered, is included. This worksheet is also very helpful when writing a letter of medical need (see algorithms).

Seating Problems Related to Skeletal Deformities

Individuals with CP often have specific deformities that are an added challenge to the design of the seating system. Good communication with the treating physician is required when designing seating systems for specific significant deformities. If this communication is overlooked, great efforts will occasionally be made to develop complex seating systems to accommodate, for example, a scoliosis deformity only to find that by the time the system has been ordered, the child no longer has scoliosis because it subsequently has been corrected. This situation has occurred on several occasions in our patients, and there is no excuse for this kind of poor communication from an adaptive seating clinic. Also, it is important for the seating team to understand that some deformities are so severe that seating is impossible. This judgment is rarely made by wheelchair vendors who have some profit motive to sell a wheelchair. Also, these vendors usually have great enthusiasm for challenges and little judgment about what is realistically feasible. The other major misunderstanding held by some members of a seating system team is that the goal of wheelchair seating is to allow children to sit comfortably for as long and with as much function as possible. The goal of wheelchair seating is never to therapeutically correct the deformity. Although there have been multiple attempts to use wheelchair seating for this purpose, these attempts have universally failed in the long term.[26]

Scoliosis

Scoliosis develops slowly in middle childhood, and during this time it is easy to maintain children in good seating posture. This sitting posture is maintained with three-point pressure by the use of offset chest laterals (Figure 5.43). Although this is a very simple and extremely functional concept, there is often great resistance by therapists and vendors due to misunderstanding the goal of the concept. First, it is important to understand that there is no great good that occurs by having chest laterals at the same height, except that it makes the wheelchair look more symmetric when it is not being

A   B

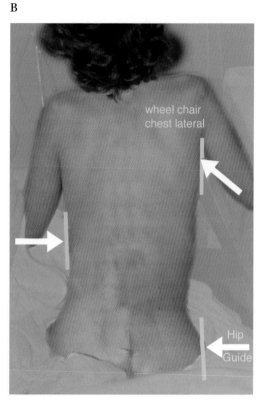

Figure 5.43. Scoliosis is a complex deformity, often including severe pelvic (A) and significant trunk rotation. In correcting this deformity, three-point pressure has to be constructed into the wheelchair with asymmetrically positioned chest laterals and a pelvic guide or block (B).

used. The side to which children fall, or the concave side of the scoliosis, needs to have the chest lateral raised until it is just below the axilla. Some therapists resist moving the chest lateral this high because of a concern that children will be hanging by the axilla. To some extent, hanging by the axilla does occur, but if the laterals are well padded, this does not cause children any harm. For children with scoliosis, even if the laterals are lowered, they will lean over until they hang on the lateral. The opposite side, or the convex side of the scoliosis, should have the chest lateral lowered to the inferior edge of the rib cage. The seat has to be constructed so children stay in the midline, and sometimes a third lateral point has to be added in the form of a lateral hip guide on the concave side of the scoliosis. As these lateral supports are brought to the midline, the scoliosis is corrected by three-point bending. The amount of correction that can be accomplished depends on the size of the curve and the stiffness of the scoliosis. At some point, the severity will increase so much that these children will no longer tolerate the pressure and this system has to be abandoned. Also, the scoliosis causes pelvic obliquity, which can lead to asymmetric seating pressure that needs to be monitored to avoid skin breakdown. For a short time as the scoliosis gets severe, children may be reclined back, and a foam-in-place back support can be used to accommodate the deformity. By this time, these children usually have very limited ability to be upright, and the next stage is to build a flat stretcher-type wheelchair in which deflatable Styrofoam bean bags are used for positioning. It is in this late stage of severe scoliosis when expensive futile attempts at seating often continue to be made after they are clearly no longer feasible (Case 5.3). Current surgical technology is such that severe scoliosis is rarely seen today, and only in children who have been medically neglected, or with parents who have chosen not to correct the scoliosis and plan to only provide comfort care with the expectation of short-term survival.

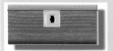

Case 5.3   Noah

Noah, an 18-year-old boy, was brought to the clinic after receiving no medical care for more than 10 years. He had not been in school. He recently had severe pneumonia, and the medical doctor referred him to the CP clinic for possible treatment. The main concern of his mother was that she needed a way to move him since she could no longer carry him, which was her main way of transporting him from room to room in the house. She never took him out of the house. The physical examination demonstrated that Noah had severe malnutrition and a severe fixed scoliosis measuring approximately 180°, although the combined physical distortion and low bone density made it impossible to measure the curve (Figure C5.3.1). There were fixed hip and knee flexion contractures of 90° each (Figure C5.3.2). Because his mother wanted no treatment except a way to move him in the house, a

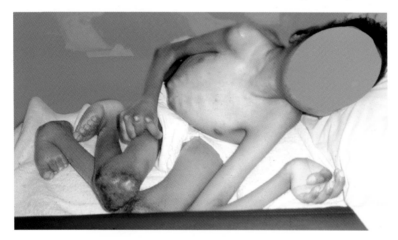

Figure C5.3.1

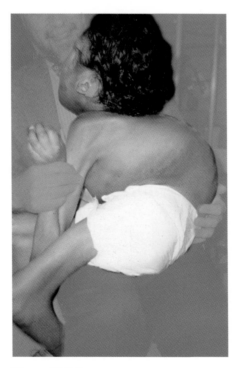

Figure C5.3.2

rolling stretcher that would go though her home doors was built on a wheelchair base, and she was given a deflatable bean bag positioning pillow to help position him (Figure C5.3.3). Noah presented in end-stage deformity in which very little else could be offered, even if his mother desired a more aggressive approach. With his re-

cent severe pneumonia, severe malnutrition, and severe end-stage scoliosis, we anticipated a very limited life expectancy, and he died 9 months later. The only seating option for such a child is some form of reclined stretcher with significant padding because seating is no longer possible (Figure C5.3.4).

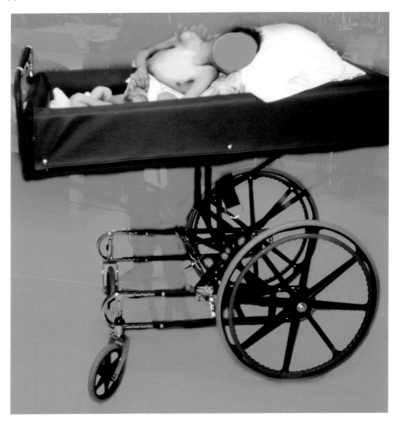

Figure C5.3.3

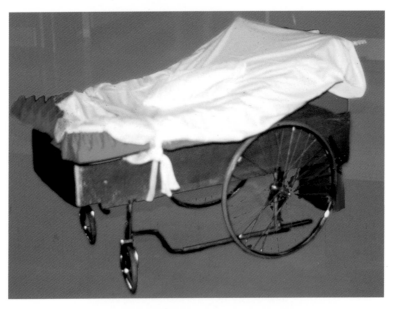

Figure C5.3.4

Kyphosis

Kyphosis in young children is relatively easy to correct because it is very flexible and easy to control with anterior trunk supports, an elevated lap tray, and 90° foot hangers. Hamstring contractures are often overlooked as a cause of kyphotic seating (Figure 5.44). These hamstrings can be inactivated by keeping the knees flexed to 90° to 100° by the use of a 90° footrest hanger and by keeping the footrests posterior. Also, it is important to keep the lap tray high enough so that the upper extremities help children to push themselves into an upright sitting position. It is reasonable to position the lap tray almost to the nipple line to keep children in a more upright position. As children get older, heavier, and the spine often becomes more stiff, this positioning correction of the kyphosis becomes more difficult. After the initial seating adaptations no longer work, serious consideration of surgical correction has to be entertained. Another seating alternative is to recline the seat back posteriorly and allow the hip to extend so children can get their heads into an upright position to look forward. This accommodation of the kyphosis, however, often feeds further into the kyphosis, and these children seem to draw forward more. Another problem with kyphosis is that children's heads drop forward into their laps. This dropping forward of the head seems to be an especially difficult problem in blind children, who have very little incentive to raise their heads and look forward.

Lordosis

Mild to moderate lordosis does not need to have any seating adaptations; however, for severe lordosis, seating is very difficult and there are few seating adaptations that are effective. Anterior elevation of the seat 20° to 30° to tilt the pelvis posteriorly may provide some short-term relief. Also, allowing the buttocks to extend posteriorly of the backrest so that children are sitting upright even with the severe lordosis makes children more comfortable and in a more functional seating position.

Hip Contractures, Dislocations, and Asymmetries

For mild cases of windblown deformity, the use of hip guides and abduction wedges can be used to obtain good positioning. Anterior knee blocks may be added, but these are usually not comfortable for the child (Figure 5.45). Severe windblown hip deformities and pelvic obliquities are very difficult to seat. For the severe deformities, surgical correction should be considered.

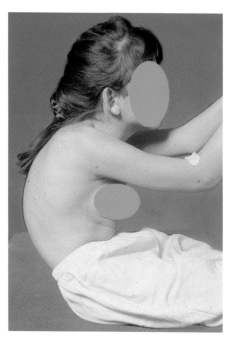

Figure 5.44. Kyphosis that occurs only during sitting and is flexible and not present while lying is often primarily caused by hamstring contracture or severe hamstring spasticity. In both, there is gentle compensatory spinal kyphosis, starting with a posteriorly tilted pelvis.

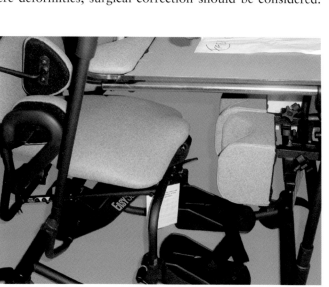

Figure 5.45. Anterior knee blocks may be used to control pelvic rotation that often occurs with windblown hip deformities. It is very difficult to get these blocks adjusted correctly so that they are comfortable for the child to use for a long period of time.

However, if surgical correction is not performed, the wheelchair needs to be significantly wider than would be needed based only on pelvic width. Typically, for these fixed deformities, 4 or more inches of additional width should be allowed to accommodate the hip deformity. These children will be seated eccentrically in the wheelchair at the side opposite the abducted hip. The abducted thigh and the adducted thigh will then extend over the midline to the opposite side of the seat. Often, attempts are made in seating clinics to keep both knees in the midline, with the result being that children's trunks spin so the adducted side of the trunk moves posteriorly, the abducted side moves anteriorly, and they end up sitting sideways in the wheelchair. Functionally, it is better to have the legs off center and the trunk centered; however, in practice a little bit of both often has to be accepted, especially when the deformities are severe. For severe pelvic obliquity, especially in heavy children, the seat may need to be built up on the side on which the pelvis is elevated.

Hamstring and Knee Flexion Contractures

Severe knee flexion contractures are usually addressed quite easily with the use of 90° footrest hangers to accommodate the knee deformities. In older and taller individuals, this may be more difficult and may require raising the seating system to allow the use of 90° footrest hangers.

Severe Foot Deformities

Severe foot deformities in adolescence can cause pressure and skin breakdown over bony prominences. Typically, these deformities are either severe varus or severe valgus foot deformities. The use of soft moccasin shoes and suspending the feet should be the primary treatment. The feet can be suspended by building an enclosed suspension-type footrest that looks like a padded open box, which prevents the lower extremities from swinging freely and swinging off to the side but does not put any pressure on the soles of the feet.

Seating During Transportation

Safe seating of individuals with disabilities has only attracted attention since the 1980s.[27] As states developed mandatory seat restraint laws for children, increased attention was directed to individuals with disabilities as well.[28] Younger and smaller children under 20 kg are most commonly transported in car seats with special seating if needed. Most young children, up to age 2 years, can be transported in standard children's car seats; then when they are too large and no longer fit, adaptive seats are required. Generally, these seats are of a similar design to regular infant car seats but are much larger (Figure 5.46). There are several companies that advertise that the standard wheelchair seat can be removed, placed on the automobile seat, and used for seating during vehicular mobility. From a practical perspective of the caretakers, this option does not work because these seats cannot be placed into the car with these children in the seats. These seating systems tend to be large and difficult to handle in and of themselves. Use of this system means that children have to be taken out of the wheelchair, the wheelchair has to be disassembled, and the seat has to be secured to the car seat, then the children have to be placed into the car seat again. The problem is that there is no place to put the children while the wheelchair is being disassembled except to lay them on the ground. Because of these difficulties, a separate car seat is required when children need this level of seating support for safe travel. For children over 20 kg in weight who have adequate trunk and head control, seating in a regular car seat is fine. The other option is to transport these children in wheelchairs; however, this requires a specially adapted van.

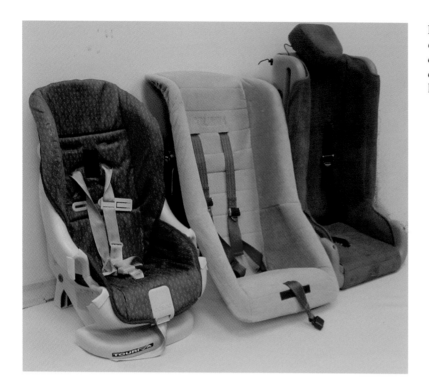

Figure 5.46. The car seats for children with disabilities are very similar to those sold for children without disabilities, except the special needs car seats are designed for much larger children.

Special Wheelchair Vans and Lifts

As children become adult sized, especially if they are fully dependent for lift transfers, routine transportation in an automobile becomes very difficult. It is easier to use a van that is equipped with a wheelchair lift or ramp. The wheelchair lift is the best solution but also is the most expensive, and this lift is not considered a medical device by medical insurance companies in the United States. Therefore, it is often difficult for families to afford to purchase a van and have a wheelchair lift installed. Also, when individuals are transported sitting in a wheelchair, approved tie-down systems and wheelchair frames that are approved for tie-down have to be used. These approved systems currently include most standard wheelchairs except for many strollers, which are typically not approved for tie-down or transportation of individuals in a vehicle.

Special Seating and Positioning

There are many different chairs manufactured to provide special seating for children with disabilities. Although there may be some functional advantage to using seats with barrel shapes in which children straddle the seat,[29] these special seats have relatively limited use. These special barrel or saddle seats are probably most beneficial if used in a school or therapy environment, where they can be shared by many children. Another problem that many parents have with all the different special seats is the limited space in the home. Before long, parents begin to feel that their house looks like a storeroom filled with medical equipment. A correctly adapted wheelchair can fill all these children's seating needs, although having other places where they can sit in the home has aesthetic value and may provide them with different levels of stimulation. The amount of additional seating should be determined by the needs of the individual child and the living environment of the family.

A   B

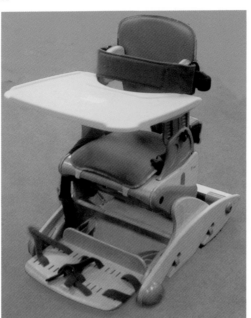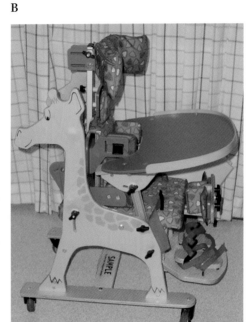

Figure 5.47. This chair is an example of a home feeding chair or a home adaptive seating chair, which provides the child an additional place to sit (A). Many of these chairs have a wooden frame and are relatively inexpensive compared with a wheelchair (B). These chairs can serve as an additional positioning device, but can never take the place of a wheelchair.

Feeding Seats

Appropriate wheelchairs should have children positioned so they can be fed easily. Some parents prefer to have a separate feeding chair because of the ease of cleaning, so the child can be at a better height for feeding, and be at the family table in a way that better incorporates them into the family. These are reasonable needs of caretakers to improve the care of children and are reasonable indications to order a feeding chair. Most feeding chairs are also relatively inexpensive (Figure 5.47).

Play Chairs

There are definite developmental benefits of allowing children to be in many different positions, such as spending time on the floor, sitting at a desk, and sitting in the wheelchair. Floor sitters and corner seats give some children this ability and are reasonable if they fit into the families' living space. This is the same for saddle seats, knee chairs, and barrel seats; however, it is inappropriate for families to get one of every kind of available chair. One or two of these special seats are reasonable. The appropriateness of these devices should be most determined by how these children function while sitting in these positions (Figure 5.48); these devices should be experienced by children in a school or therapy environment before they are ordered for the home. It is inappropriate to order these chairs just because parents saw a nice picture in a catalog. Equipment should not be ordered out of a catalog sight unseen unless a company will guarantee that they will take the devices back with a full refund within a certain time period if they do not meet these children's needs.

Toilet Seating

Children with CP who are cognitively able to understand the concept should be toilet trained by middle childhood. Toilet training children with spasticity and poor trunk control requires an adaptive seat with good trunk support and good footrests so they are comfortable sitting and not afraid of falling. Many different types of toileting seats are available. When children are ap-

A

B

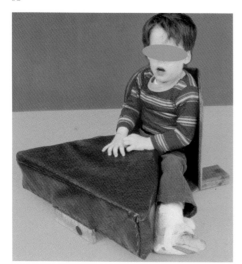

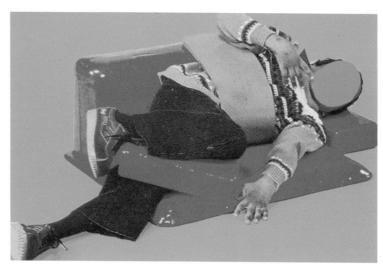

Figure 5.48. Other home positioning devices may include floor sitters (A) or side liers (B). The indication for these different positioning devices requires consideration of the benefit to an individual child and the available home space to use the device.

proximately 4 years of age, an appropriate toilet seat should be obtained for families based on a trial-and-error evaluation of the individual child's comfort on the toilet seat. These toilet seats can be tried either in school environments if they are available, or through an occupational therapy evaluation in a pediatric hospital (Figure 5.49). As children reach adolescent size, most can use a standard toilet with some assistance. The availability of handrails in a bathroom is very helpful for many individuals.

Bath Chairs

Children who are not able to sit independently by 3 years of age should be measured for a bath chair. The simplest bath chair that works well for young children is an open-mesh sling seat that can be set into the bathtub (Figure 5.50). When children get too large to lift out of the bathtub, a shower chair can be used. Bath chairs, which are powered by the pressure of tap water, are available. These bath chairs allow children to sit in a sling seat in the water in the bathtub, but then can be raised to chair height to assist caretakers in lifting the children out of the tub. Another option for heavier children is to use a mesh-covered stretcher that sets above the bathtub and the caretakers can use a shower nozzle for bathing. This option works well for larger adolescents who are unable to assist with sitting. For individuals who are able to sit independently but are not able to stand independently, the use of a shower stall with a bench seat is the best alternative.

Desks

The use of adaptive desks in school is often a difficult issue. For children with good seating ability, which means most ambulatory children, sitting at a regular desk at school is expected. Sometimes the height of the desk may need to be adjusted. Children who require full trunk support should be seated in their wheelchair and not placed in a desk, which universally provides poor trunk support. Children who fall in between need individual evaluations. Children who are able to sit at regular desks often feel more included with their peers in the classroom. However, for children who are unable to support themselves and do not have good trunk stability, there is often decreased functional ability for fine motor skills, such as writing. For children who are between definitely needing the trunk support and definitely being able to sit

A

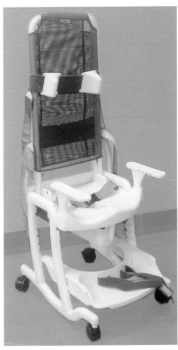

B

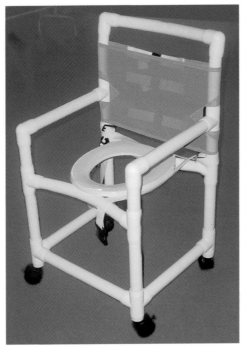

C

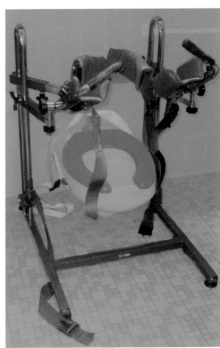

Figure 5.49. There are many variation of adaptive toilets seats available; however, toilet training is difficult if the child does not have a comfortable seating chair. Some devices are stand-alone potty chair designs with armrests and foot supports (A), while others have a more typical chair design but roll over a normal toilet (B). Good trunk stability imparted by armrests is important and, for some children, is all that is required (C).

at a desk, there is some advantage of them doing both. In this situation, children will spend some time sitting at the desk to stimulate balance and trunk control mechanisms, and then will spend time sitting in the wheelchair working on fine motor skills.

Floor Positioning Devices

Individuals with severe quadriplegic pattern involvement with no head or trunk control need some position changes throughout the day. These position changes should include getting children out of the wheelchair into different lying positions, such as side lying and prone positioning (see Figure 5.48). These individuals often need pillows or supports for side lying and prone lying. Wedges are often helpful to position these children into the prone position, which allows them to still have interaction with others in the room. These lying supports are most beneficial in school environments; however, some parents find them helpful in the home environment as well. For individuals with severe deformity, especially those with severe scoliosis, deflatable Styrofoam bean bags are the ideal positioning device. These bags can be reconfigured every time children are placed in different positions, and when they are deflated, they are very stable.

Standers

Children who are not able to ambulate with a device still benefit from being in a position other than sitting and lying. An upright standing posture will provide stimulation to the bones in the lower extremities, encourage children to work on head and trunk control, improve respiratory function by aerating different parts of the lungs, and stimulate gastric motility. In addition, children would be placed in a position to experience the world from the perspective of standing upright instead of sitting or lying. There is no research that specifically and objectively quantifies each of these benefits or defines how much standing is required to gain these benefits. The exact position and amount of weight bearing and time of weight bearing is an especially problematic concern for children with severe osteoporosis and osteopenia who have an increased risk of fracture. The major cause of the decreased bone stock results from the bones getting no weight stimulation; however, how much stimulation is required and at what level has not been documented. Like most biological systems, a little stimulation presumably is better than none, but there probably is a therapeutic dose that needs to be reached to make a measurable impact. We recommend that the minimal goal is to get children to stand with as much weight bearing as possible for a minimum of 1 hour per day. For children who can tolerate standing, moving to 2 hours per day is desirable. The standing program should be initiated between 24 and 30 months of age. Some children do not like standing and parents need to encourage standing in connection with activities that they enjoy. For example, children may be allowed to watch a favorite video, television, or listen to specific music only while in the stander. As children get heavier and near adult size, placing them in standers may become too difficult for families. Continuing standing in the school environment is encouraged so long as standers that fit these individuals are available and the caregivers can get them into the stander (Figure 5.51). The specific stander that is most appropriate for a specific child depends on the child's level of function. Children who walk with walkers do not need to spend time standing as well unless the amount of walking is extremely limited to minimal therapy walking.

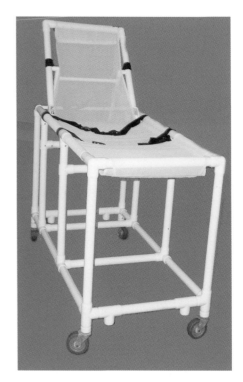

Figure 5.50. Bath chairs or bathing frames can be constructed from PVC pipe or purchased from vendors. There are many types available.

Prone Standers

Standers in which children lean forward and are supported on the anterior aspect of the body are called prone standers. This is the preferred stander for children who have acquired head control sufficient to hold their heads up while engaged in activities. Children should be inclined forward 10° to 20° with a tray on the front of the stander. This is the ideal position for children to use their hands for fine motor skills, such as writing and coloring. The main posterior restraint for the prone stander is a belt at the level of the buttocks and chest to hold children in place. These standers are also available with wheels, with the goal being that children can self-propel the stander around the room while being in an upright position. Self-propelling seldom works with individuals with CP who need to use a prone stander because few have sufficient arm coordination or strength to push themselves. These wheeled walkers are convenient for some caregivers who may use the wheels to push the stander with the children in place to different areas in the home, but they provide little direct functional benefit to the children.

Supine Standers

Standers in which children lean back for support are called supine standers. This design is used for children who do not have head control. In the supine stander, children's heads can be supported posteriorly as well. The principal anterior restraints are at the level of the knees, hips, and chest. As much upright positioning as can be tolerated is encouraged, usually with the stander reclined 10° to 20°. In this reclined position, it is not possible for children to do any significant fine motor functioning with the upper extremities; however, most children who require a supine stander do not have any upper extremity function (see Figure 5.51).

Parapodiums

Standing boxes or standers in which children are in an upright position and supported only at the pelvis, abdomen, or lower chest are called parapodiums.

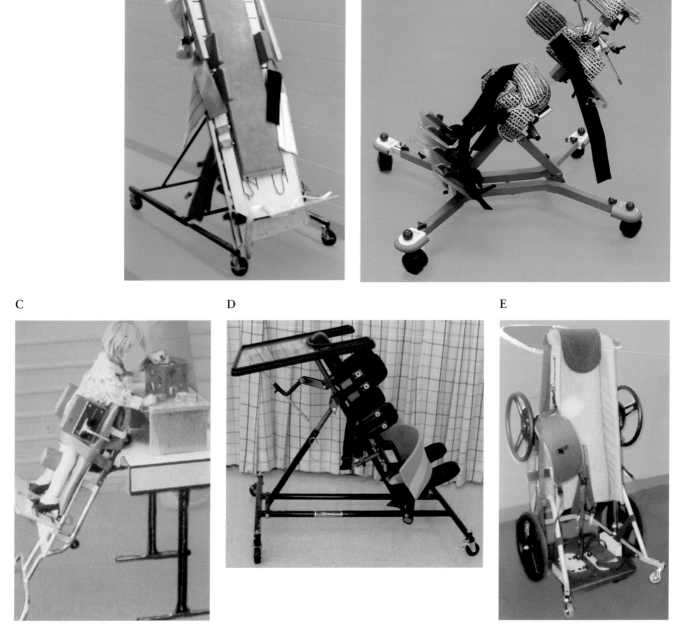

Figure 5.51. Standers come in either supine or prone patient position. The standers may also be called "tilt boards" because many started as flat stretchers that could be tilted up at one end providing a basic supine stander (A). Newer designs hold the child with a few well-placed pads; however, the effect is still the same supine standing (B). For children with hand function and head control, the prone stander is preferred because it places the child in a more functional position. This can be a simple frame that leans on a regular table (C), or a more sophisticated free-standing device with its own attached tray (D). Standing boxes, or mobile standing boxes that the child can push, have been developed and work well for children with spinal cord dysfunction who have normal arm function; however, these devices have little role for children with CP, because if their arm function is that good they are even more functional in a walker (E).

These were specially designed for children with spinal cord paralysis who have good upper extremity and upper trunk control and function. Parapodiums are almost never appropriate for children with CP who require a stander. Children with CP who stand in the paraopodium tend to collapse into the device until they are hanging on its most proximal support. Parapodiums and standing boxes should not be ordered for children with CP.

Walking Aids

Most children with CP will, at some time during their growth and development, use a walking device. Most children who become independent ambulators will start ambulation with the use of a walker. Also, many children who can do standing transfers only will have a period of time when they can do some walking with a walking aid. Most children start standing by pulling to stand and holding onto furniture or toys. Most children are cognitively not able to effectively use a walker until approximately 2 to 2.5 years of age; however, many will be pushing toy baby buggies, wheeled chairs like office chairs, or other toys. As children start to do this type of assistive walking, a walker should be introduced, usually at 24 to 30 months of age. As children gain confidence, and through work in therapy, the use of the walker will increase. For children who have excellent lower extremity control and functional gait but are not able to walk independently, crutch use is introduced in therapy at approximately 5 years of age. Developmentally, even normal children can seldom learn to use crutches until approximately 5 years of age. Therefore, it makes little sense to try to get children with CP to use crutches much earlier. As children get to early adolescence, crutch use should be more strongly encouraged if the physical functional ability is present. There are very few young adults with CP who continue to use walkers for a significant amount of ambulation. Most individuals who use an assistive device and are functional community or full independent household ambulators will do so with crutches and not a walker. The walkers tend to be clumsy and difficult to transport. For a full-sized adult, the walker is often so wide that it does not easily fit through standard home doors.

Walkers

Walkers are available in a complex array of shapes and options; however, there are some basic styles that are important to consider when deciding which walker is appropriate for individuals. Even for therapists or physicians with significant experience, finding the best walker for children is still a combination of trial and error to see which walker these children prefer and which they can handle best. The most basic difference in walkers is they are either back- or front based. The front walker, or anterior-based walker, is pushed in front of children and the back or posterior walker is pulled along behind children. These walker styles are available in all sizes and many different frame constructs. In general, for children with CP, the posterior walker encourages a more upright posture and may improve walking speed. The posterior walker is the most common design used for children in early and middle childhood (Figure 5.52). The two exceptions are blind children and those with mental retardation who often cannot functionally use a posterior walker. Children with severe mental retardation may not be able to understand that the walker, which they cannot see, will still provide support. A developmental age of approximately 24 to 30 months is required to use a posterior

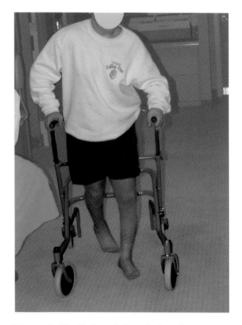

Figure 5.52. Gait assistive devices have many designs, each that tend to have benefits for an individual child. The most common posterior walker encourages children to stand more upright and may increase walking speed.

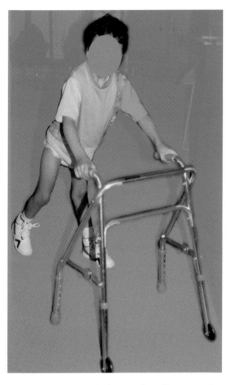

Figure 5.53. Simple forward walkers are also easier for children who have severe mental retardation to learn to use, but tend to encourage children to lean forward too much.

walker. For children with lower cognitive ability, the front-based walker works better (Figure 5.53). Blind children also tend to do better with a front walker. As children get older and heavier, the posterior walkers become very wide. If individuals cannot functionally use crutches by adolescence, conversion to an anterior walker allows for a more narrow based design and is often smaller and easier to transport. The variations between the benefits of children being in a more upright position are more obvious in childhood than in adolescence.

These anterior-based walkers for adolescents and adults may be fitted with articulating wheels and brakes, and some even have flip-down seats so individuals have a place to sit when stopped (see Figure 5.52). The standard height of walkers should be between the top of the iliac spine and the lumbosacral junction. The standard height of the handgrips between the iliac spine and the lumbosacral junction level can be altered based on an individual child's needs. The position of the handgrips is another optional element when ordering walkers. These handgrips may be either horizontal handgrips at the top of a standard walker height or elevated vertical handgrips. In a few children, even using a walker that allows leaning on the elbows works (Figure 5.54). In a population of individuals with CP who use walkers, the position of these handgrips makes no functional difference[30]; however, there are individual children for whom this handgrip position can make an important functional difference. The simplest handgrip, if children can hold comfortably to this handhold, is the horizontal grip at the top of the walker. For children who want to have their arms in the high or midguard position and who cannot get their arms to their side, elevated vertical handgrips, often positioned somewhat toward the midline, are required. For children with a hemiplegic posturing upper extremity, an elevated arm platform with a vertical handgrip is required on the hemiplegic side.

The floor interface for walkers may be wheels or simple crutch tips. For children who have started to walk, the walker should start with crutch tips on all legs. As children gain confidence and speed of walking, posterior wheels may be added. These wheels usually lock in reverse so they can only turn when the children move forward. As children gain more ability, front wheels may be added. As children gain even more ability, free-turning front caster wheels can be added. The need for this different level of support has to be determined through trial and error based on how children are functioning and how the functional ambulation is changing. A major aspect of ongoing physical therapy treatment should be monitoring of children's changing development and ambulation ability. As this ambulation ability increases, the support provided by the walker should be decreased sequentially by the use of wheels that provide less resistance and stability of the walker on the floor. The advantage of these wheels is that they allow children to move faster. As more children are mainstreamed into neighborhood schools where there are fewer experienced physical therapists and where there is little equipment available, this kind of sequential support reduction as children are gaining ambulation skills often gets overlooked. Therefore, ambulation skills have to be more diligently evaluated by CP physicians during routine clinic visits.

Hip guides are another optional attachment that can be added to a walker. Some children continue to have difficulty with medial to lateral instability of the pelvis. Adding hip guides to keep the pelvis in the midline is a method to address this problem. These hip guides should be used only when children have a tendency to be very unstable or to consistently be pushing to one side of the walker.

Gait Trainers

Another type of walker that has many different variations is the gait trainer. Conceptually, this device works exactly like the infant ring walker, which would allow 8- to 9-month-olds to walk around the house before they have independent walking ability. Gait trainers by definition have some kind of seat that will support children if they do not hold themselves in a standing position (Figure 5.55). These walkers provide enough support so that children will not fall over even if completely relaxed. Many children seem to enjoy the movement ability in a gait trainer much more than being restrained in a stander. There is great controversy among some physical therapists with a concern that these walkers foster poor posture and do children great harm. This same view has been expressed about infant walkers.[31] There is no objective evidence that a gait trainer can cause any harm or limit development of children. The major risk of children who can actually move the walkers is for the walkers to go down stairs, drop off a step, or tip over. Parents must be warned about these risks, especially if there are other children in the home who may open and not close basement doors or outside doors where children in walkers could go down stairs. These dangers are exactly the same as for infants in ring walkers. There are no clear documented benefits from the use of gait trainers; however, some children enjoy them very much and it does give them a chance to move in a way that they are not able to do otherwise (see Figure 5.52). These walkers may help provide some force on the bones and improve respiratory and gastrointestinal function similar to a stander.

Typically, the gait trainer is used for children from age 4 to 10 years with widely varying degrees of success. Parents are often very enthused about seeing children upright in a position where they are moving themselves. There is a sense among parents that this is the first step in children developing more independent gait; however, children almost never gain additional ability. It is very rare for children to move from a gait trainer to independent use of an unsupported posterior or anterior walker. At this time, there is no documented benefit that gait trainers help or harm children's functional motor development. Because of the many styles and shapes of gait trainers, a trial use should confirm that it functions before it is ordered for an individual child. If this is not possible, the company should give a guarantee that they will take the gait trainer back within a certain time frame if the child is not able to use the device. The gait trainer design should allow older and heavier children to be positioned in the walker without having to lift them up and over, as with the infant ring walker design. Also, many children seem to do better if positioned with a slight anterior tilt to the trunk similar to being in a prone stander. There are some large commercial gait trainers available that allow adolescent young adults to be placed directly from the wheelchair seated position and then raised to standing with a mechanical lift (see Figure 5.55). These gait trainers are mostly used in special schools that have a special movement educational program for adolescents with severe motor and cognitive limitations. The adolescents seem to enjoy this mobility and do very well with this kind of extensive motor stimulation. Other direct benefits of this kind of motor stimulation for cognitively limited adolescents are more difficult to quantify (Figure 5.56).

Crutches and Canes

Most adolescents who use assistive devices and are full community ambulators use single-point forearm crutches. These crutches are primarily used to

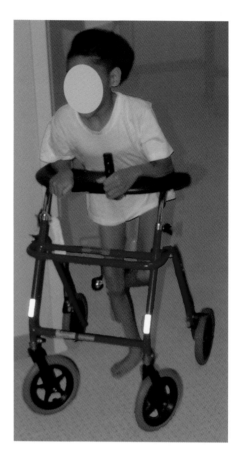

Figure 5.54. The forward-based walker allows better weight bearing on marginally functioning upper extremities.

A

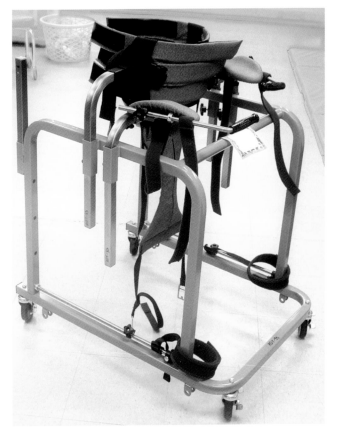

B

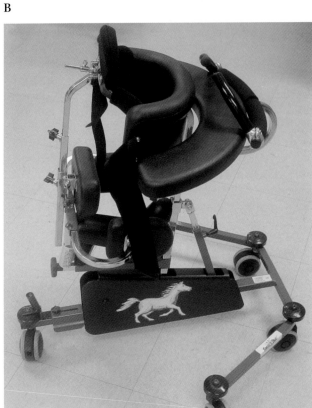

Figure 5.55. For children with more limited motor or balance function, there are many styles of gait trainers, from relatively simple walking frames (A) to frames with good armrests (B) and those with sophisticated armrests, hip guides, and foot guides (C).

augment individuals' poor balance and not to unload weight from the legs (Figure 5.57). The amount of weight applied to the crutches varies greatly. Lightweight forearm crutches are the best walking aids to assist with balance because they are easy to maneuver and, with the forearm strap, can even be held by the forearm while the hand is used for other functions, such as holding cups. Many of these individuals walk around the home holding on to furniture or using only one crutch. A fairly large group of excellent walkers with forearm crutches have a period of time in middle childhood, often between the ages of 7 and 10 years, when they have walked independently in the community without assistive devices. During this middle childhood period, the children fall often, but are able to keep up with their peers because going at a relatively fast speed works well with their poor balance, although their instability causes the frequent falls. As individuals grow heavier and much taller, there is often a period in adolescence when they may find walking more difficult and have to start using crutches. Using crutches may seem like a setback to children and parents; however, when it is pointed out that these adult-sized individuals with crutches are now walking without falling all the time, the parents and the adolescents can see the major benefit of crutch use for community ambulation. Using crutches does not mean that these individuals' walking ability has deteriorated, it primarily means that the walking functions and actions of 8-year-olds are not socially acceptable for 16-year-olds. Also, falling at age 16 years hurts much more than falling at age 8 years, when children are much smaller. It is a grave mistake to put a falling child in wheelchair without trying to teach them crutch use. This

C   D

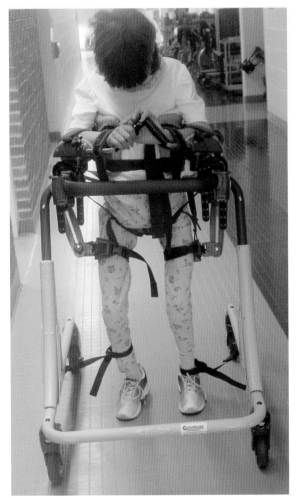

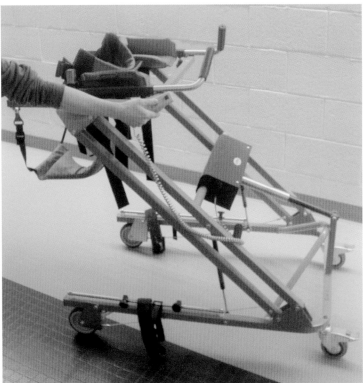

Figure 5.55 (continued). Gait trainers are also available with built-in hydraulic lifts, which allow use by larger and heavier adolescents (D).

step sometimes causes the child to become a permanent wheelchair user when she could well have been a community ambulator with crutches had she been given the appropriate therapy training with the crutches before becoming psychologically wheelchair dependent (see Case 5.1).

Other assistive devices, such as single-point or three-point canes, may be used on occasion in physical therapy to stress the balance development of growing children. The same function can be applied to the use of three- or four-point forearm crutches. Individuals with CP can seldom use one or two single-point canes effectively, and when they try to use three- or four-point canes or crutches, gait slows greatly. Also, with these three- or four-point canes or crutches, there is great postural instability unless the surface is perfectly level and flat, which is exactly the major problem with which these individuals are struggling. Individuals who cannot use single-point forearm crutches in general need to stay with walkers and often are switched to anterior walkers at adolescence.

Standard axillary crutches have no use for children with CP because the fixed position required of the upper extremities is often difficult to maintain, and it is very difficult for individuals with CP not to just hang on the axillary bar.

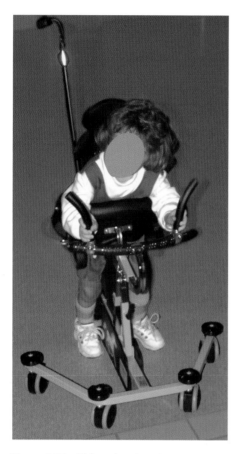

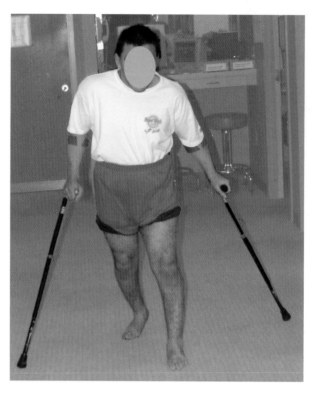

Figure 5.56. Although gait trainers may pose some safety risk to children with CP and there is not good documentation of long-term benefit, many children really enjoy the opportunity to be able to move under their own force.

Figure 5.57. Forearm crutches are the most versatile assistive devices that an adolescent with CP can use if they are not independent ambulators. These are available in various colors and are lightweight.

Patient Lifts

A major problem occurs when adolescents grow to the point where parents can no longer lift them. If children's physical disabilities require a full dependent lift, this often creates a significant strain on the caretakers, especially during rapid adolescent growth. One solution that is often requested by caretakers is to obtain a patient-lifting device. There are two general types available One is a lift that rolls on the floor and has to roll underneath the device from which the children are being lifted. These lifts usually lift children with a sling that has been placed underneath them. After children are lifted by the device, the lifting device can then be rolled to a different location where they can be lowered. The second patient lifting system is attached to a ceiling and runs on tracks mounted on the ceiling. Patients are lifted using a similar sling seat but then rolled along the tracks. The system that rolls on the floor requires a hard surface with no carpet. Also, the device from which individuals are lifted has to be open to allow the lifting device to roll underneath. This means beds and wheelchairs are usually appropriate; however, individuals cannot be lifted out of bathtubs with this type of lifting device. Also, these floor rolling devices have wheels that are very small and are often very hard to push, especially if the individuals lifted are very heavy. Most caretakers find this style of floor rolling lift very difficult to use and often more trouble than beneficial, unless there is absolutely no other way to move the individuals. The ceiling-mounted system is very easy for caretakers to use and to push; however, it is limited to the location where it is installed. In general, the ceiling-mounted lift system is highly praised by caretakers. The ceiling-mounted system can be installed so that individuals can be lifted out of the bath, onto the toilet, out of the wheelchair, and onto the bed. This system can be installed in a bathroom and bedroom combination and is very functional. Another disadvantage with the ceiling-mounted patient lift is that it can be installed only if families own their homes and if they are willing to make significant structural changes to allow the installation of the system into the ceiling. Another major disadvantage for families is that this system, because it is installed in the home, is considered a home modification by insurance companies and is usually not a covered benefit. In comparison, the floor rolling system, which does not work very well, is not attached and therefore can be considered a medical device and not a home modification.

Other Durable Medical Equipment

There are other devices for which physicians may be asked to write prescriptions: these include communication devices, home environmental controls, home modifications, and diapers. Augmentative communication is a large complex area, which is almost impossible for physicians to keep up with. There are augmentative communication specialists who are usually specially trained speech therapists. Many of these systems are obtained through school systems so there is no need for a medical prescription. If requests for prescriptions are made and physicians believe, on the basis of their knowledge level, that the children have the cognitive ability and physical need for the device, physicians should obtain a full evaluation. This evaluation should include a description of the testing that was performed and the rationale for the specific devices requested. This report should also document that the children have demonstrated an appropriate physical and cognitive ability to use the system. Home environmental control switches, stair lifts, and home modifications such as door widening and special bathroom installations are very appropriate methods of ameliorating the disability from motor impairments. Physician are seldom in positions to make specific recommendations; however, prescriptions or letters of medical need that such modifications are appropriate because of these children's motor impairments may help families obtain resources to get this work done. These modifications are never covered by medical insurance; however, with a letter of medical need families can deduct the cost as a medical expense in some cases on their tax returns. These deductions should only be made on the recommendation of a tax specialist. Some insurance plans will cover the cost of diapers after a certain age if children are not toilet trained. These diapers need a prescription, which is an annoyance because the need is self-apparent; however, families have to get this paperwork and a family physician or other physicians caring for these children to provide this prescription to help families access the appropriate supplies. Another area where families often ask for recommendations or prescriptions are special play equipment such as tricycles. Some of these can be set up as therapeutic devices (Figure 5.58); however, it is often difficult to find adequate documentation to get medical coverage for these devices. A device such as a wheel swing may add to children's normal childhood experience, but again it is very difficult to justify these as medical devices (Figure 5.59).

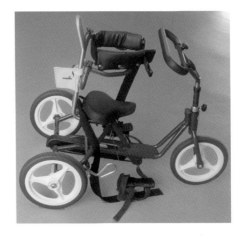

Figure 5.58. Other devices that tend to bridge the gap between therapy and play are therapeutic tricycles, which may provide excellent endurance training and balance development.

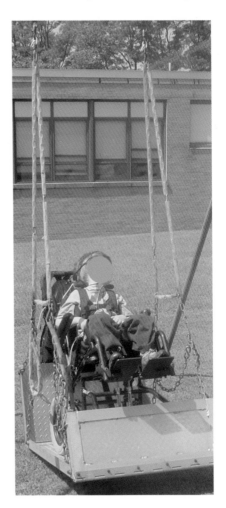

Figure 5.59. A wheelchair swing can also provide excellent stimulation for some children who have little chance for such normal childhood activities as experiencing a swing.

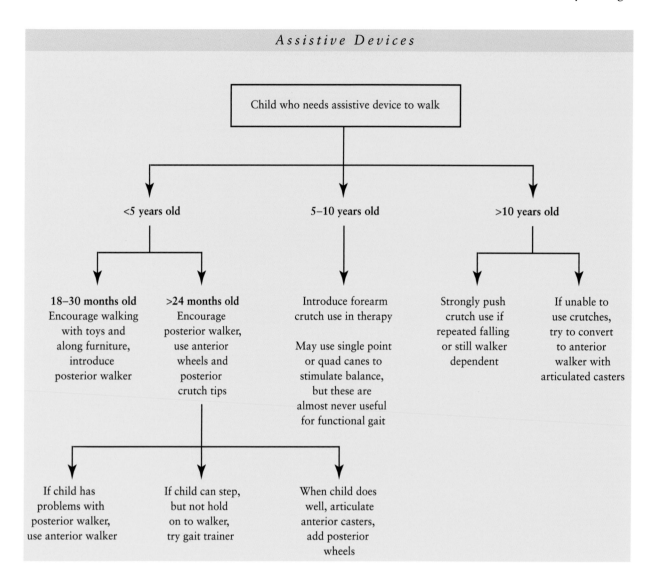

Assistive Devices

Child who needs assistive device to walk

<5 years old

5–10 years old

>10 years old

18–30 months old
Encourage walking
with toys and
along furniture,
introduce
posterior walker

>24 months old
Encourage
posterior walker,
use anterior
wheels and
posterior
crutch tips

Introduce forearm
crutch use in therapy

May use single point
or quad canes to
stimulate balance,
but these are
almost never useful
for functional gait

Strongly push
crutch use if
repeated falling
or still walker
dependent

If unable to
use crutches,
try to convert
to anterior
walker with
articulated casters

If child has
problems with
posterior walker,
use anterior walker

If child can step,
but not hold
on to walker,
try gait trainer

When child does
well, articulate
anterior casters,
add posterior
wheels

Prescribing a Wheelchair

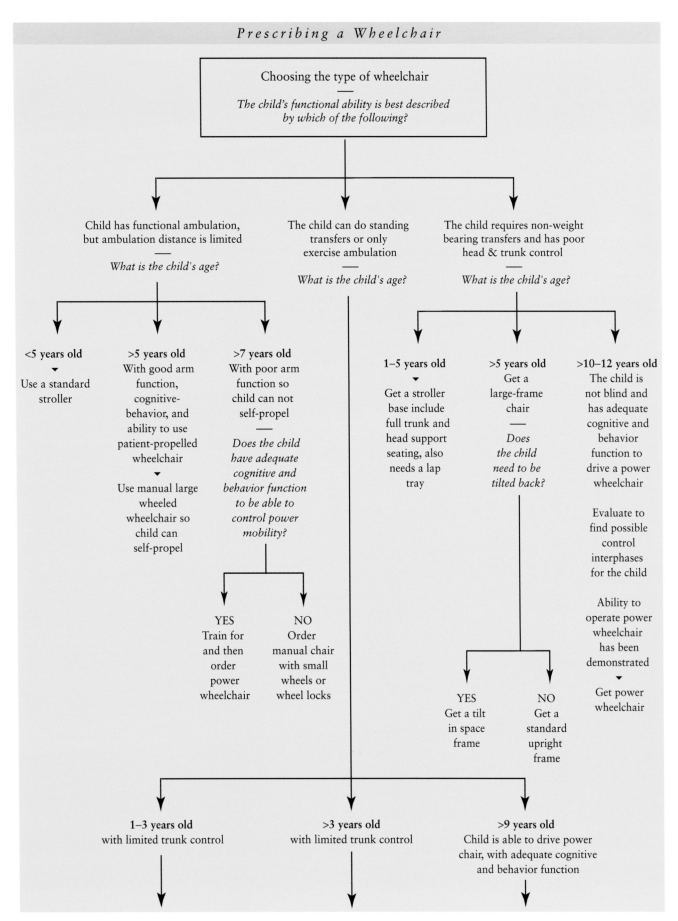

Choosing the type of wheelchair
—
The child's functional ability is best described by which of the following?

Child has functional ambulation, but ambulation distance is limited
—
What is the child's age?

The child can do standing transfers or only exercise ambulation
—
What is the child's age?

The child requires non-weight bearing transfers and has poor head & trunk control
—
What is the child's age?

<5 years old
▼
Use a standard stroller

>5 years old
With good arm function, cognitive-behavior, and ability to use patient-propelled wheelchair
▼
Use manual large wheeled wheelchair so child can self-propel

>7 years old
With poor arm function so child can not self-propel
—
Does the child have adequate cognitive and behavior function to be able to control power mobility?

1–5 years old
▼
Get a stroller base include full trunk and head support seating, also needs a lap tray

>5 years old
Get a large-frame chair
—
Does the child need to be tilted back?

>10–12 years old
The child is not blind and has adequate cognitive and behavior function to drive a power wheelchair

Evaluate to find possible control interphases for the child

Ability to operate power wheelchair has been demonstrated
▼
Get power wheelchair

YES
Train for and then order power wheelchair

NO
Order manual chair with small wheels or wheel locks

YES
Get a tilt in space frame

NO
Get a standard upright frame

1–3 years old
with limited trunk control

>3 years old
with limited trunk control

>9 years old
Child is able to drive power chair, with adequate cognitive and behavior function

continued

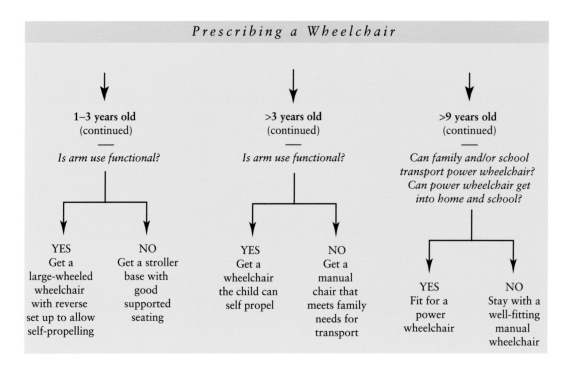

Prescribing a Wheelchair

1–3 years old
(continued)
—
Is arm use functional?

YES
Get a
large-wheeled
wheelchair
with reverse
set up to allow
self-propelling

NO
Get a stroller
base with
good
supported
seating

>3 years old
(continued)
—
Is arm use functional?

YES
Get a
wheelchair
the child can
self propel

NO
Get a
manual
chair that
meets family
needs for
transport

>9 years old
(continued)
—
*Can family and/or school
transport power wheelchair?
Can power wheelchair get
into home and school?*

YES
Fit for a
power
wheelchair

NO
Stay with a
well-fitting
manual
wheelchair

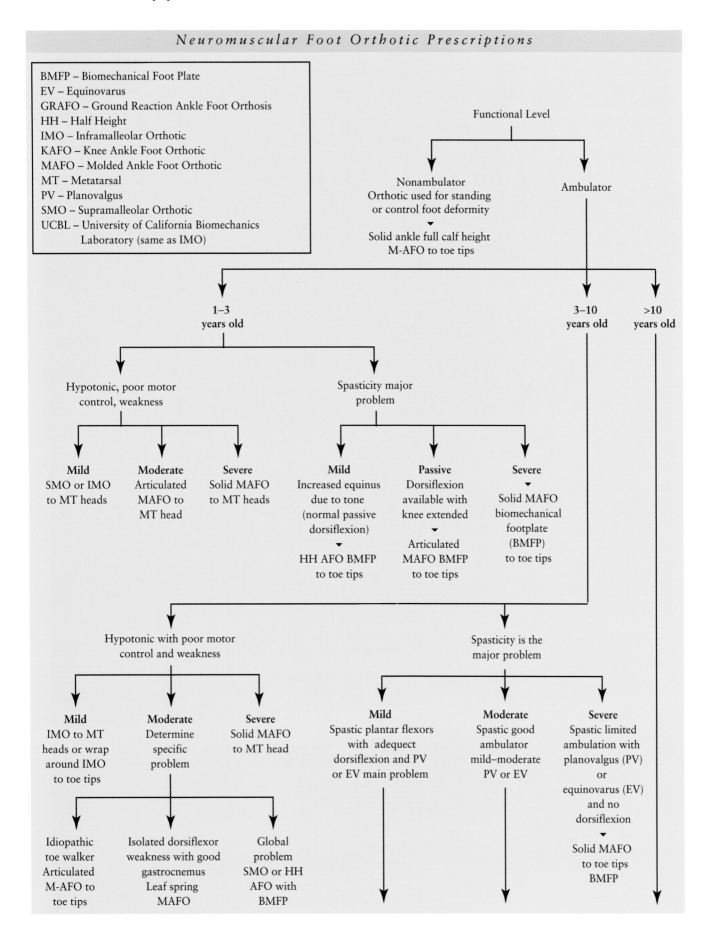

Neuromuscular Foot Orthotic Prescriptions

BMFP – Biomechanical Foot Plate
EV – Equinovarus
GRAFO – Ground Reaction Ankle Foot Orthosis
HH – Half Height
IMO – Inframalleolar Orthotic
KAFO – Knee Ankle Foot Orthotic
MAFO – Molded Ankle Foot Orthotic
MT – Metatarsal
PV – Planovalgus
SMO – Supramalleolar Orthotic
UCBL – University of California Biomechanics
          Laboratory (same as IMO)

Functional Level

Nonambulator
Orthotic used for standing
or control foot deformity
▾
Solid ankle full calf height
M-AFO to toe tips

Ambulator

1–3
years old

3–10
years old

>10
years old

Hypotonic, poor motor
control, weakness

Spasticity major
problem

Mild
SMO or IMO
to MT heads

Moderate
Articulated
MAFO to
MT head

Severe
Solid MAFO
to MT heads

Mild
Increased equinus
due to tone
(normal passive
dorsiflexion)
▾
HH AFO BMFP
to toe tips

Passive
Dorsiflexion
available with
knee extended
▾
Articulated
MAFO BMFP
to toe tips

Severe
▾
Solid MAFO
biomechanical
footplate
(BMFP)
to toe tips

Hypotonic with poor motor
control and weakness

Spasticity is the
major problem

Mild
IMO to MT
heads or wrap
around IMO
to toe tips

Moderate
Determine
specific
problem

Severe
Solid MAFO
to MT head

Mild
Spastic plantar flexors
with adequect
dorsiflexion and PV
or EV main problem

Moderate
Spastic good
ambulator
mild–moderate
PV or EV

Severe
Spastic limited
ambulation with
planovalgus (PV)
or
equinovarus (EV)
and no
dorsiflexion
▾
Solid MAFO
to toe tips
BMFP

Idiopathic
toe walker
Articulated
M-AFO to
toe tips

Isolated dorsiflexor
weakness with good
gastrocnemus
Leaf spring
MAFO

Global
problem
SMO or HH
AFO with
BMFP

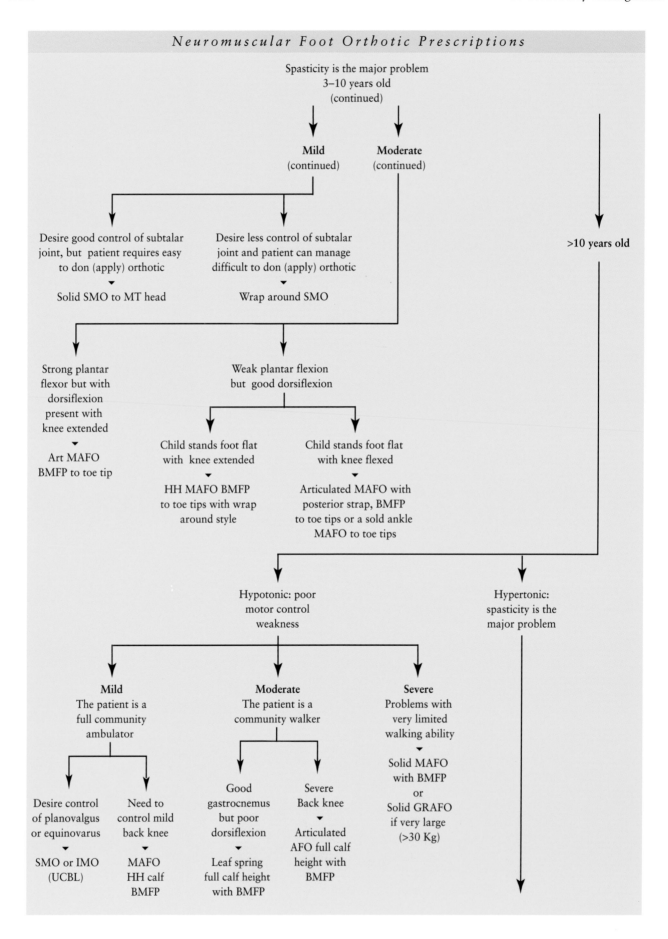

Neuromuscular Foot Orthotic Prescriptions

Spasticity is the major problem
3–10 years old
(continued)

Mild
(continued)

Moderate
(continued)

>10 years old

Desire good control of subtalar
joint, but patient requires easy
to don (apply) orthotic

Solid SMO to MT head

Desire less control of subtalar
joint and patient can manage
difficult to don (apply) orthotic

Wrap around SMO

Strong plantar
flexor but with
dorsiflexion
present with
knee extended

Art MAFO
BMFP to toe tip

Weak plantar flexion
but good dorsiflexion

Child stands foot flat
with knee extended

HH MAFO BMFP
to toe tips with wrap
around style

Child stands foot flat
with knee flexed

Articulated MAFO with
posterior strap, BMFP
to toe tips or a sold ankle
MAFO to toe tips

Hypotonic: poor
motor control
weakness

Hypertonic:
spasticity is the
major problem

Mild
The patient is a
full community
ambulator

Moderate
The patient is a
community walker

Severe
Problems with
very limited
walking ability

Solid MAFO
with BMFP
or
Solid GRAFO
if very large
(>30 Kg)

Desire control
of planovalgus
or equinovarus

SMO or IMO
(UCBL)

Need to
control mild
back knee

MAFO
HH calf
BMFP

Good
gastrocnemius
but poor
dorsiflexion

Leaf spring
full calf height
with BMFP

Severe
Back knee

Articulated
AFO full calf
height with
BMFP

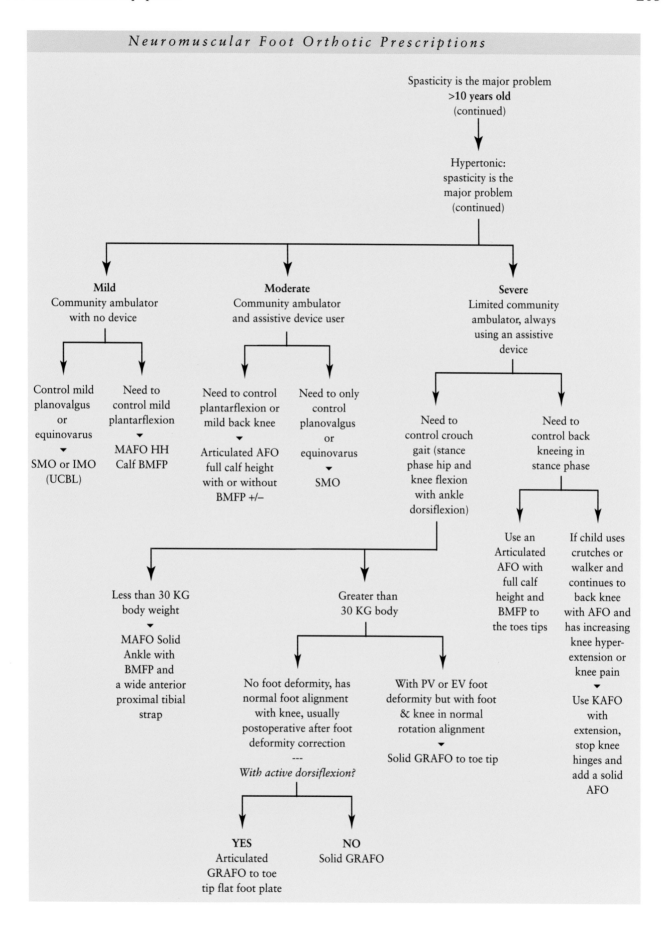

Neuromuscular Foot Orthotic Prescriptions

Spasticity is the major problem
>10 years old
(continued)

Hypertonic:
spasticity is the
major problem
(continued)

Mild
Community ambulator
with no device

Moderate
Community ambulator
and assistive device user

Severe
Limited community
ambulator, always
using an assistive
device

Control mild
planovalgus
or
equinovarus

SMO or IMO
(UCBL)

Need to
control mild
plantarflexion

MAFO HH
Calf BMFP

Need to control
plantarflexion or
mild back knee

Articulated AFO
full calf height
with or without
BMFP +/−

Need to only
control
planovalgus
or
equinovarus

SMO

Need to
control crouch
gait (stance
phase hip and
knee flexion
with ankle
dorsiflexion)

Need to
control back
kneeing in
stance phase

Use an
Articulated
AFO with
full calf
height and
BMFP to
the toes tips

If child uses
crutches or
walker and
continues to
back knee
with AFO and
has increasing
knee hyper-
extension or
knee pain

Use KAFO
with
extension,
stop knee
hinges and
add a solid
AFO

Less than 30 KG
body weight

MAFO Solid
Ankle with
BMFP and
a wide anterior
proximal tibial
strap

Greater than
30 KG body

No foot deformity, has
normal foot alignment
with knee, usually
postoperative after foot
deformity correction

With active dorsiflexion?

With PV or EV foot
deformity but with foot
& knee in normal
rotation alignment

Solid GRAFO to toe tip

YES
Articulated
GRAFO to toe
tip flat foot plate

NO
Solid GRAFO

References

1. Miller A, Temple T, Miller F. Impact of orthoses on the rate of scoliosis progression in children with cerebral palsy [see comments]. J Pediatr Orthop 1996;16:332–5.
2. Leopando MT, Moussavi Z, Holbrow J, Chernick V, Pasterkamp H, Rempel G. Effect of a soft Boston orthosis on pulmonary mechanics in severe cerebral palsy. Pediatr Pulmonol 1999;28:53–8.
3. Miller F, Slomczykowski M, Cope R, Lipton GE. Computer modeling of the pathomechanics of spastic hip dislocation in children. J Pediatr Orthop 1999;19:486–92.
4. Szalay EA, Roach JW, Houkom JA, Wenger DR, Herring JA. Extension-abduction contracture of the spastic hip. J Pediatr Orthop 1986;6:1–6.
5. Carlson WE, Vaughan CL, Damiano DL, Abel MF. Orthotic management of gait in spastic diplegia. Am J Phys Med Rehabil 1997;76:219–25.
6. Crenshaw S, Herzog R, Castagno P, et al. The efficacy of tone-reducing features in orthotics on the gait of children with spastic diplegic cerebral palsy. J Pediatr Orthop 2000;20:210–6.
7. Radtka SA, Skinner SR, Dixon DM, Johanson ME. A comparison of gait with solid, dynamic, and no ankle-foot orthoses in children with spastic cerebral palsy [see comments] [published erratum appears in Phys Ther 1998;78(2):222–4]. Phys Ther 1997;77:395–409.
8. Burtner PA, Woollacott MH, Qualls C. Stance balance control with orthoses in a group of children with spastic cerebral palsy. Dev Med Child Neurol 1999;41:748–57.
9. Ricks NR, Eilert RE. Effects of inhibitory casts and orthoses on bony alignment of foot and ankle during weight-bearing in children with spasticity. Dev Med Child Neurol 1993;35:11–6.
10. Abel MF, Juhl GA, Vaughan CL, Damiano DL. Gait assessment of fixed ankle-foot orthoses in children with spastic diplegia. Arch Phys Med Rehabil 1998;79:126–33.
11. Hainsworth F, Harrison MJ, Sheldon TA, Roussounis SH. A preliminary evaluation of ankle orthoses in the management of children with cerebral palsy. Dev Med Child Neurol 1997;39:243–7.
12. Ounpuu S, Bell KJ, Davis RB III, DeLuca PA. An evaluation of the posterior leaf spring orthosis using joint kinematics and kinetics. J Pediatr Orthop 1996;16:378–84.
13. Wilson H, Haideri N, Song K, Telford D. Ankle-foot orthoses for preambulatory children with spastic diplegia. J Pediatr Orthop 1997;17:370–6.
14. Nwaobi OM, Smith PD. Effect of adaptive seating on pulmonary function of children with cerebral palsy. Dev Med Child Neurol 1986;28:351–4.
15. Hulme JB, Bain B, Hardin M, McKinnon A, Waldron D. The influence of adaptive seating devices on vocalization. J Commun Disord 1989;22:137–45.
16. Hulme JB, Shaver J, Acher S, Mullette L, Eggert C. Effects of adaptive seating devices on the eating and drinking of children with multiple handicaps. Am J Occup Ther 1987;41:81–9.
17. Nwaobi OM. Seating orientations and upper extremity function in children with cerebral palsy. Phys Ther 1987;67:1209–12.
18. Reid DT. The effects of the saddle seat on seated postural control and upper-extremity movement in children with cerebral palsy. Dev Med Child Neurol 1996;38:805–15.
19. Medhat MA, Redford JB. Experience of a seating clinic. Int Orthop 1985;9:279–85.
20. Rang M, Douglas G, Bennet GC, Koreska J. Seating for children with cerebral palsy. J Pediatr Orthop 1981;1:279–87.
21. Colbert AP, Doyle KM, Webb WE. DESEMO seats for young children with cerebral palsy. Arch Phys Med Rehabil 1986;67:484–6.
22. Trefler E, Hanks S, Huggins P, Chiarizzo S, Hobson D. A modular seating system for cerebral-palsied children. Dev Med Child Neurol 1978;20:199–204.

23. Trefler E, Angelo J. Comparison of anterior trunk supports for children with cerebral palsy. Assist Technol 1997;9:15–21.
24. McPherson JJ, Schild R, Spaulding SJ, Barsamian P, Transon C, White SC. Analysis of upper extremity movement in four sitting positions: a comparison of persons with and without cerebral palsy. Am J Occup Ther 1991;45:123–9.
25. Nwaobi OM. Effects of body orientation in space on tonic muscle activity of patients with cerebral palsy. Dev Med Child Neurol 1986;28:41–4.
26. Gibson DA, Albisser AM, Koreska J. Role of the wheelchair in the management of the muscular dystrophy patient. Can Med Assoc J 1975;113:964–6.
27. Stout JD, Bandy P, Feller N, Stroup KB, Bull MJ. Transportation resources for pediatric orthopaedic clients. Orthop Nurs 1992;11:26–30.
28. Paley K, Walker JL, Cromwell F, Enlow C. Transportation of children with special seating needs. South Med J 1993;86:1339–41.
29. Cristarella MC. Comparison of straddling and sitting apparatus for the spastic cerebral-palsied child. Am J Occup Ther 1975;29:273–6.
30. Levangie PK, Guihan MF, Meyer P, Stuhr K. Effect of altering handle position of a rolling walker on gait in children with cerebral palsy. Phys Ther 1989;69:130–4.
31. Holm VA, Harthun-Smith L, Tada WL. Infant walkers and cerebral palsy. Am J Dis Child 1983;137:1189–90.

Gait

Treatment of the motor effects on ambulatory ability are the most common musculoskeletal problems that the orthopaedist has to address when treating children with cerebral palsy (CP). There are only a minority of patients whose motor function is so limited that ambulation is of no concern. From children with the most mild effects of hemiplegia to children with quadriplegia who are just able to do standing transfers, lower extremity function for mobility is usually a major concern of parents. The first task in the orthopaedic treatment plan is to individually identify how significant the gait impairment is to a child's whole disability. The second task is to determine if treatment of the impairment is likely to improve this child's function. The final goal is to explain the treatment plan to the parents and children and to inform them of the specific functional gains that can be expected and the associated risks. Normal human gait is one of the most complex functions of the human body, and gait is clearly the most complex impairment treated by pediatric orthopaedists. To understand and develop a specific treatment plan for children with gait impairments due to CP, orthopaedists have to have a good understanding of normal gait, understand measurement techniques used to evaluate gait, and be able to evaluate pathologic gait.

This discussion starts with an overview description of the basic scientific concepts required to understand gait. This basic science background is crucial to understanding normal gait and is even more important to understanding the pathologic gait of children with CP. The goal of this text is not to provide a comprehensive review of all the basic science of gait. For individuals who have had limited exposure to the scientific understanding of human gait, more detailed texts with much more information are available. To understand normal gait, the textbook *Gait Analysis,* written by Jacquelin Perry, is strongly recommended.[1] For a better mathematical understanding, the text *Human Motion Analysis,* edited by Harris and Smith, is recommended.[2] *Gait Analysis in Cerebral Palsy,* written by James Gage, is directed more specifically at the treatment of CP.[3]

Basic Science

The basic science of gait involves neuromotor control; global mechanics of the musculoskeletal system; and the mechanics and physiology of the structural subsystems including connective tissue, muscles, and bones. The basic concepts of motor control are discussed in Chapter 3 on motor control and tone. The concepts from that section, which will be used to understand motor control of gait, focus predominantly on the theory of dynamic motor control, in which the system may express some level of fuzzy control but is drawn to chaotic attractors of differing strengths. This discussion will also use the underlying assumption that there is a central program generator with a combination of feed-forward and feedback control. A basic assumption of gait treatment includes the concept that little can be done to selectively influence the central program generator, although providing an improved biomechanical environment should allow the central program generator to provide the best possible control of gait. Another assumption is that most of the primary pathology in gait abnormalities in CP is located in the central program generator, and because it cannot be affected directly, the outcome of gait treatment is not expected to be a normal gait pattern. Therefore, the defined goal is always to improve the gait pattern functionally toward normal. With these underlying assumptions, the mechanics of how this central program generator's directives become the physical motion of walking will be examined.

Biomechanics

To understand a discussion of biomechanics, a clear and concise understanding of the terms has to be present (Table 6.1). Motion or movement, can mean either physical translation of a person or a segment of a person through space. Motion is also used to define angular rotation around a point. Temporal spatial measurements are related to movement of the whole person and include velocity, which is the amount of motion per unit time, usually defined in centimeters per second (cm/s). Temporal spatial measurements also separate elements of whole-body movement by the phase of gait defined by global mechanics. Angular motion around the individual joints is defined as kinematic measures. Usually, these measures are plotted as degrees of joint motion in clinically defined joint planes, such as degrees of flexion. The first derivative with respect to time of angular rotation per unit time is joint velocity, the second derivative is joint acceleration, and the third derivative is joint jerk.

The forces and their characterizations involved with gait are called kinetic measures. The kinetic measures include the force measured in newtons (N). The weight of an object measured in kilograms (kg) is similar to mass measured in newtons (N) as defined by Newton's second law. This definition states that a given external force (F) is required to move a given mass (m) at a specific acceleration (a) ($F = ma$). Gravity, which is the attraction of two bodies toward each other, is a force we call weight, which has an important impact on human movement. Force is also generated by chemical reactions in muscle and may be absorbed by a chemical reaction of muscle and the elastic action of soft tissues and bone. To change the state of a mass from rest to motion, a force has to be applied to satisfy Newton's second law. In mechanics, this means there is a force that causes a predictable reaction of an acceleration for a given mass. Constant velocity does not require a force, except to overcome friction and other negative forces acting on the body. The application of force over a distance is defined as work and is usually measured in joules. The capacity to perform work is called energy. The capacity of a moving body to perform work is called kinetic energy, which is released when there is a drop in the velocity. An example is a 1-kg weight lifted 1 m, and then allowed to drop; gravity will produce work through the acceleration and kinetic energy will be released when the object strikes the ground. This principle of force being applied over a distance is used to define the angular motion that occurs at joints as well. With angular motion, a force

Table 6.1. Description of biomechanical terms.

Term	Description
Temporal spatial characteristics:	Changes in the body or body segments related to the gait cycle.
Gait velocity:	Change in distance per unit time of the whole body during gait.
Step:	The gait cycle of one limb; the distance one foot moves with each gait cycle.
Cadence:	The number of gait cycles per unit time.
Stride:	Gait cycle of the whole body that equals two steps.
Stance phase (support time):	The time as a percent of time the foot is in contact with the floor during one step cycle.
Swing phase:	The time as a percent of time the foot is *not* in contact with the floor during one step cycle, or if there is toe drag, the time when the foot starts to move forward.
Initial double support:	Starting at heel strike or foot contact, time until the opposite limb starts swing phase.
Second double support:	Starting at heel strike or foot contact on the opposite limb, time until the index limb starts swing phase. Each step has two double supports; however, each stride also has only two double supports.
Step width:	The distance in the transverse plane of how far the feet are separated during double support.
Kinematics:	Measurement of the displacement of the body segments during gait, usually defined as angular change of the distal segment relative to its proximal articulated segment, or motion relative to a global coordinate system.
Joint velocity:	Amount of joint motion per unit time.
Joint acceleration:	Change in the velocity per unit time.
Joint jerk:	Change in the acceleration per unit time.
Kinetics:	Measurement of the forces acting upon the body segments.
Joint moments (torque):	Force applied at a defined distance from a point that generates rotation motion if it is not opposed (force times distance).
Joint force (joint reaction force):	The force a joint experiences defined in three planes and three moments.
Joint power:	Net joint moment times the joint's angular velocity.
Normalized kinetics:	Dividing the kinetic measure by the body weight in kilograms to obtain a number that can be compared over growth and to different-sized individuals.

of a specific magnitude is applied at a distance from the center of the angular motion, and is called a moment or torque. Unless an equal and opposite moment is applied, a joint motion occurs. This distance from the center of the joint motion to the application of the force is called the moment arm. Joint power is the application of the moment over a specific distance per unit time, which is defined in units called watts. Angular joint power is defined as being positive when motion, which is produced by concentric or shortening contractions of muscle, occurs. Angular joint power is negative when the motion is being controlled by an eccentric or a lengthening contraction. Absorption of power is the typical term used instead of negative power.

The term strength is very confusing as it is used in clinical care related to muscles. Often, strength is used in some combination to mean how much force a muscle can apply, how much work it can do, or how much angular power it can generate. All these definitions of strength are very confusing in the clinical literature. For the remainder of this discussion, the term strength is be used unless it is used to mean force unrelated to any time or distance parameters. The best way to use strength is to define the total limit of stress (force per unit area) or strain (length change per unit length) in a specific given environment. For example, it would be technically correct to say that a board of the same size and shape is stronger if it is made of steel rather than wood. Application of these mechanical concepts of understanding the function of the mechanical subsystems will be important to combine all parts into a functional, whole musculoskeletal system.

Muscle Mechanics

Energy Production

Based on the understanding of Newtonian physics, a change in movement state cannot occur unless there is an output of energy. In the human body, this output of energy occurs through the muscles, which are constructed of small subunits called sarcomeres (Figure 6.1). Sarcomeres have actin and myosin subunits that form chemical bonds, causing the actin and myosin subunits to overlap when they are stimulated by electrical depolarization produced by the motor neuron. The chemical energy needed for this shortening action of the sarcomere may be produced by aerobic metabolism, where

Figure 6.1. The microanatomy of the muscle fiber starts with sarcomeres, which are the building blocks of the muscle fibers. The sarcomeres are made of thin actin molecules that slide over the thicker myosin. With maximum elongation, there is only a small area of overlap. At rest, the fibers have approximately 50% overlap, and at full contraction, there is complete overlap. The chemical reaction causing this overlapping of the actin and myosin is the force-generating mechanism of muscle. In cross section, the fibers are stacked to provide a maximum number of contacts of the actin to the myosin fibers.

A

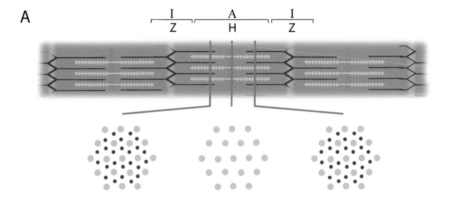

B

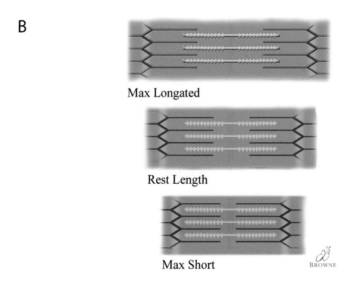

Max Longated

Rest Length

Max Short

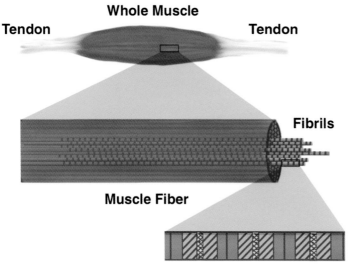

Whole Muscle
Tendon   **Tendon**

Fibrils

Muscle Fiber

Isolated Muscle Fibril

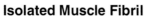

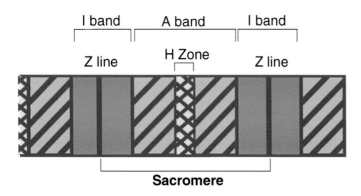

I band   A band   I band

Z line   H Zone   Z line

Sacromere

Figure 6.2. The sarcomeres are then combined end to end to form myofibrils, which are combined parallel to each other to form muscle fibers. Many muscle fibers are then combined into a single muscle attached at each end to a tendon.

oxygen is consumed through glycolysis of glucose in which adenosine triphosphate (ATP), carbon dioxide, and water are produced. Alternatively, energy can be produced by anaerobic metabolism using glycolysis of glucose in which ATP and lactic acid are generated as by-products. Another mechanism allows the enzymatic breakdown of phosphocreatine with the production of ATP and creatine. The chemical directly used by the sarcomere is ATP, which binds to the myosin and provides the energy for the cross-bridging to actin. The chemical details of sarcomere function and the energy production are well understood from a biochemical perspective; however, this energy production process is seldom a basic problem for children with CP. Sarcomeres are then combined into muscle fibers; the specific diameter of the fiber is determined by how many sarcomeres are placed together in the transverse plane (Figure 6.2). The diameter of muscle fibers varies from approximately 20 micrometers (μm) in hand intrinsic muscles to 55 μm in leg muscles.[1] The length of the fiber is the length of the muscle. Many muscle fibers are combined into one motor unit, which is controlled by a single motor neuron. The number of muscle fibers per motor neuron varies from approximately 100 in hand-intrinsic muscles to 600 in the gastrocnemius muscle. Thus, a hand-intrinsic muscle may contain approximately 100 motor units and the gastrocnemius contains approximately 1800 motor units.[1] Each motor unit is controlled by one motor neuron. The muscle fibers in each individual motor unit are dispersed throughout the whole body of the muscle.[4] Each motor

Figure 6.3. The length of the muscle fiber is determined by the number of sarcomeres placed end to end. This muscle fiber length determines the muscle excursion length and therefore the active range of motion of the joint. For example, if the gastrocnemius usually produces 60° of active ankle joint range of motion, and the muscle loses 50% of its fiber length, it can generate only 30°of active ankle range of motion.

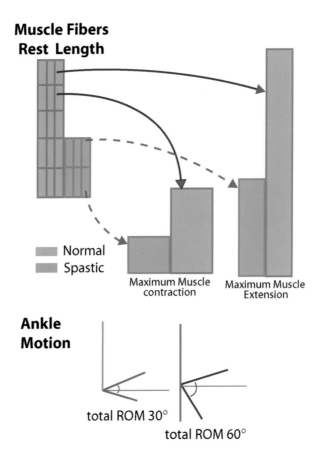

unit has only one mechanism of action, which is either contraction or no activity. The large number of motor units present mutes this all-or-nothing response in the whole muscle. Therefore, the level of muscle force that can be generated is based on how many motor units can contract simultaneously.

Force Production

The amount of force that a muscle can generate is based on the cross-sectional area of the muscle; however, the amount of work and power a muscle can generate is based on the total mass of the muscle. Adding sarcomeres side to side and expanding the diameter of the muscle fiber builds up the cross-sectional area, thereby increasing the force-generating ability of the muscle. However, by adding sarcomeres end to end, the total excursion of the muscle fiber increases so the force can be applied over a longer distance. Another way to understand this is a muscle with a longer muscle fiber allows greater joint range of motion (Figure 6.3). At the next level of the micro-anatomy, the addition of more muscle fibers to the whole muscle adds to the force-generating capacity of the muscle because it increases the cross-sectional area. However, this increased cross-sectional area does not increase the excursional length of the muscle or the joint range of motion through which the muscle can function. Selective control is improved by reducing the number of muscle fibers per motor unit. In normal individuals, the difference between 100 fibers per motor unit in the hand-intrinsic muscles compared with 600 fibers in the gastrocnemius demonstrates why there is much better fine motor control of the hand intrinsics than of the gastrocnemius muscle. Many things affect muscle fiber size in both length and cross section. These complex effects are magnified during the growth years.

Fiber Types

Another aspect of muscle physiology is the presence of different muscle fiber types. The fiber types are defined by histochemical staining. Type 1 fibers are slow twitch, with a high capacity for oxidative metabolism. Type 2 muscles are divided into two subtypes, types 2a and 2b. Type 2a also has a high capacity for oxidative metabolism and type 2b is primarily anaerobic metabolism. Type 1 fibers are slow twitch and type 2 fibers have a faster twitch response.[4] Fiber types 1 and 2a are more fatigue resistant than type 2b fibers. In other words, aerobic metabolism provides for better endurance, but anaerobic metabolism provides for better short bursts of high force with fast fatiguing, although not all the data support a clear distinction in fatigue ability between the histochemically defined fiber types.[5] The strength or ability to generate force is not significantly different between the fiber types.[6] Each motor unit is made up of similar fiber types.[6] The slow-twitch oxidative type 1 muscle fibers are ideal for submaximal force generation required over long periods of time. Type 2 fibers are ideal where high bursts with maximal contraction are required for short periods of time. For example, long-distance runners have increased type 1 fibers and weight lifters have increased type 2 fibers.

Muscle Anatomy

All the muscle fibers are combined into motor units, which are structured to make whole single muscle units. The individual muscle fibers can be anatomically combined to make an individual muscle with varying degrees of fiber orientation. The fibers may be oriented with a pennation angle relative to the tendon, or the fibers may be aligned straight with the line of action of the tendon (Figure 6.4). An example of a bipennate orientation is the deltoid muscle or gluteus muscle. A unipennate structure is most common in other muscles of the lower extremity. The pennation angle is another way in which the force is increased, but it works over a shorter distance. For a few muscles, the pennation angle is important in considering the amount of muscle force generation, but for most muscles that cause problems in children with CP, there is no need to worry about the pennation angle because it is small and has relatively little effect. The muscle can generate force while it shortens, while it lengthens, or while its length is static. The mechanism of force generation is the same for all situations and involves an all-or-none response by many motor units within the muscle. However, for example, if the same 100 motor units contract, the amount of energy required is very different depending on the effect in the muscle. A concentric contraction, in which the muscle is shortening and doing positive work, has the highest energy demand. Eccentric contraction, in which the muscle is lengthening and doing negative work or absorbing power, requires three to nine times less energy than a concentric contraction. Isometric contraction uses an intermediate amount of energy.[3] As a general rule, muscles that do the work of moving have to produce angular joint acceleration and do active work by concentric contraction. Muscles that decelerate, or act as shock absorbers or transfer energy, are eccentric acting muscles in which power is absorbed. Isometric muscle contraction predominantly works to stabilize a joint or to help with postural stability.

Muscle Length–Tension Relationship (Blix Curve)

Another important aspect of a muscle's ability to generate force is the length position in which the muscle fiber is stimulated relative to its resting length.

Figure 6.4. The arrangement of the muscle fibers in the muscle is another variable in determining the excursion length of the muscle and the amount of force the muscle can generate at the joint level (A). The angle at which the muscle fiber inserts into the tendon is called the pennation angle, which can be very high for a muscle such as the deltoid. For most muscles of ambulation that have long muscle fibers, the pennation angle is so small that it has little impact on the force generated (B).

A

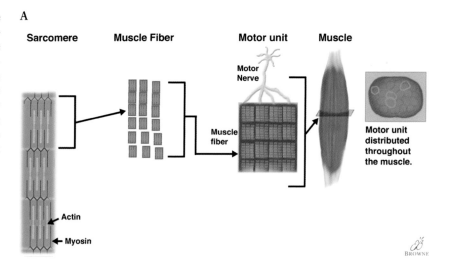

B

Muscle Fiber Orientation

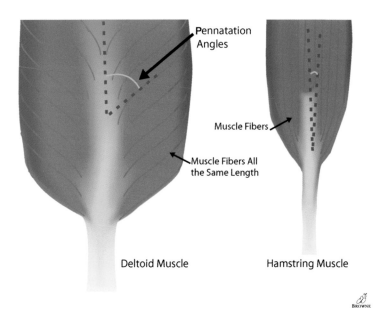

Thus, when a muscle is at resting length, the actin and myosin are in the relaxed position with slight overlap, and in this position, the muscle can generate its maximum force. If the muscle is distracted so that the sarcomeric subunits have less overlap, the muscle strength will decrease. Also, if the muscle is at an increased shortened position, it will use maximum force-generating ability because of too much overlap at the sarcomere level. This phenomenon has been defined by the Blix curve, or the muscle length–tension curve, and has been presented in many textbooks as a key mechanism to understand a muscle's response in generating force (Figure 6.5). An understanding of a muscle's length relative to the Blix curve is especially important when planning muscle-lengthening procedures. Although less clearly

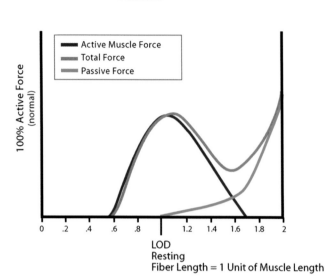

Figure 6.5. The muscle fiber length–tension curve (Blix curve) is crucial to understanding the muscle force-generating ability. At rest length the muscle has the ability to generate the highest amount of active force. As the muscle shortens, this ability to generate force decreases to zero at approximately 60% of rest length. As the muscle lengthens, the active force-generating ability also decreases and reaches zero at approximately 170% of rest length. However, as the muscle lengthens, the passive collagen elements provide a passive restraint to further lengthening, thereby increasing tension as the muscle is lengthened. This increases until approximately 200% of rest length, when the muscle starts to physically fail.

defined, increased resting tone in a muscle will also increase the amount of force the muscle can generate when it is stimulated.[7]

The biomechanical response that the muscles in children with CP develop affects the force-generating ability. This force-generating ability is altered by changes in muscle fiber size, fiber pennation angles, length of the fiber relative to its resting length, and the cross-sectional size of the whole muscle.[8] The longitudinal excursion of a muscle depends primarily on the length and the pennation angle of the muscle fibers. Endurance or fatigability of a muscle depends on the muscle fiber type, especially its primary metabolic function, which is either oxidative or anaerobic, and the muscle fiber's velocity of contraction, meaning specifically whether it is concentric, eccentric, or isometric. A muscle's selective control is altered mainly at the muscle level by the size of motor units. This means that an individual muscle has less selective control when its motor units increase in size, such as expanding from 500 to 800 fibers per motor unit. The amount of angular joint force produced by a given muscle is further defined by the mechanical anatomy, such as the course of the tendon, the moment arm length from the center of motion to the tendon insertion, and the angular velocity of the motion.

Alteration of Muscle Mechanics

Normal mechanics of a muscle unit change over time under the influence of many factors. Areas that are of specific concern in the treatment of children with CP are the influence of growth and development, the impact of muscle tone change, and the impact of stretching and strengthening stimuli.

Muscle Control

Each group of motor units is controlled by one motor neuron that can only contract or not be active. Variable control of muscle contraction is gained by how many motor units are contracting in concert. In normal individuals, each gastrocnemius has approximately 1800 motor units; therefore, the brain, via the central program generator, has a choice of how many motor units to fire at a specific time.[1] If the central program generator is damaged, it cannot handle as many input and output choices. The number of motor units can be decreased, but the muscle stays the same size if the muscle fibers are enlarged and the number of fibers per motor neuron is increased. The central program generator also has to consider any change in fiber types, from fast twitch to slow twitch, as to the muscle's impact on activation of a specific motor unit. These fiber types are determined through motor neuron interaction.[3] The strength generated by each fiber is about the same.[6] It is not clear how this feedback occurs or what the factors are that cause the motor neuron to switch fiber types; however, there is documentation suggesting that in spastic muscles there is also a decrease in the number of mechanoreceptors within the muscles.[9] It is clear in children with CP and spasticity that there is reorganization with an increase of type 1 muscle fibers and a decrease in type 2 muscle fibers.[10, 11] There is an especially large loss of type 2b fibers, which are the anaerobic metabolism fibers. Therefore, the muscles in children with spasticity organize toward slower-twitch, fatigue-resistant fibers, which are organized into larger motor units having fewer mechanoreceptors. All these motor units add together to form a situation with fewer variables that the central program generator needs to control. Although the physiologic drivers for these changes are not well defined, this change of fewer variables and fewer inputs is very sensible in the context of dynamic motor control. There is no evidence that any of these changes can be reversed in children with CP because the real problem resides in the central program generator, which probably cannot be impacted. The primary pathology is in the central program generator; therefore, there is less control available, so secondary muscle alterations are of primary benefit to children's overall function.

Muscle Force-Generating Capacity

In young children, the cross section of the muscles is much larger compared with their body size than in adults. For example, a 2- to 3-year-old child who is 90 cm tall may have a gastrocnemius with a radius that is approximately one half of what it will be at maturity when he is 180 cm tall (Figure 6.6). At age 2 years, this child may have a radius of 2 cm in his gastrocnemius for a cross section of the gastrocnemius of approximately 12 cm². By maturity, the radius will double and he will have a cross-sectional area of approximately 50 cm². The muscle can generate 2 kg tension force per square centi-

Figure 6.6. Muscle shortening seen in children with spastic CP leads to the frequently observed decreased joint range of motion. This shortening of the muscle fiber also leads to significant changes in the length-tension response of the muscle. The impact of decreasing the muscle fiber length is seen to cause a great narrowing of the length–tension curve, meaning that the muscle can generate effect force over a much shorter range as well. This change concentrates the muscle force-generating ability into a very narrow range of joint motion (A). In addition, many children have decreased muscle diameters, causing muscle weakness defined as having a decreased ability to generate maximum force. This atrophy or weakness causes the peak tension of the length–tension curve to be decreased (B).

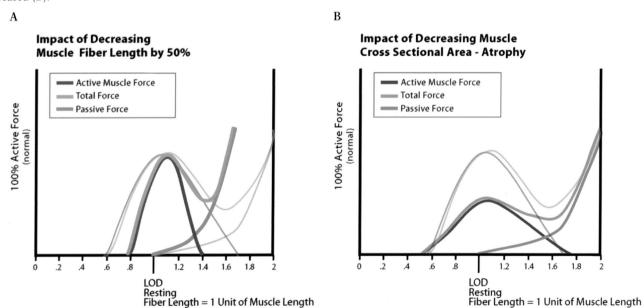

meter. Therefore, the 90-cm-tall boy weighing 12 kg generates 25 kg of force in his gastrocsoleus, whereas by adulthood he will generate only 100 kg of force for a 70-kg weight. This means the power of his gastrocsoleus will drop from more than 200% of body weight to 140% of body weight. This percent drop also demonstrates the importance of avoiding severe obesity because this same individual will only generate the same amount of gastrocsoleus force if he weighs 70 kg or 100 kg; this has significant implications when comparing toe walking in a 3- or 4-year-old with toe walking in an adult-sized individual. This force discrepancy is one reason why adults are not long-distance toe walkers in the same way many younger children are. As children grow, the cross-sectional area of their calves grow at approximately the same rate as height, and the area of muscle is defined by the radius. However, weight is defined by the expansion in length and width, which mathematically means it is the cube of expansion. Therefore, most young children generate high force for their weight, and as they grow older and heavier, their force-generating strength-to-weight ratio gradually decreases. Here, muscle strength is defined as the force-generating ability of a muscle, which is also impacted by repeated heavy loading. As a muscle experiences load, it increases the cross-sectional area of the muscle fibers as the primary mechanism of increasing muscle diameter. If a muscle is not used, the diameter of the muscle decreases as it thins the muscle fiber. This change implies that the body wants to avoid carrying extra muscle mass that is not needed. Therefore, muscle strength is increased with resistive weight training in which work and power are expended, although isometric contractions also increase muscle girth.

Children with CP are generally weaker, specifically meaning they have an inability to generate tension in the muscle.[12] The cause of this weakness is multifactorial; however, the lack of repeated maximal loading from play and activities of daily living is one significant factor. The inability of the neurologic system to cause coordinated contraction of all motor units in the same muscle may be another reason. As these children grow and the effect of increased mass becomes more problematic, there is a major boost in muscle mass and cross-sectional area development with the onset of puberty. Only at this time is there a measurable difference in the strength of the muscle. The growth hormones and androgens stimulate this development, which occurs at some level in nonambulatory children as well. The impact of testosterone is more dramatic than estrogen; therefore, males have larger and stronger muscles. Muscle-strengthening exercises as a treatment of muscle weakness, which is present in almost all children with CP, have traditionally been contraindicated because the effects of spasticity might be worse. This theory is clearly false and is related in part to misunderstanding strength. The strength of a contraction of a muscle or joint defined as the ability to move the joint against resistance during a physical examination has little relationship to the active force generated by an isolated contraction of a specific muscle. Recent work by Damiano and associates has shown that it is possible to do weight resistive training with children with CP, and also that there is a measurable increase in muscle force-generating ability with no recognizable side effects.[13, 14] Therefore, children who have functional deficits related to strength have no contraindication to strength training with resistive exercise. Some functional gain may develop, which is true especially for situations such as following surgery or casting where children have developed disuse atrophy.

Muscle Excursion

Muscle excursion is the difference between the maximum shortening and maximum lengthening of a muscle. The midpoint is called the rest length.

Muscle excursion is directly related to the available joint range of motion. As a muscle's physical length shortens, the associated joint loses range of motion. Also, as children grow, muscle length has to keep up with the increasing length of bone for it to continue to generate the correct amount of force. There is no known condition in which a muscle grows too long. The problem in CP is that muscles do not grow enough. As a consequence, the associated joints lose range of motion, which is called a muscle contracture. Contracture is a poor word because it leaves the impression that a muscle has somehow pulled into itself such that it could be pulled out of its contracted position. This concept is wrong, and what the term really means is that the muscle fibers are too short and have a decreased level of excursion. The stimulus for in vivo growth of muscle is poorly defined, but it is some combination of stretching to the maximum over a frequency or time period. This stimulus is almost exclusively a mechanical factor that is altered by an increase in muscle tone. The increase in muscle tone probably prevents children from stretching the muscle in a relaxed state during activities such as position changes in bed during sleep. If a joint is immobilized, the muscle will shorten, but it will lengthen again after release of joint immobility if the joint has a good range of motion. The length growth of a muscle occurs by muscle fibers adding sarcomeres at the muscle–tendon junction, very similar to the growth plate in bone.[15, 16] A muscle can also shorten by removing sarcomeres in this growth plate area, a trick the bone growth plate has not learned.

Increasing Excursion

The clinical treatment of shortened muscles known as contractures has traditionally focused on stretching range-of-motion exercises done with passive and active stretching. There is no doubt that children with no ability to do self-movement need to have their joints moved and these muscles stretched. For ambulatory children who are active ambulators and are growing fast, the goal of trying to avoid the muscles getting shorter and shorter by stimulating muscle growth through stretching is reasonable; however, the objective data to support the efficacy of this are minimal. Based on our examination of children in patterning therapy where they receive many hours of passive range-of-motion exercises, we believe it is possible to make muscles grow. However, the amount of passive range-of-motion stretching required is so disruptive to the lives of families and the other activities of these children that muscle contractures are far less disabling than the therapy to prevent the contractures. Stretching is like many exercise programs done for general health, meaning a little is better than none; however, there is an amount that makes a significant difference. We do not know how much stretching in the relaxed position is required; however, it is probably in the range of 4 to 8 hours per day.

Other treatments to make muscles grow are poorly documented. There are reports in the literature that claim that muscle growth occurred based on increased range of motion after Botox injections[17]; however, others, with careful assessment, have not found this to be the case.[18, 19] Muscles in spastic mice have been demonstrated to lose half their length as the spastic limbs grew.[16] Static stretch in a brace or a cast probably has some effect; however, this is not well documented. In an unpublished study, we tried to stretch hamstring muscles in children with the use of knee immobilizer splints. A splint was used every night on one leg but not the other. There was a measurable improvement in the popliteal angle, suggesting increased length in the muscle. However, the major problem was that only 30% of the children could follow through a 12-week wearing time on one leg only, which suggests that nighttime splinting does not have good acceptance with families or children.

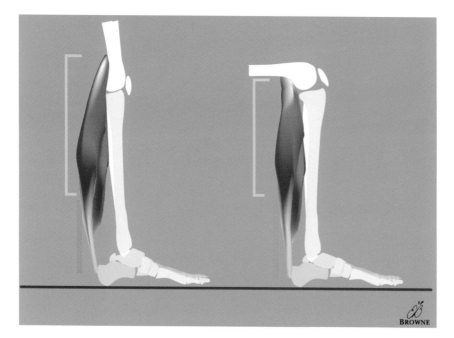

Figure 6.7. When the goal is to stretch the gastrocnemius, it is very important to realize that this cannot be done without also keeping the knee extended. This means nighttime ankle bracing without bracing the knee into extension is worse than not bracing because it only stretches the soleus, which is usually not contracted, and allows the gastrocnemius to further contract because the child will sleep with severe knee flexion.

Also, the splinting has to stretch the muscles. Many therapists believe children should wear ankle-foot orthotics (AFO) at night to stretch the contracted gastrocnemius. However, if only AFOs are used, children will flex the knee and only the soleus gets stretched, further increasing the length difference many children already have between the gastrocnemius and soleus muscles (Figure 6.7). Stretching the gastrocnemius requires the use of a knee extension splint and a dorsiflexion splint, a combination that is bulky and adds to the poor acceptance. The use of casting adds other problems, especially muscle atrophy. One of the most efficient ways to shrink the size of a muscle is to rigidly immobilize the joint in a cast so the muscle has no motion possible. No documentation is available to show that a muscle grows longer if immobilized under tension in a cast; however, based on knowledge of how muscle grows, it probably does grow longer in addition to developing severe atrophy. The severe atrophy and temporary nature of the clinical length gain make the use of casting for chronic management of short muscles in children with CP a poor choice. The major problem in the research of muscle growth is the difficulty of measuring muscle growth separate from tendon growth. The mechanical stimuli for growth of these two different anatomic structures, muscles and tendons, somewhat overlap and the effort to cause muscle growth probably causes tendon growth as well.

Connective Tissue Mechanics

Short muscles in CP are clinically well recognized; however, the problem of excessive length of the tendons is often not recognized. The high-riding patella is an exception. However, surgeons who operate on the tendons frequently see tendons that are much too long, as if these tendons were trying to make some adjustment for the very short muscles (Figure 6.8). Tendons grow by interstitial growth throughout, but most of the growth seems to occur at the tendon–bone interface.[20] Tendons also increase their cross-sectional area through growth, which increases the strength of the tendons. The stimulus for increased tendon growth and tendon cross-sectional area growth is not well defined, but depends heavily on the force environment. The regulation of length growth is heavily influenced by tension, but the

Figure 6.8. Tendons have a growth plate-like structure at the tendon–bone interface and at the muscle–tendon interface, this structure is a high concentration of satellite cells that contribute to muscle growth. In addition, the muscles and tendons also have some interstitial growth ability.

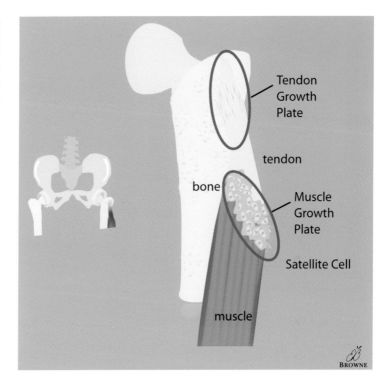

specific stimuli that cause growth are not well defined. Tendons contain mechanoreceptors called Golgi tendon organs, which give feedback to the brain and also influence the sensitivity of muscle spindles.[21] This scenario suggests that tension on a tendon makes the motor neuron more sensitive to fire through its modulation by the muscle spindle. In the presence of spasticity with continuous low-level tension, this system may be altered to accommodate for chronic stimulation, possibly by the system dropping mechanoreceptors.[9] Therefore, the stimulus for growth may also cause the response to decrease the number of mechanoreceptors so that the stimulation of a muscle is decreased.

Another connective tissue effect that has been long recognized and recently better quantified is the increase in connective tissue in the muscle in the presence of spasticity.[22] This increase is responsible for the increase in the stiffness of the muscle and may also be related to decreased excursion. This process of increasing connective tissue seems to get worse with increasing magnitude of spasticity, increasing exposure time to spasticity, and increasing age of the patient. This is another component of what is defined as the contracture, but is the least understood element of this pathology. We know of no treatment to impact this process.

Growth of the Muscle–Tendon Unit

The current understanding of growth regulation of a muscle–tendon unit is that the muscle fibers grow in response to stretching of the sarcomeres while they are not actively firing. This stretch has to occur for some amount of time each day. The tendon grows in length by summation of the total tension over time. The specific pattern of maximum to minimum tension is unknown. Another factor that is important but not well understood is the influence of motion, which both muscles and tendons need to have for healthy growth. Defining the specific stimulus for growth of tendons compared with muscles would be a useful research project. These two structures balance themselves

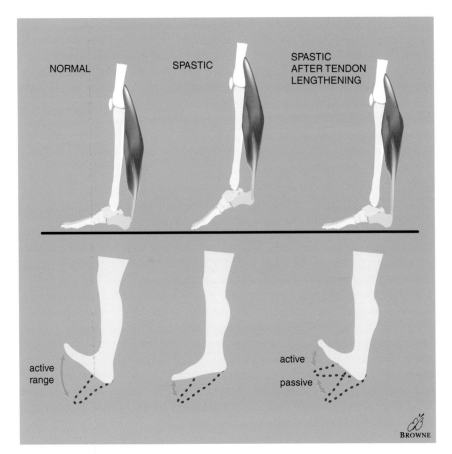

NORMAL

SPASTIC

SPASTIC
AFTER TENDON
LENGTHENING

active
range

active

passive

BROWNE

Figure 6.9. The length of the muscle fiber directly determines the active total joint range of motion; however, the muscle rest length plus tendon length defines where that active range of motion occurs. Therefore, if the active range of the ankle is from −20° of dorsiflexion to 60° of plantar flexion, there is no definitely known mechanism to lengthen the muscle fiber and create an active range of muscle activity from 30° of dorsiflexion to 60° of plantar flexion. However, by lengthening the Achilles tendon, we can move the 40° active range to 10° of dorsiflexion to 30° of plantar flexion, a much more useful position of the muscle's active range of motion. This is the principal function of tendon lengthening in short spastic muscles.

out as if one were trying to make up for the other's deficiency. The physical impact of a short muscle is to decrease joint range of motion. The physical impact of tendon length is to determine the anatomic range in which a muscle can apply its reduced range-of-motion activity. For example, a 50% decrease in the muscle fiber length of the gastrocsoleus will reduce the available range of motion from 60° to 30°. The length of the tendon then will determine if active range of motion occurs from −15° dorsiflexion to 45° plantar flexion or if the active range of motion will occur from 10° dorsiflexion to 20° of plantar flexion. The tendon length is the surgically approachable aspect of this problem (Figure 6.9). By lengthening the tendon, surgeons can choose where to place the active range of motion; however, there is no way of increasing the active range of motion, which would require increasing muscle fiber growth. Usually, if the tendon is found to be shorter than would be functionally ideal, the opposing tendon will be long. For example, with the short gastrocsoleus, the tibialis anterior almost always has a tendon that is causing its active range of motion to also function in equinus. By lengthening the short tendon of the gastrocnemius, the too-long tibialis anterior tendon will spontaneously decrease its muscle fiber length and tendon length. Shortening tendons is seldom required, and except for a few upper extremity tendons, does not work well. This also means if surgeons do a little too much lengthening, the body will adjust the tension by altering the muscle fiber length and, to a lesser degree, the tendon length. This mechanism can function only if the muscle–tendon unit is intact, and it cannot function if the tendon is completely transected. If the tendon is transected and becomes thin from experiencing no force, the muscle will become severely atrophied with very short fibers.

The ideal goal of treatment in children with spastic CP would be to make muscles grow and tendons shrink. The muscles are normal, and as the bones grow, the muscles grow too, but not enough to keep up with bone growth. The tendons make up the difference. The strong flexor muscles usually develop relatively short tendons, which are still longer than normal, and the extensor muscles, which are short, develop excessively long tendons. The only treatment with confirmed efficacy is surgical lengthening of the relatively short tendons. Other treatments, such as passive range of motion, splinting, and Botox injections, may have short-term benefits that can delay the need for surgical lengthening.

Bone Mechanics

Bones are the strong, supportive structures that provide the structural frames on which all mobility depends. Ambulatory children have few problems with the strength of bones; however, this is a major concern for nonambulatory children. Osteopenia and osteoporosis are major problems and are largely related to decreased force experienced by the bones. These problems were discussed at length in the metabolic bone discussion. The stimulus for length growth occurring at the growth plates is the result of hormonal, genetic, and mechanical factors. The hormonal factors may be abnormal for children whose apophyseal pituitary axes were involved in their original CP lesions. This involvement primarily occurs in children who are nonambulatory; however, we have several patients who ambulate independently and were found to have growth hormone deficiency. Children's height should be routinely measured, and when they fall below the fifth percentile on the growth chart or have no growth over 1 year, referral for full endocrinologic evaluation is recommended. A much more frequent effect causing diminished growth in one leg is the decreased force exposure, which occurs in the involved limb of children with hemiplegia. The hemiplegic limb is usually 1 to 2 cm shorter by the conclusion of growth. If this difference is more than 2 cm, a leg equalization procedure may be needed.

Another area of force effects on bone is the prevention of infantile bone shape maturation into adult-shaped bone configurations. This bone maturation occurs through the influence of the muscle action, causing remodeling effects on the growing bone through Pauwel's law.[23] The lack of remodeling frequently leaves children with an infantile bone shape, such as increased femoral anteversion or tibial torsion. Although unclear, there are suggestions that in very young children, under age 5 years, abnormal forces can cause the bones to develop abnormal torsion.[24] Careful attention to correcting the abnormal forces in early childhood is especially important to prevent recurrence or a new deformity. However, there is no evidence to suggest that correcting these forces can cause correction of infantile torsional deformities.

Joint Mechanics

The joints require motion for normal development during childhood. The ligament and joint capsules, which provide stability to the joints, have interstitial growth throughout their entire length.[25] However, over time if there is no motion, the structures tighten and restrict joint range of motion. In children with CP, this occurs very slowly. For example, hamstring contractures, which prevent full knee extension, only very slowly allow the development of a fixed knee contracture; however, by adolescence and after puberty, this process occurs much faster. Also, these flexion contractures are much more amenable to stretching out in young children. During childhood growth, many joints are very sensitive to abnormal joint reaction forces. These abnormal forces may cause substantial abnormalities in the development of the joints and, in some cases, lead to joint dislocation. Joint dislocation is a prominent problem at the hip and is a lesser problem in the other joints. The specific joint problems are addressed in the sections devoted to those joints. Children with spastic CP have a tendency to have short muscles, which translates into decreased joint range of motion. The decreased range of motion subsequently leads to fixed joint contractures, even when there are no structural joint deformities.

Joint Motor Mechanics

Often, the mechanics of a single joint are based on the specifics of the involved joint; however, the only active way to move a joint is by the muscle attached to that joint. These muscle–tendon units attach in the bone and work by creating a moment through a moment arm. An excellent example of this is the knee, where the hamstring muscles attach to the tibia by being posterior to the joint's center of motion. A moment arm is created and a tension force is applied to create a moment that may cause motion. The moment created is called the strength of the hamstring in clinical scenarios (Figure 6.10). The amount of strength, or joint moment, that is created includes the percent of the muscle's contraction, the cross-sectional area of the muscle, the position of the muscle fiber length on the Blix curve, the direction and velocity of the change in the muscle fiber, and the moment arm of the muscle. Another variable is muscle fiber configuration with the degree of pennation of the fibers to the line of action of the muscle. In the hamstring muscles, this variable is of no significance because of a very low pennation angle. Some of these variables can be actively altered, and others are structural variables. The variables that can be actively altered are the percent of muscle firing, the moment arm length, the position on the Blix curve, and the velocity of length change. The variables with the structural characteristics that can change over time are the diameter of the muscle through muscle

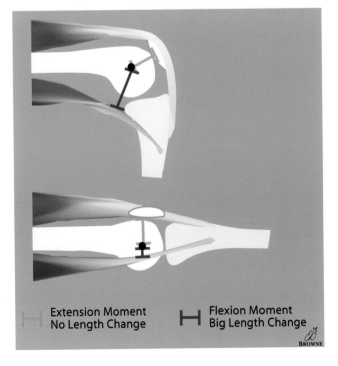

**Extension Moment
No Length Change**   **Flexion Moment
Big Length Change**

Figure 6.10. To understand the force-generating ability of the muscle, it is very important to understand the concept of stable versus changing moment arms. An example is the quadriceps, which has a relatively consistent moment arm length independent of the joint position. The hamstrings, on the other hand, have a moment arm that is very dependent on joint position with the moment arm being very short at knee extension and very long at full knee flexion. Thus, the impact of a hamstring contracture very quickly becomes more significant as the degree of knee flexion increases.

hypertrophy or growth, the position on the Blix curve by the addition or sub-
traction of sarcomeres, and the moment arm length by bone shape change
and tendon length.

Single-Joint Muscles

From the perspective of the central program generator, muscle activation
that crosses a single joint requires consideration of the impact of at least three
variables, including the percent of motor units to activate, the current length
of the fiber that will define the moment arm and the Blix curve location, and
the velocity of muscle fiber shortening. The system also has to consider its
longer-term organization caused by structural alterations. From the treatment
perspective, the major alterations are made in the structural variable. A major
element in the clinical assessment of children is trying to understand if these
structural changes are positive to the function of the joint and the whole-
body motor system or if this structural change is now part of the pathology
of the impairment that is increasing the disability. The intellectual understanding of muscles that cross single joints, such as the short head of the
biceps femoris, is relatively easy. The force generated is easily modeled, leading to a clear understanding of the effects; however, in children with CP, these
single joint crossing muscles cause far fewer problems than the muscles that
cross multiple joints.

Multiple-Joint Muscles

Multiple-joint muscles, such as the rectus femoris and the gastrocnemius,
comprise most of the problematic muscles. With these muscles, it is extremely hard to conceptualize a clear understanding of an individual muscle's
function at a specific time in the gait cycle of a child. For example, the long
head of the biceps femoris crosses the hip and knee joints; therefore, the
number of variables in the control algorithm more than doubles, because
now the hip position and knee position have to be considered for each variable (Table 6.2). This complexity is relatively apparent, and it is easy to
understand why control of these muscles is most problematic for the central
program generators of children with CP. These multiple-joint muscles tend
to function predominantly as energy transfer muscles and in deceleration;
this means multiple-joint muscles are used predominantly in situations that
require eccentric contraction. In approaching these muscles as a treating
physician, an attempt needs to be made to understand as many of the variables in the control scenario as possible. However, dynamic control theory
seems to work better to understand the process. The easy example of this is

Table 6.2. Factors that have to be controlled during a contraction of the semitendinosus compared with the vastus.

	Semitendinosus	Vastus
Active change	Eccentric or concentric or isometric Muscle fiber length Muscle tension Tendon length Moment arm at the knee that changes Position of the knee joint to determine moment arm Moment arm of the hip that moves Position of the hip joint to determine moment arm Position of the hip and knee to determine muscle fiber length Direction and velocity of hip and knee joint motion	Eccentric or concentric or isometric Muscle fiber length Muscle tension Tendon length Moment arm at the knee that is static Position of the knee joint only to determine muscle fiber length Direction and velocity of only knee joint motion
Long-term changes	Fiber types Muscle resting fiber length Size of the motor unit	Fiber types Muscle resting fiber length Size of the motor unit

the spastic rectus muscle, which may contract too long in the swing phase, causing knee stiffness and subsequent toe drag. Although this is the most common cause of toe drag in children with CP, there are many other variables in the cause of knee stiffness related to other abnormal contraction patterns and to the amount of power output to cause knee flexion. However, in clinical study, we see patients who have no problems with decreased or delayed knee flexion in swing phase, whereas other children who have almost the same examination and input data demonstrate a significant knee stiffness in swing phase with toe drag as a major complaint. This scenario suggests that there is a strong attractor to walk with enough knee flexion to be functional or, alternatively, fall into the stiff knee gait pattern. Although this pattern varies, it is unusual to see children in whom it is unclear if the pattern is present. If children have a stiff knee gait, it may be harder to decide if the problem should be treated, which basically means making a decision about how strong the attractor is to keep the stiff knee gait pattern of these children. Most muscle pathomechanics in the treatment of gait in children with CP involves trying to understand the complex interactions of these multiple-joint muscles.

Global Body Mechanics of Human Gait

Human walking is a complex interaction between the central nervous system and the peripheral musculoskeletal system. Understanding the combined function of the mechanical components of the musculoskeletal system in a way that produces functional gait requires an assessment of what the whole organism has to accomplish to be able to ambulate. For example, it is not enough to understand how the muscle generates tension and then translates it into joint power. This joint power has to occur in a well-orchestrated fashion. The elements of the whole body that are important in the production of functional gait require individuals to have the ability to conceptualize where they want to move. Individuals have to have sufficient energy available for mobility, their bodies have to be able to balance themselves, their central program generators have to be able to provide motor control, and their mechanical structures have to be stable to support the force output. The airplane can serve as an analogy to human walking in which the determination of where the airplane should fly is an administrative decision made during the creation of flight schedules. The crew arrives on the airplane after being given the information of where to go, and it is the responsibility of the crew to make sure that they have enough fuel that can get to the engines to use as energy. While the airplane is sitting on its wheels, it is very stable; however, this stability has to shift into a stability of momentum of air flight controlled by gyroscopes, which monitor the in-flight balance. The crew, through the available computer, has to control the engine speed and airplane direction as the most direct control of the system. Each mechanical component of the airplane has to function or the crew has to make adjustments for a malfunction. For instance, if one engine stops, the plane can still fly, but appropriate adjustments have to be made. Just as with airplane flight, the musculoskeletal subsystems have to always be considered when evaluating the global gait function of individuals.

Cognitive Subsystem

Occasionally, children will present with the question from parents of why they do not walk. After a full history, it may be determined that these children

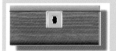 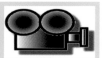

Case 6.1   Caleb

Caleb, a 4-year-old boy with mild diplegia, was brought in for an evaluation because of his parents' concerns that he was not able to advance to independent ambulation. He had no contractures on physical examination, had walked with a reverse walker for 2 years, but was unable to stand without holding on with his arms. He appeared to be cognitively age appropriate. He used articulated AFOs with a dorsiflexion posterior strap, which limited him to 10° dorsiflexion. In physical therapy he worked to learn to use quad canes that were weighted. His parents were mostly interested that he progress to independent ambulation. After the evaluation, his parents were told that the primary problem was his poor balance, and he was old enough to learn to use crutches, which would likely be the assistive device he would use at maturity. Continuing to use the canes is a good stimulus for balance development but these devices are never functional ambulatory aids. Two years later, after training in therapy and a lot of practice, he was very proficient with crutches.

have severe mental retardation, which may be the reason for not walking. These children may not have conceptualized the idea of getting from one place to another or be willing to try new ways of mobility such as getting up off the floor. For example, a child with a cognitive level of 3 to 6 months will not even try to walk, even though this same child's motor development may be such that he could walk from a motor perspective. Many of these children will slowly develop insight with stimulation to the point where they will stand up suddenly and start walking. The oldest child in whom we have seen this occur was just short of her 13th birthday. This kind of dramatic late beginning of walking never occurs if the major impairment limiting walking is in any other subsystem except the cognitive system.

Balance Subsystem

Balance is required for children to ambulate, and this is often the difference between independent bipedal ambulation and ambulation in a quadruped pattern with a walking aid. Balance is a complex function, in which most of the research has been reported with standing[26] or sitting balance studies.[27] The concept of balance during ambulation is hard to define, but it is primarily measured by high variability in step lengths, step widths, and joint range of motion. Often, the transitions in movement, such as stopping and standing or starting from a sitting position, are especially difficult when balance is a major impairment (Case 6.1).

Energy Production

Ambulation always requires an output of energy as fuel for the muscles. Even downhill walking, which in many mechanical systems can generate energy, requires more energy than it generates with human gait. Children must have the energy available for the musculoskeletal system to use or walking is not possible or comfortable (Case 6.2). A typical reason for low energy supply is a walking pattern that consumes more energy than children can generate (Case 6.3). Another common cause is poor cardiovascular conditioning, which limits the amount of energy available to the musculoskeletal system.

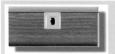

Case 6.2   Kimberly

Kimberly, a 12-year-old girl with significant hypotonia, was evaluated because her parents complained that she had decreased walking endurance. On physical examination, general muscle weakness and hypotonia were noted. Her videotape demonstrated a gait pattern typical of hypotonia. On assessment of her energy requirements of walking, she was found to have walking velocity of 85 cm/s with an oxygen cost of 0.12 ml oxygen per kilogram of body weight per meter of distance covered. This was 2.3 standard deviations below the mean, indicating that her energy efficiency was much better than normal children of her size. In spite of this energy-efficient gait, her main complaint was decreased endurance. Although there was no known diagnosis in Kimberly except hypotonia, we made the presumption based on her energy use that there was a deficiency in the way the muscle used energy; therefore, her limited endurance was due to primary muscle pathology, not mechanical inefficiency.

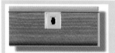

Case 6.3   Collette

Collette had severe diplegia, and during middle childhood and adolescence, had many operative procedures to correct femoral anteversion, crouched gait, and stiff knee gait. She attended a regular high school, which required long walks between classes. In middle childhood she used a posterior walker and was later switched to Lofstrand crutches, which she used exclusively by high school. During high school, in the period of her adolescent growth, she developed knee pain and complained about increased fatigue. An oxygen consumption test showed that she walked with a very slow velocity of 78 cm/s with an oxygen cost of 0.52 ml O_2/kg/m (0.27 normal predicted), which was 3.9 standard deviations above the normal mean. Based on the complete analysis, there were no mechanical inefficiencies that could be corrected, and it was recommended that she get a wheelchair to use for long-distance ambulation. She obtained a wheelchair and used it in school for many months until her knee pain resolved. However, she was very unhappy in the wheelchair because she believed she was gaining weight, felt herself becoming more deconditioned, and did not like to sit when talking to friends who were standing. She decided to walk with her crutches, which she did throughout high school, and she completed a university nursing degree walking with her crutches. As a young adult in her mid-twenties, she said she still had a wheelchair somewhere, but she did not quite remember where it was because she never needed it.

Motor Control

Motor control is an extremely important aspect of developing good walking skills. Individuals with significant motor control disorders, or the inability to develop motor control, will have significant problems with gait. This aspect is discussed at length in Chapter 3 on neurologic control.

Structural Stability

The mechanical mobility system includes the muscles, bones, and tendons. The interaction of these structural elements is the primary focus of much of the remainder of this chapter because it is the area where the most opportunity is present to make alterations in the system to functionally improve children's gait. As understanding of the mechanics of walking in individual children is gained from a clinical perspective, the defined methods of measuring the effects of different subsystems also have to be understood.

Measurement Techniques Used in Gait Analysis

Measuring human walking with techniques that delineate the functional components is called gait analysis. This analysis is a critical process in understanding the problems of children with abnormal gait. The analysis needs to be performed with the same scientific understanding and organization upon which modern medical practice is based. For example, physicians treating hypertension have to understand the physiologic basis of hypertension, do a workup to determine the specific etiology of hypertension in an individual patient, then plan the treatment, which is followed by an ongoing evaluation of the response to the treatment. Usually, this means the patient is given medication and the response of the medication is monitored by periodically measuring his blood pressure. This same workup and treatment outline is applied to the treatment of gait abnormalities in children with CP. This process can only be done with an appropriate understanding of the physiology of each of the subsystems involved in the creation of human gait. For this reason, descriptions of the response of the central nervous system, muscles, connective tissue, and bones are detailed. The next step in this process is to understand gait as a functional entity, which requires an understanding of the components of the gait evaluation process. This evaluation process follows the modern medical evaluation model currently used in almost all medical disciplines, which means physicians always start with a history and physical examination, then order additional tests as indicated by the initial data. With gait, the additional tests include recording of a videotape, kinematic and kinetic evaluation, understanding muscle activation patterns with electromyogram (EMG) and pediabarograph, and measuring the energy demands of walking.

History

Patients' histories should include an understanding of the etiology of the CP if one is known. A history of the developmental milestones related to ambulation, such as when did these children start cruising and when did independent ambulation start, should also be included. The recent functional history is important, and it should include issues such as how frequently do the children fall, how often do they wear through shoes, and have they gotten better, worse, or stayed the same in the last 6 to 12 months. The parents or caretakers should always be asked what their concerns are relative to the children's ambulatory problems (Table 6.3).

Physical Examination

The physical examination needs to focus on the aspects that are important in understanding the etiology of the gait problems, including evaluation of global functions, such as balance, independent motor control ability, muscle strength, muscle tone, muscle contractures, and bone alignments (Table 6.4).

Global Function Measures

In routine clinical evaluation the specific measurement of global gait function is recorded by noting functional abilities such as children's ability to walk

Table 6.3. Elements of the history that are important in gait treatment decision making.

History questions	Information applications
Was the child premature?	Prematurity has more predictable spasticity, usually with diplegic pattern involvement.
What is the known cause of the CP?	Some causes, such as middle childhood trauma, have a different course.
How has the child changed in the last 6 to 12 months?	It is important to consider if the child is improving, static, or diminishing in physical skills.
What is the child's level of cognitive function?	This can give a level of expectation of future improvement with therapy or the ability to do self-directed therapy.
Does the child wear orthotics and for how much time each day?	If the orthotics are being worn but are ineffective, other treatment is indicated.
Does the child object to orthotic wear?	Some adolescents refuse orthotic wear because of cosmetic concerns and this has to be considered.
Does the child use an assistive device in the home?	A good idea of the child's function at home and in the community is important to consider.
Does the child use an assistive device in the community or school?	A good idea of the child's function at home and in the community is important to consider.
Does the child use a wheelchair? If yes, when?	This, again, is a part of understanding the function of the child, and a child using a wheelchair as primary ambulation is hard to change to ambulation.
Does the child complain of pain? If yes, when and where?	This can be a major limitation on function.
What are the concerns of the family?	The family will not be happy with any treatment outcome if their concerns are not addressed.
What are the child's concerns if he or she is mature enough to have an opinion?	Also, addressing the child's concerns, especially if he or she is an adolescent, is important. These concerns are often different from the parents' concerns.
What have been the previous musculoskeletal surgeries and treatments?	Future treatment has to consider prior treatment.

independently, to walk with one hand held, or to hop on one foot. A specific set of parameters that also relate to motor development should be monitored (Table 6.5). For a more in-depth gait analysis, the use of the Gross Motor Function Measure (GMFM) is recommended. The whole GMFM measure can be used, but we prefer to use only the fourth dimension, which is the standing dimension of the GMFM that focuses on standing and transitional movements. These movements are of most interest to orthopaedists, especially in children who are being evaluated for gait problems. This measure gives a numerical score and is useful as a general measure of children's balance, motor control, and motor planning. Other more specific tests of balance or motor planning are available, but currently these are mainly used for research purposes and not for standard diagnostic clinical evaluations.

Motor Control

Individual muscle motor control is tested on routine evaluation by noting in general terms if children can make steps on command, move the foot on command, and stand on one leg with the hand held. For more detailed gait analysis, an assessment of each major muscle group in the lower extremities should be made. For example, a child is asked to extend the knee, and if knee extension is performed as an isolated movement, it is rated as good. If the knee can be extended, but only associated with joint motion, such as hip extension or plantar flexion with the knee extension, it is rated as fair. If no voluntary focal movement of the specific joint occurs, it is rated as poor motor control (Table 6.6). Children with cognitive limitations that are so severe that they do not understand the concept cannot be rated.

Table 6.4. Physical examination parameters.

Parameter	Full gait analysis	Routine clinical evaluation
Global Motor Function Balance (GMFM)	GMFM may use only standing dimension.	Record what general functions, such as single leg and standing, hopping, or running, a child can do.
Muscle strength	Do manual muscle testing of the major muscles of the lower extremity.	Record general comments of good to poor strength.
Passive joint range of motion	Do goniometer measurements of all major joint motions in lower extremity. Record ROM of hip abduction, rotation, popliteal angle, knee extension, ankle dorsiflexion with knee extended and knee flexed.	Record ROM of hip abduction, rotation, popliteal angle, knee extension, ankle dorsiflexion with knee extended and knee flexed at each outpatient clinic visit.
Motor control	Record active motor control of major lower extremity motions.	Make a general comment of motor control, such as good or poor.

	Motor Control
Grading Score	Description
Good	Patient can isolate individual muscle contractions through the entire available passive range of motion upon command.
Fair	Patient is able to initiate muscle contractions upon command, but is unable to completely isolate the contraction through the entire available passive range of motion.
Poor	Patient is unable to isolate individual muscle contractions secondary to synergistic patterns, increased tone, and/or decreased activation.

	Muscle Strength
Grading Score	Description
1	Contraction visible in the muscle but no visible movement of the joint.
2	Can do partial arc of motion with gravity reduced.
3−	Can do complete arc of available joint motion with gravity reduced.
3	Can move joint through available range against gravity.
3+	Can move joint through available range against gravity with minimum additional resistance.
4−	Can move joint through available range against gravity with definite additional resistance.
4	Able to move joint through available range against moderate resistance.
4+	Able to move joint through available range against increased moderate resistance.
5	Able to move joint through maximum resistance expected for the specific muscle.

Table 6.5. Level of ambulatory ability.

Mobility Function:

1. Independent community ambulation, uses no assistive device or wheelchair
2. Ambulation with assistive device such as walker or crutches, uses a wheelchair less than 50% of the time for community mobility
3. Household ambulation, uses a wheelchair more than 50% of the time for community mobility
4. Exercise ambulation, uses a wheelchair 100% of the time for community mobility
5. Primary wheelchair user in home and the community, does weightbearing transfers in and out of wheelchair
6. Wheelchair user, dependent for transfer

Table 6.6. Motor control grading.

Good	Patient is able to isolate individual muscle contraction through entire available passive range of motion upon command.
Fair	Patient is able to initiate muscle contraction upon command, but is unable to completely isolate contraction through entire passive range of motion.
Poor	Patient is unable to isolate individual muscle contraction secondary to synergistic patterns, increased tone, and/or decreased or absent activation.

Muscle Strength

Strength of each major muscle or muscle group in the lower extremity is tested with a 0 to 5 rating scale (see Table 6.4). Testing the muscle strength in children with spasticity can be difficult. We use the standard term of resistance until children cannot sustain the load. The strength levels of moving against gravity may be difficult to determine with spasticity present, as co-contraction severely limits motion, not in the technical sense of muscle weakness, but because the agonist cannot overpower the co-contraction of the antagonist. It is best to stay with a narrow definition of strength assignment, but make comments if the strength is strongly affected by spasticity or co-contraction. Strength testing depends on voluntary motion of children who can give their full effort. If the children's behavior or severe mental retardation preclude this level of cooperation, strength testing cannot be completed. When strength testing children weighing 15 kg compared with adolescents weighing 80 kg, a subjective assessment of their appropriate strength has to be made by the examiner. This makes the strength examination somewhat more subjective and focuses on the importance of the examiner having extensive pediatric experience.

Muscle Tone

Muscle tone is another important aspect in monitoring the assessment of gait impairments. In routine clinical evaluations, gastrocnemius and rectus spasticity provides a general overview. Also, subjective comments about the relative importance of the spasticity and the children's support, as well as problems that the spasticity is causing, should be noted. For more detailed assessments, the major motor groups in the lower extremities should have numerical assessment of spasticity. The modified Ashworth scale is preferred because it provides more options and allows notation of hypotonia (Table 6.7).

Passive Range-of-Motion Assessment

Muscle contractures are monitored by routinely recording specific measures made in the same fashion. These measures often include specific joint range of motion as accurately as the clinician can determine. Notation should also be made with regard to the source of the contracture, especially if it is believed to be a muscle contracture or a fixed joint-based contracture. Bone deformities and length should be noted as well. The specific joint examination should include a back examination with comments of scoliosis as determined by the forward bend test, significant lordosis, or kyphosis present in standing or sitting. At the hip, knee, ankle, and foot, standard joint ranges of motion are recorded.

Table 6.7. Modified Ashworth scale.

00	Hypotonic.
0	No increase in tone.
1	Slight increase in tone manifested by a catch and release or by minimal resistance at the end of range of motion.
1+	Slight increase in muscle tone manifested by a catch followed by minimal resistance throughout the remainder (less than half) of the range of motion.
2	More marked increase in muscle tone through most of the range of motion, but affected part easily moved.
3	Considerable increase in muscle tone, passive movement difficult.
4	Affected part rigid.

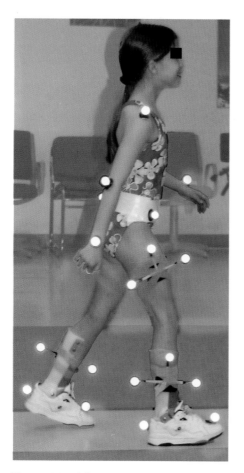

Figure 6.11. The most common gait measurement system requires that the individual being measured is instrumented with retroreflective markers that are imaged by multiple video cameras. The markers define specific anatomic body points, which the computer program uses to calculate joint motion.

Videotaping

In the assessment of gait in developing children, the simplest and cheapest method also provides the most data needed for routine clinical decision making. A videotape of these children should be made in an open area with a predetermined format. The format requires that the children be undressed to only thin underwear or swimming suits. The videotape is made with a frontal and a rear view, then with both right and left lateral views. The videotape should include gait with bare feet, with the shoes and orthotics that are typically worn, and the children should be asked to run. Also, different assistive devices are included as appropriate. Usually, the videotape is 1 to 2 minutes long and is seldom more than 3 minutes long. A storage and retrieval system for the videotapes must be available so they can be retrieved for each clinic visit. At each visit, the video is reviewed as the children's gait is observed. On routine evaluations, a videotape is always made at the first evaluation, and a new videotape is added as changes are noted with each examination. When children are under age 3 years, a new videotape is typically made every 6 months. From 3 to 12 years of age, a new videotape is made every 12 months, and over 12 years of age, approximately every 2 to 3 years. This time table is individualized to each child and a new videotape is made only when some change is noted based on a subjective clinical evaluation of the child and of previous videotapes.

Kinematics

During kinematic evaluations, the motion of each joint is measured as the children walk. These measurements are used to provide additional information to help make major interventional decisions, such as surgery or difficult orthotic decisions. Also, the kinematic evaluation is important as a measure of children's response to treatment. Kinematic evaluations are performed only as part of a full gait analysis. The modern interest in measurements of human motion started in the first half of the 1900s with the use of stop-frame video pictures from which each angle could be drawn to assign measures from one frame to the next. With improvement in camera technology and computers, this same concept is still the primary method of measuring joint range of motion during gait. The process is now completely automated, so it is fast, efficient, reliable, and accurate (Figure 6.11). Other technology, such as the use of accelerometers or electronic goniometers, have been explored for kinematic measurements; however, the optical system is the only system widely used in clinical diagnostic laboratories.

Optical Measurement

The modern optical kinematic measurement is based on dividing the body into segments. The most commonly used clinical systems divide the body into 7 or 13 segments (Figure 6.12). Each of the segments is defined by an embedded Cartesian coordinate system related to the specific segment's bony anatomy. The motion of each of these segments relative to its adjacent segment is marked by placing retroreflective markers on specific anatomic landmarks within the segment. Each segment must be defined by a minimum of 3 markers, which means that for a full body assessment 39 markers are required. Then, each of these markers is imaged by a minimum of two cameras simultaneously. With the same marker being imaged from two cameras separated in space, the exact position in three-dimensional space for the marker can be defined. This is the same method our brain uses to give us three-dimensional vision. Because of visual obstruction, most current kinematic

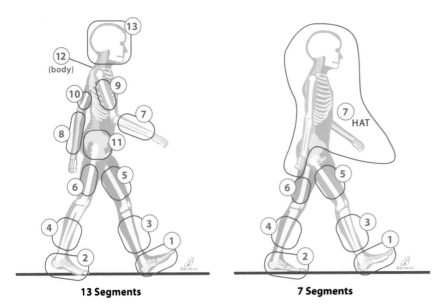

13 Segments **7 Segments**

Figure 6.12. To calculate body motion in space or kinematics, mechanical models of the human body have to be developed. In current clinical gait analysis, the 7-segment model of two feet, two shanks, two thighs, and the HAT (head-arms-trunk) segments has been in use the longest. As computer power has increased, there has been a movement to the 13-segment model, which includes two feet, two shanks, two thighs, two forearms, two upper arms, a pelvis, a trunk, and the head.

analysis systems use five to eight cameras placed circumferentially around a child. These cameras are focused on a fixed space in the room, which is assigned a room coordinate system. All cameras are synchronized to take images at the same time, for gait usually at a rate of 60 frames per second. With current clinical gait analysis systems, this process of identifying the marker and calculating its precise position in three-dimensional space is all automated; however, some error still occurs requiring each patient to be reviewed by a technical person who has experience with the system, usually an individual trained in biomechanics. Once the marker is identified in space, specialized software defines the specific assigned segment whose motion can then be calculated into clinically defined joint range of motion.

The specific joint motion is calculated from the motion of each segment. A problem that occurs in this reduction process is that the motion of the markers includes soft-tissue motion because the markers are not fixed to bones, but are attached to the skin. To counteract soft-tissue movement, the marker path is smoothed to remove high-frequency motion and the segments are assumed to be attached at points that represent accurate anatomic structure, because joints rarely have any measurable motion in translation or distraction. These two data manipulations help decrease the soft-tissue artifact; however, soft-tissue motion still has to be considered as a possible measurement error in some children if unexplained motion is found. The next major task in the kinematic data reduction is to assign specific clinically recognizable joint positions, such as degrees of flexion or rotation. This task requires choosing a method to reduce the three-dimensional data. Understanding this system is important for clinicians because it may explain the size of some of the numbers that do not correlate with physicians' own assessments.

Data Reduction Algorithms

All commercially available clinical data reduction software algorithms currently in use reduce the data using Euler angles.[2] In this approach, each coordinate system is rotated to neutral with respect to its adjacent coordinate system in a predetermined order. This process mimics what clinicians routinely do in physical examinations. For example, when a physician measures a specific contracture of the hip, he would say there is so much abduction, so much flexion, and so much rotation present. The mathematical concepts

Figure 6.13. The use of Euler angle calculations is very order dependent; therefore, the order of the calculations has to be understood. For example, the position of the shoulder with a calculation order of 45° internal rotation, 45° abduction, and 45° flexion (A) is very different from the position obtained with 45° flexion, 45° abduction, and 45° internal rotation (B).

A

B

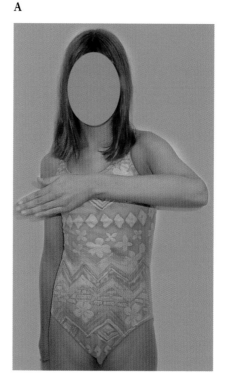
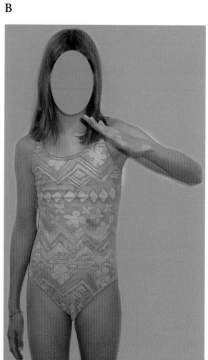

of the Euler angles were initially applied to biomechanics because they closely mimic clinical practice.[28] The problem with this mathematical system that clinicians must be aware of is that Euler angle reduction is very sensitive to the order of reduction in joints with large, 3° freedom of movement. These joints include the hip, shoulder, and subtalar joints. For example, a shoulder position of 45° flexion, 45° abduction, and 45° internal rotation is very different from 45° internal rotation, 45° abduction, and 45° of flexion (Figure 6.13). All current kinematic systems have adopted the convention of flexion and extension followed by abduction and adduction, then rotation as the order of derotation in the coordinate systems. Based on personal experience, most clinicians seem to rotate out rotation first, or, alternatively, they rotate out the largest plane of motion first. There has been no evaluation of what order clinicians cognitively use for visual or physical examinations; however, the difference is sometimes large enough to make clinicians uncomfortable with the kinematic numbers. There are no right or wrong numbers, as these only reflect the measurement algorithm, and clinicians need to understand that their impression suffers the same faults.

Although the Euler angle transformations are currently in primary clinical use, other coordinate transformation systems are used for research and may gradually find a role in clinical practice. The Grood–Suntay technique[29] sets up a global coordinate system in each segment with defined positions of the adjacent coordinate system. The easiest but oversimplified explanation of this system is that it functions similar to the assignment of latitude and longitude in the global surface position assignment systems. The advantage of this system is that it is independent of the order of rotation and may better reflect how clinicians look at children; however, we do not think it reflects how clinicians mentally, or by physical examination, assign degrees of deformity. Another system that is independent of the order of rotation is the finite helical screw approach in which the motion of the mobile coordinate system is defined as motion along a vector, which has a radius and a length.[30] This system may have special appeal for complex motion, such as that of the subtalar joint, and to define motion in space of the pelvis and the trunk. It is important to recognize that the significance of these rotation orders are only important with larger motion changes in three planes; therefore, in relatively normal gait and in most joints they have little relevance.

Measurement Accuracy

The accuracy of the kinematic measures is a separate issue and depends on the specific motion and joint measured. This variation is due to the residual problems of markers attached to soft tissue and the problem of clearly defining bony anatomical landmarks. For example, defining the center of the hip joint is much more difficult and error-prone in large, obese adolescents than in children in middle childhood with a thin body habit. Also, the clinically significant changes are reflected much more reliably for large movements, such as hip and knee flexion, than for rotation or abduction and adduction of the knee joint. These specific joint issues are discussed later.

Kinetics

The measurement of forces at each joint is called a kinetic evaluation. For maximum clinical utility, kinetic measures should give a measure of the muscle force of each muscle; however, this is not clinically possible. Therefore, net joint forces, which are indirectly measured as the opposite of the force required to counteract the momentum and ground reaction force, have to be relied upon. Momentum is measured by assigning each segment a mass and a center of mass, and by the velocity and acceleration of the mass through the use of kinematic measurement. The ground reaction force is measured with sensitive and accurate force plates fixed to the floor, over which children walk (Figure 6.14). The function of these force plates is very similar to bathroom scales; however, in addition to the vertical vector measurement of weight, they can also measure forward and sideways forces on the floor, as well as moments about each of these axes. The residual of the ground reaction force at each joint has a direction and distance from the defined center of the joint. By knowing where the joint's center is in space and the direction of the ground reaction force vector, the moment arm can be calculated. With knowledge of the moment arm and the ground reaction force vector, the

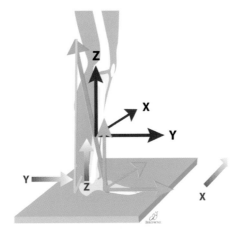

Figure 6.14. The force plate or force platform measures the contact force of the foot to the floor as a single force vector with direction and magnitude. This allows decomposition of the force into orthogonal vectors in the vertical, mediolateral, and anteroposterior planes. Torsional moments can also be measured around each of the principal vectors, but for gait analysis, only the torsional moment around the vertical vector has significance.

GRF - Ground Reaction Force

Figure 6.15. Calculation of joint moments and powers is called kinetics. The joint moment is calculated by the magnitude and direction of the ground reaction force measured from the force plate combined with the momentum component calculated from the kinematic motions of the joint segments.

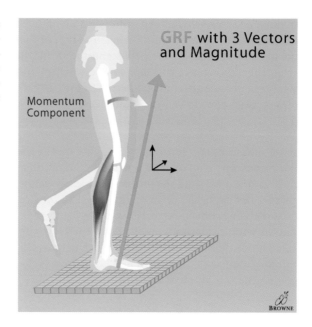

moment generated by the ground reaction force vector can be calculated. The moment from the ground reaction force vector is then added to the moment of momentum and the total external joint moment is measured. Therefore, it can be assumed that the muscles, ligaments, and bones must create an equal and opposite internal force because the system is stable in the instance in which the measurement was made. Once the moment has been calculated, joint power is calculated by multiplying moment times velocity (Figure 6.15). The software technique used to reduce the moment and ground reaction force data into joint moment and powers is known as inverse dynamics. Moments are typically measured in units of Newtonian meters (Nm), which are then divided by a child's body weight for a unit of Nm/kg to allow comparison with a normal mean and range. Joint powers have units of watts and again, to compare them with a normal mean, are divided by a child's body weight; therefore, the units typically plotted are the watts per kilogram of body weight.

Measurement Accuracy

The accuracy of kinematic measures is impacted by various measures, with the error of the kinematic system coming along to the kinetic measures. Also, there is error in determining the segment mass and the center of the mass. However, the kinetic measures are far more accurate overall than the kinematic measure. The increased accuracy of kinetics occurs because the contribution from the momentum side of the equation is usually substantially less than the ground reaction force contribution. The ground reaction force measure is extremely accurate and reliable. There are other theories for determining joint forces with forward dynamics being studied extensively, but this presently has no direct clinical application. With forward dynamics, a mathematical model of the musculoskeletal system is developed, then inputs using EMG to define activity times, segment motion from kinematics, and ground reaction force from the force plates are used with the assumption that the body is trying to walk with the least possible energy. This technique can theoretically give, in addition to joint forces, the force of each individual muscle, and by further refinement, where on the length–tension curve the muscle is functioning. The forward dynamic model has many appealing benefits; however, there are currently so many assumptions required that the model provides no useful individualized information for specific patients. The model has been useful to understand the forces around a specific joint, such as what muscles are important in producing internal rotation about the hip.[31] There have been attempts to use this model to understand hamstring muscle forces in individual patients.[32, 33] The problem with this focus on the hamstring muscles and tendon length, as measured by the model's origin to insertion of the muscle–tendon unit, is that there is no consideration for where on the length–tension curve the muscle functions. This crucial information is important for deciding whether or not the muscle should be lengthened. Although these models are being used in a few centers to evaluate muscle origin to insertion length, clinical application of the information is of marginal value in diagnostic decision making.

Electromyography

Electromyography is a summation of all the individual muscle fiber action potentials. This complex waveform varies by the number of action potentials and the distance the recording is from the action potential. If the EMG is recorded from the surface of the skin, the signal is decreased by the subcutaneous fat and skin. Electromyography recorded from the skin has the advantage of recording over a larger area of big muscles, but with small muscles or small children, cross talk from adjacent muscles may occur. Another method for recording EMG is with the use of an indwelling wire electrode that is inserted percutaneously through a needle. The needle is then withdrawn and the wire is left implanted. The location of the wire is confirmed by testing a muscle EMG response to a specific isolated activity of that muscle. The advantage of using the indwelling wire electrode with the EMG is the ability to localize recording from a small or deeply located muscle. The wire electrodes also have less cross talk from neighboring muscles. The main problem with wire electrodes is pain that may make normal walking not as relaxed as normal. Also, children are often scared of needles and will not cooperate after insertion of the wires. The EMG recording contains information on the magnitude of the electrical activity and the timing of the activity in the gait cycle. The magnitude of the EMG relates in complex ways to the force of the muscle contraction.[34] However, for children with CP, it is not possible to get reliable maximum voluntary contractions, which are required as part of the calculation to relate muscle force to EMG magnitude. In addition, there is great variation in the resistance of soft tissues and strength of individual motor potentials, all making the relationship of force to EMG magnitude very unreliable. Therefore, the only clinically useful data obtained from EMG are timing data. The EMG has to be closely correlated to the gait cycle either by synchronizing the EMG to the kinematic measurements or by adding foot switches to the feet to assess gait cycles. By using the EMG as timing, a muscle can be determined to have a normal pattern, to be on early or late, to turn off early or late, to be continuously on or never on, or to be completely out of phase (Table 6.8). Using EMG in this fashion was suggested by Perry[1] and is widely used in clinical diagnostic assessment; however, the consistent evaluation of the terminology is less widespread. Usually, EMG assessment is used with kinetics and kinematics for a complete analysis of the gait cycle. Surface EMG is used in most patients for most muscles. Specific muscles, such as the tibialis posterior, soleus, iliacus, and psoas can be reliably measured only with the use of percutaneous wires. These muscles are recorded only in specific indications for children who are able to cooperate.

Table 6.8. Clinical definitions of electromyography activity.

Terminology	Definition
Early onset (premature):	Activity of the muscle begins before the normal onset time.
Prolonged:	Muscle activity continues past the normal cessation time.
Continuous:	The muscle is always on with no turn-off time (constant activity may be hard to distinguish from no activity that generates background noise).
Early off (curtailed):	Early termination of the muscle activity.
Delayed:	Onset of muscle activity is later than normal.
Absent:	No muscle activity, which can be hard to separate from continuous activity.
Out of phase:	The muscle is active primarily during the time it would normally be silent and is silent when it should be active.

Pedobarograph

The force plate measures the force the floor applies to the foot. This force is measured as a summated force vector with a specific point of application. However, the foot does not contact the floor physically as a point, but as a flat surface. The measurement of the pressure distribution on the sole of the foot in contact with the floor is called a pedobarograph. These devices are mats that contain a whole series of pressure sensors (Figure 6.16). Currently, several systems are available, with the major difference being a choice between larger sensing area with less accuracy for the absolute measurement or a smaller sensing area with greater accuracy for the absolute measurement. The use of this system in children with CP is a way of quantifying planovalgus or equinovarus foot deformity as well as heel contact times. There is little need to focus heavily on the absolute pressure measurement for a specific area. If children are developing pressure sores on the feet, such as children with insensate feet from diabetes or spinal cord dysfunction, the more sensitive systems are probably better. Regardless of which system is used, the information on foot position as children walk over the measurement plate without targeting the plate is reliable and the best way currently available to monitor childhood foot deformities. The test is quick and easy to understand, mainly through pattern recognition, and allows quantifying varus, valgus, and heel contact positions. The test can be used as a yearly follow-up tool for children with foot deformities and is especially useful to assess planovalgus feet in young children as radiographic imaging is of little use in this age group. Although the pedobarograph is not available in every laboratory, most pediatric laboratories have it available and use it routinely.

Oxygen Consumption

The most recent addition to the tools of gait analysis is the measurement of whole-body energy consumption. The current mechanism for measuring energy relies on indirect calorimetry, which measures the amount of oxygen used and carbon dioxide produced. Indirect calorimetry works under the assumption that the final pathway, which burns fuel to release energy, comes from a process that consumes ATP and oxygen. For anaerobic metabolism, carbon dioxide production increases; however, there is no increase in oxygen consumption. The instruments currently available for oxygen consumption measurement are small telemetry face masks, which can be worn during normal gait (Figure 6.17). This device gives output of continuous oxygen use,

A

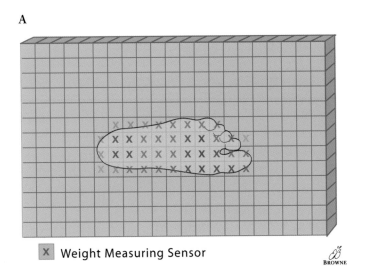

☒ Weight Measuring Sensor

BROWNE

Figure 6.16. Measurement of the distribution of the force on the sole of the foot is done using a pedobarograph. This device has a series of sensing cells that measure vertical load only (A). These areas of pressure measurement can then be plotted together to represent an image of a footprint that shows which area of the foot has the highest force. Segments of the foot can be divided, and the total segments are plotted (B) Other specific data can be calculated, such as the relative distribution of force on the medial side versus the lateral side of the foot; this provides a measure of the varus (increased force over the lateral foot segments) or valgus (increased pressure on the medial side of the foot) foot deformities.

B

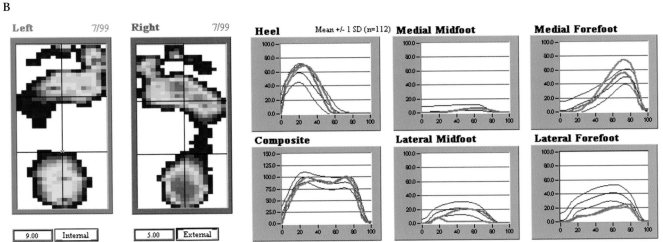

	Left	Comment	Right	Comment	Normal
Time of Heel Rise	65.0	normal	63.0	normal	46.7 - 69.7
Heel Impulse	37.8	normal	35.7	normal	23.3 - 39.8
Varus-Valgus Foot Postition	28.8	Valgus	5.1	Normal	-15 to +15
Foot Progression	9	Internal	5	External	0 to 10 external

carbon dioxide excretion, respiratory rate, volume of inspired and expired air, and the heart rate. Walking speed is added to these measures. A typical way to measure oxygen consumption is to have children sit comfortably and relax for 3 to 5 minutes, then ask them to get up and walk in a specific predetermined gait pattern for 5 to 10 minutes. The amount of time they are required to walk on a walkway is recorded, and by knowing the distance they have walked, the velocity can be calculated. Typically, the oxygen consumption has to be normalized for body size. There is a significant reduction in milliliters of oxygen per kilogram of body weight as children get older and heavier. We normalized this measure to the body surface area and used a Z-score or a number of standard deviations from the normal mean to define a child's relative function.[35] The heart rate and respiratory rate are evaluated

Figure 6.17. Measuring the energy cost of walking requires measuring the amount of oxygen consumed and the amount of carbon dioxide generated. This measurement is currently performed with a self-contained unit that fits over the child's face and has a data collection system that can telemeter the data to a local computer (A) The system also records breath rate and heart rate. If the velocity of walking is also recorded, oxygen cost in milliters of oxygen per meter walked per kilogram of body weight can be calculated (B).

A

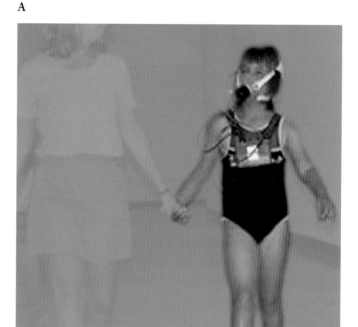

B

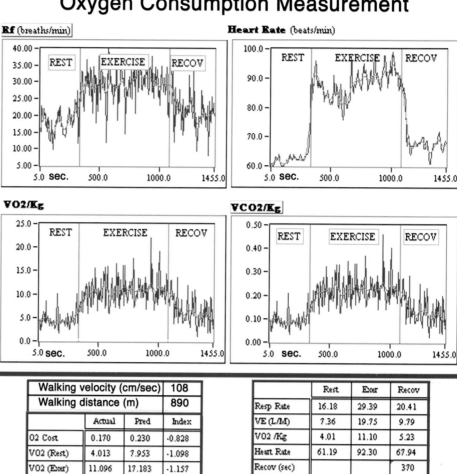

Oxygen Consumption Measurement

Walking velocity (cm/sec)		108	
Walking distance (m)		890	
	Actual	Pred	Index
O2 Cost	0.170	0.230	-0.828
VO2 (Rest)	4.013	7.953	-1.098
VO2 (Exer)	11.096	17.183	-1.157

	Rest	Exer	Recov
Resp Rate	16.18	29.39	20.41
VE (L/M)	7.36	19.75	9.79
VO2 /Kg	4.01	11.10	5.23
Heart Rate	61.19	92.30	67.94
Recov (sec)			370

as well. Oxygen cost is defined as the amount of oxygen burned per kilogram of body weight per meter of movement. Speed is not considered as a variable factor, and for walking in the normal range of 80 to 160 cm per second, there is little impact of velocity.[36]

Another measure is oxygen consumption, which is defined as the amount of oxygen consumed over time, and is expressed as milliliters of oxygen per kilogram of body weight per second. Oxygen consumption is seldom abnormal in children with CP because they have normal muscles, hearts, and lungs. However, children with muscle disease have oxygen consumption and cost that may be very low.[37] The measurement of oxygen cost has been promoted as an excellent outcomes measure in gait treatment in children with CP.[3] A definite goal in treatment is to improve the efficiency of gait; however, as demonstrated in comparison with children with muscle diseases, similar functional gait impairments can have even more efficient gaits than normal children as demonstrated by decreased oxygen costs. Oxygen costs should not be used as a lone outcome measure; other functional measures of gait improvement have to be considered as well. Children who seldom walk may have such severe deconditioning that this is the major impediment to their walking. These data are hard to obtain in any way except with oxygen consumption. Oxygen consumption measurement is not available in all laboratories, and because it is the most recent addition, it has the least clear clinical benefits. We routinely measure oxygen consumption with full assessments if children can cooperate and their gait is thought to be substantially abnormal.

There are many older oxygen consumption systems that require using a pushcart to push along as children walk. All these systems give the same information and it is only the issue of convenience and ease that defines the modern devices. Another technique for measuring energy use that has been promoted is the energy cost index, which is a measure in the change in heart rate with increased activity.[38] There is a rough correlation of energy consumption with increased heart rate over a resting heart rate. This measure, which is also known as the physiologic index, is almost useless in assessing children with CP over time because of the many variables that impact heart rate. The correlation to the actual measure of oxygen consumption is poor.[36] Even if the equipment to measure oxygen consumption is not available, poor reliability of the energy cost index makes it not worth the effort to collect.

Gait Analysis

Diagnosing the Gait Impairment

After the discussion on techniques and methods of assessing gait impairments in children with CP, there is a need to have a focused and goal-oriented methodology to apply these tools in the care of children. The medical treatment of gait follows the same order as followed in other medical care. For example, the evaluation of a child seen by an orthopaedist for a lump on the thigh would start with a history of how and when it was noted, any history of trauma or surgery in the area, and questions as to whether there is pain or are there functional problems. The next step is to do a physical examination, which may be all that is needed if this lump is thought to be a superficial hematoma; otherwise, the next investigation would be a radiograph. The radiograph may show a typical osteochondroma and the treatment can be planned, but if a lesion with periosteal elevation is seen, the next step would be to get a magnetic resonance imaging (MRI) scan of the thigh. Because of uncertain diagnosis with periosteal elevation, testing would likely include a computed tomography (CT) scan and a bone scan before biopsy. Then, after all the data have been collected, a diagnosis and plan of treatment is offered to families and children.

To follow the same analogy of the thigh lump, when children with gait impairments are initially seen, the history should include questions about the etiology of the CP to confirm to the physician that this is CP and not some other as yet undiagnosed condition. Also, the age of the children, when they started walking, and how specifically the walking has changed in the last 6 to 12 months are important in the evaluation. Questions about orthotic wear, how long the children have had them, do they object to brace wear, and are the braces worn every day are also important. After the history is obtained, the physical examination is performed focusing on joint range of motion, joint contractures, muscle tone, and gross motor function. Following the physical examination, children are observed walking in an area that is big enough to walk a distance. This area should be a hallway at least 10 meters long and wide enough (2 to 3 meters) so that a lateral view of the gait can be observed. It is impossible to see a typical gait pattern in a small examination room, and additionally, children must be undressed to underwear or swimsuits so the legs can be observed in their entirety. The observational assessment of gait should focus on joint position at various parts of the gait cycle, overall motor control and balance, and children's motivation and comfort with ambulation. Barefoot and orthotic shoe combinations used by children should also be assessed. This assessment should include a wheelchair evaluation if one is used. Parents must be instructed to bring all orthotics and walking aids to the appointment because these devices cannot be examined if they are left at home. The first visit with a child is similar to the initial evaluation for the thigh lump. Most of the information has been gained from a history and physical examination, which allows an assessment that further specific treatment is not indicated at this time. Cerebral palsy gait impairment for most children is an evolving condition that is heavily impacted by growth. For these children, there has to be a determination that there should or should not be significant change in treatment; however, children need to be followed to monitor the gait. In this situation, which is similar to that following an asymptomatic osteochondroma, a gait video is ordered.

This video is equivalent to a radiograph for a benign bone lesion. Typically, most children with CP gait impairments should be followed every 6 to 12 months, with the younger and more severe problems monitored every 6 months and the milder, older adolescent patients monitored every 12 months. For each repeat visit, the interim history of change is obtained, the examination is completed again, and gait is observed and compared with the videotape taken previously. The videotape also provides the parents and children the ability to see for themselves what the physicians are seeing. Many parents remember very poorly how their children walked earlier. Home videotapes show these gait patterns poorly because the children are frequently dressed in clothes that mostly obscure the lower extremities and the angles of the views are often very oblique and are not standard frontal or lateral views. Also, most of these home videotapes do not contain activity, such as normal walking, but often involve the children at play, at some other activity, or just standing. If during an examination the determination is made that an additional major change in treatment, such as surgery or major medication or orthotic treatment is indicated, a full gait assessment is ordered. This is the analogy of ordering an MRI scan, a CT scan, and bone scan for the lump on the thigh. The data from the full gait analysis are then used to make a definitive treatment recommendation. The results of the evaluations are combined with the history and physicians' examinations to make the final treatment plan to present to families. Having videotapes available of similar children and knowledge of how they responded to the treatment are very helpful to the parents and children to understand what to expect.

Is Full Gait Analysis Really Needed to Decide Treatment?

The role of full instrumented gait analysis in the treatment planning of children with CP serves exactly the same function as advanced tests for a mass of uncertain etiology in the femur. In geographic locations where these tools are not available, the treatment of the femoral mass should proceed based on the available data. This means the bone would typically be biopsied and surgery is planned. It has been the experience of the medical community that additional tests help provide more information and therefore treatment can be more specific with possible better outcome. For the treatment of bone tumors, the outcome is easy; either the tumors return and the children die, or they are tumor free on long-term follow-up. Children with a gait impairment from CP will not have such dramatic success or failure. In spastic gait, the good versus bad result is less clear as compared with tumor follow-up. However, as with tumor surgery, there has to be an aggressive follow-up program. Tumor surgeons do not sit back and wait and see if the children will die, but perform periodic tests to find early recurrence by using bone and MRI scans. This same approach is used with gait treatment. A full evaluation should be performed 1 year after surgery, and ongoing clinical follow-up every 6 months is indicated until significant change occurs. The next level of treatment is then initiated. This use of regular periodic physician evaluations and when needed, the use of other available gait measurement tools, gives children the best chance for an optimal outcome.

There are still a few physicians who take the view that no one has shown that gait measures improve the outcome of gait treatment, and from some level of strict scientific perspective, this may be true. It is also true that there is no scientific documentation to prove that the use of radiographs improves the outcome of treating forearm fractures. This scientific documentation for gait analysis could be obtained. We know of one attempt to do a preoperative and postoperative gait analysis but not use the results of the analysis in deciding the surgical treatment. This study could not get Institutional Review Board approval because it was thought that useful information cannot ethically be withheld in the decision-making process. Withholding available information from physicians could potentially harm children. We doubt that ethically this type of study could be performed today. Studies comparing different approaches based on gait analysis measurements are more ethical and more scientific in approach than saying doctors can make better decisions with less information. It is true that more information is not always better, especially if the information is not understood; however, it is also true that in most situations, too little information is worse than too much.

How Should Gait Analysis Be Applied?

The modern scientific medical approach is to evaluate and measure the measurable elements, then try to understand the problem and construct a solution to the problem based on the physical facts. The application of these principles to the treatment of gait impairments demands gait measurement. So, are all the tools of full gait analysis really needed? Yes, in the same way MRI, CT, and bone scan are needed to treat bone tumors. Can physicians treat gait impairments of children with CP without gait analysis? Yes, they should definitely treat the gait impairments to the best of their abilities, just the same as physicians should treat children with osteosarcoma of the femur if only regular, plain radiographs are available as the only imaging technique.

The application of measurement methods, especially those used in instrumented gait analysis, requires more than just measurement. The data must be combined and clinically analyzed by individuals who understand the data. This understanding of the data is a much greater obstacle for many physicians than getting the measurements done. Understanding the gait data requires a good understanding of normal human gait and the adaptations that the body makes. For those with little background in normal gait, we would recommend the book *Gait Analysis, Normal and Pathological Function* by Jacquelin Perry.[1] Because understanding normal gait as a whole-body function is crucial to understanding and planning treatment for abnormal gait, a review of normal gait is included here.

Normal Gait

Normal human walking is bipedal, which makes the balancing function more crucial than in quadruped ambulation. Bipedal gait is extremely versatile and energy efficient for short-distance mobility. This extremely complex function requires a large dedication from the central nervous system to fulfill the functions of balance, motor control, and cognitive decision making. However, the functions of balance and motor control, which emanate entirely from the brain, can act only through the mechanical components of the musculoskeletal system. When the motor control of gait is abnormal, the mechanical systems still respond directly to the command from the motor control. For example, if the brain can no longer maintain the body in the bipedal stance because of its limited function, it will still try to make the system work, and the muscles will contract normally when a contract command is sent. The attempt to accommodate for limitations due to the brain's decreased ability is not only a one-way street from the brain to the musculoskeletal system, there also seem to be accommodations occurring as the muscles, tendons, and bones make adaptations. In growing children, the musculoskeletal system is responsive over the long term and in trying to accommodate structurally to the brain's impairment. The accommodation by the musculoskeletal system largely follows rules of mechanics and is not always an accommodation that makes a positive impact on the global gait ability. An example of this principle is increased spasticity, or muscle tone, which serves a useful function by stiffening the body and allowing easier control. However, with increased tone, the muscles do not grow as fast, which at a mild level may also help motor control by decreasing joint range of motion over which the muscles can function. Both the increased tone and the decreased range at one level can allow the gait function to improve with a given level of brain functional ability. However, both increased tone and decreased range can get so severe that each becomes part of the impairment in itself. The third element needed for balance is energy output. In normal gait, the brain tries to keep the energy cost of walking low so individuals do not tire out. Understanding the mechanical components of the musculoskeletal system and how this system responds to brain impairments is crucial to clinical decision making, which is directed at producing functional improvement in a specific abnormal gait. In the end, the brain, with its given ability, tries to find a pattern of movement that allows individuals to be stable, mobile, and move with the energy available.

Gait Cycle

Gait is a cyclic event just like the beating heart, and just as understanding the cardiac cycles is important to understanding the heart, all the understanding of human gait falls into understanding the cycles of gait and the function of each cycle (Figure 6.18). Clinical descriptions of gait events follow the general pattern and naming convention popularized by Perry.[1] The basic separation of the gait cycle is in the stance and swing phases called periods by Perry.[1] The role of stance phase is to support the body on the floor and the role of swing phase is to allow forward movement of the foot. This two-phase function of gait is analogous to the heart, which fills with blood during its first phase and empties itself of blood during its second phase. The tasks of each phase of gait are simple; however, each of these phases is broken down further. The gait cycle of one limb is called a step and the right and left concurrent steps are known as a stride. The step of a walking cycle has two phases in which both feet are on the ground, a time called double support. The step cycle of running has two periods in which neither foot is in contact with the floor, called float or flight times. Therefore, the difference between running and walking is that walking has double support and running has flight time (Figure 6.19). This also means that walking always has a longer stance phase than swing phase and running always has a longer swing phase than stance phase.

Some basic quantitative definitions of the phases of gait are called the temporal spatial characteristics of gait. The temporal spatial characteristics include the step length, which is the distance the foot moves during a single swing phase measured in centimeters or meters, and the stride length, which is the combination of the right and left step length. Stance phase is measured as support time by the amount of time the foot is in contact with the floor. Swing phase is measured as the swing time, or the amount of time the foot is moving forward, usually equal to the time the foot is not in contact with the floor. The amount of time in seconds or minutes is measured, and both support and swing times are given as a ratio of total step time. For normal walking, the support time is 60% and swing time is 40%. The time when both feet are in contact with the ground is called double support, and each double support is 10% of the cycle. Each step has an initial double support and a second double support. Each stride also has only two double support times because the right initial double support is the same as the left second double support. Also, the time when only one foot is in contact with the ground is called single limb support time, and in normal gait, it is 40% of the step cycle. By knowing the time in seconds of a stride, the number of strides per time unit can be calculated, which is called cadence and is measured as strides per minute. By knowing the stride length and the cadence, the velocity of gait can be calculated, usually expressed as centimeters per second (cm/s) or meters per minute (m/min). There is still large variation between the use of cm/s or m/min; however, for the convenience of staying with a consistent numeric system for the remainder of this text, cm/s is the format used. The final temporal spatial measure is step width, measured from some aspect of the foot as the medial lateral distance between the two feet during the gait cycle.

Stance Phase

The role of stance phase in gait is to provide support on the ground for the body. This support function includes complex and transitional demands. The transition from swing phase to stance phase is called initial contact and is important in defining how the limb will move into weight bearing. The first time component of a step cycle is the loading response, which requires the limb to obtain foot stability on the floor, preserve forward progress of the body, and absorb the shock of the sudden transfer of weight. Loading time is equivalent to initial double support time and ends with the beginning of single limb support. Middle stance is the first half of the single support time

A

Step Cycle

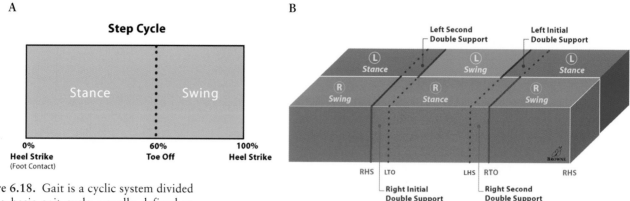

Figure 6.18. Gait is a cyclic system divided into a basic gait cycle, usually defined as going from foot contact (heel strike) to foot contact. This basic cycle has a stance phase and swing phase. The basic gait cycle of one leg is called a step (A). The basic gait cycle with the right and left limbs combined is called a stride (B). Besides breaking down a step into stance and swing phase, additional specific events break down the phases of gait into smaller phases. Stance phase is divided into loading response, midstance, terminal stance, and preswing (C).

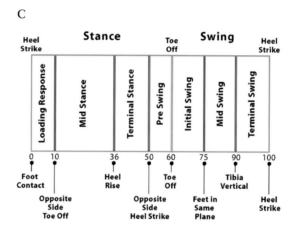

and is the time when the body is progressing over the stable foot fixed on the floor. Late stance, or terminal stance, is the last half of single limb support, and is the time when the body is in front of the planted foot when the foot can put energy into causing forward progression of the body. Preswing is a period corresponding to the second double support time just before swing phase. This is the time when the foot rapidly transfers weight to the other side and prepares for swing phase.

Swing Phase

Swing phase has the requirement of moving the foot forward. The time of initial swing phase takes up approximately the first third of swing phase. This period lasts from toe-off until the foot is opposite the planted foot. The role of the initial swing is to bring the limb from a trailing position to the position of the stance foot, with the swing foot clearing the floor. Midswing begins with the swing foot even with the stance foot, and ends when the tibia is vertical to the floor. At this point, the hip and knee flexion are approximately equal. Midswing takes up approximately 50% of the swing phase. Terminal swing occurs with the knee extending and the limb preparing for foot contact.

Body Segments Important in the Gait Cycle

To understand the gait cycle in more detail, the body has to be considered as segments linked together. The concept popularized by Perry is to consider the passenger, or cargo segment, and the locomotor segments.[1] This is equivalent to thinking of an automobile as having a power train and a body mounted on top of the power train. The passenger, or cargo element, con-

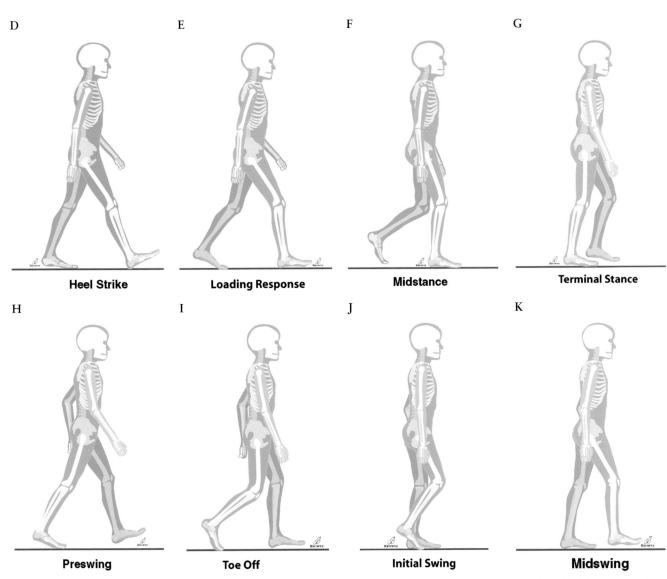

D Heel Strike **E** Loading Response **F** Midstance **G** Terminal Stance

H Preswing **I** Toe Off **J** Initial Swing **K** Midswing

tains the head, arms, and trunk and is abbreviated as the HAT segment (Figure 6.20). The locomotor segments are the foot, shank, thigh, and pelvis, which are articulated by the ankle, knee and hip, and lumbosacral junction. The HAT segment is moved during gait with the goal of its motion being as straight a line as possible in the direction of the intended motion. The HAT segment can be defined by a center of mass that is somewhat higher than the center of gravity of the whole body. The center of mass of the HAT segment is also somewhat dynamic because this segment allows motion of the head and arms independently. The focus on the influence of this changing position of the center of mass of the HAT segment has not been well defined for the application of clinical gait analysis. The concept of the center of mass means that the body mechanically acts as if all its mass were at that point. The center of gravity is approximately the point on the body where the center of mass is located. The center of gravity is also dynamic and can be changed by a change in body shape, but in an upright standing position, the center of gravity is typically just anterior to the first sacral vertebra.[1] During gait, each of the locomotor segments has its own center of mass, which is fixed because each segment is an approximate rigid body that cannot significantly change

Figure 6.18 (continued). The stance phase events that make up these divisions are foot contact (heel strike) (D), opposite limb toe-off (loading response) (E), forward roll of the tibia (midstance) (F), initiation of heel rise (terminal stance) (G), opposite side foot contact (preswing) (H), and toe-off (I). Swing phase is broken down into initial swing, mid-swing, and terminal swing smaller phases (C). The swing events are toe-off (I), both feet in the same transverse plane (initial swing) (J), shank is vertical to the room (midswing) (K) and terminal swing ending with foot contact (L). Another breakdown can be related to the ankle rockers, in which the events are foot contact (K) to foot flat (E), to define first rocker. Foot flat (E), to heel rise (G) defines second rocker, and heel rise (G) to toe-off (I) defines third rocker.

Figure 6.19. The basic cycles of running are very similar to walking, except there is no double limb support and there is, instead, float time. Running is defined as a gait pattern in which there is a period of time that the body is not in contact with the ground.

Running Gait Phases

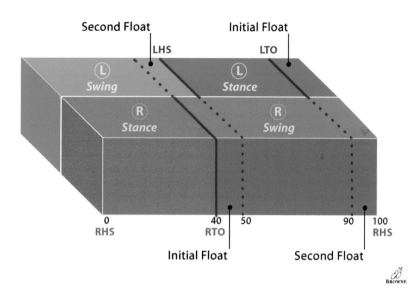

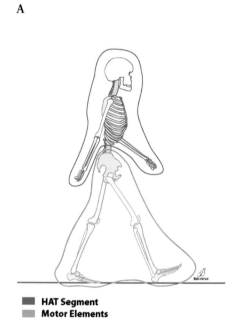

HAT Segment
Motor Elements

Figure 6.20. As a mechanism for understanding gait, the body can be divided into a motor segment that includes the pelvis and lower limbs, on which rides the cargo segment of the HAT segment (A). The goal of gait should be to move this cargo segment forward with as small a vertical oscillation of the cargo mass as is possible. Lifting this mass vertically and letting it drop with each step is very energy consuming (B).

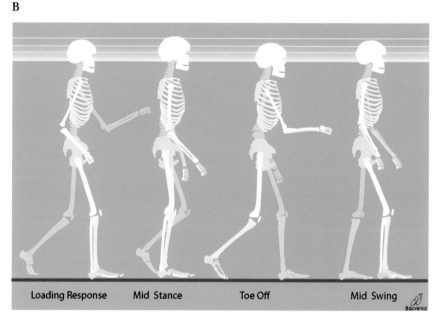

its shape. This concept holds true consistently for the pelvis, thigh, and shank segments, but is much less stable for the foot and HAT segments. The center of mass can be changed significantly by swinging arms, trunk bending, and head movement in the HAT segment. For the foot segment, the change in center of mass is less dramatic than the problem of the foot not being a rigid segment, as assumed in gait modeling. Flexibility of the supposed rigid segment can cause additional problems for gait measurement.

For the gait cycle to have maximum efficiency, the center of mass of the HAT segment should move in a single forward direction of the intended motion only; however, this is not physically possible. Therefore, the goal is to minimize the vertical and side-to-side oscillation of the center of mass of the HAT segment (Figure 6.21). This is accomplished primarily by central

A

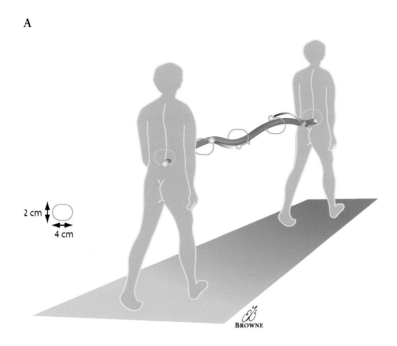

2 cm
4 cm

B

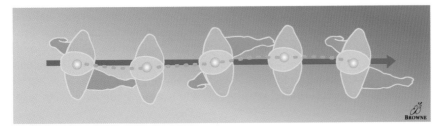

Figure 6.21. The body's center of mass is located just anterior to the sacrum. The most energy-efficient gait requires the least movement of this center of mass out of the plane of forward motion. In actual fact, the motion of the center of mass is really a path that looks like a screw thread in which there is vertical and sideways oscillation (A). There is a significant component of side-to-side movement (B).

motor control adjusting limb lengths through sagittal plane motion of the joints connecting the locomotor segments. Understanding these relationships is easier by looking at the individual joints and at how each joint functions in normal gait throughout the full gait cycle.

Ankle

The ankle is mechanically modeled as the joint that connects the foot to the shank. The ankle is modeled as a single axis of motion in flexion extension, with mechanical perspective of the gait measurement. However, this description is a great oversimplification and the measures of rotation around the vertical axis and varus–valgus motion are recorded as well. The ankle joint measurements of rotation and varus–valgus motion are primarily reflections of motions in the foot itself through the subtalar joint; therefore, these measurements are not very useful because of the inaccuracy associated with marker placement and mathematical assumptions of the foot as a single rigid segment. Therefore, it is better to think of the ankle as having only plantar flexion and dorsiflexion ability and then separately consider flexibility and stability issues of the foot as a segment.

Motion of the ankle joint starts at approximately neutral in initial contact with heel strike. At heel strike, the ankle starts plantar flexion controlled by an eccentric contraction of the tibialis anterior. This motion of the ankle from heel strike to foot flat is called first rocker. During first rocker, there is a dorsiflexion moment at the ankle joint. All moments will be defined as internal moments, or moments that are being produced by the muscles to counteract the external moments produced by the ground reaction force. After the foot is flat on the floor, the tibia rolls anteriorly as the ankle goes into dorsiflexion, a motion controlled by eccentric contraction of the gastrocnemius and soleus. This motion produces a gradually increasing plantar flexion moment, but with only a small power absorption. This period of dorsiflexion, which is controlled by the eccentric plantar flexor contraction, is called second rocker. Then, as the ankle reaches maximum dorsiflexion at approximately 10° to 15° at the end of late stance phase, a rapid plantar flexion motion occurs under the influence of a strong concentric plantar flexor contraction from the gastrocnemius and soleus. This period is called third rocker and is the main power generation for forward progression in normal gait. The important element of this power burst is to have the plantar flexors pretensioned on the slightly elongated segment of the Blix curve. This power burst also requires the foot to be stable, at right angles to the axis of the ankle joint, and aligned with the forward line of progression. The third rocker continues through preswing until toe-off when the dorsiflexors, by concentric contraction, produce dorsiflexion at the ankle to assist with foot clearance (Figure 6.22).

Maximum ankle dorsiflexion occurs in middle swing phase, and only a slight amount of plantar flexion occurs in terminal swing as the foot is prepared for initial contact. The primary dorsiflexor of the ankle is the tibialis anterior and the secondary dorsiflexors of the ankle are the extensor hallucis longus and the extensor digitorum longus. The primary plantar flexors at the ankle are the soleus, which is the largest muscle, and the gastrocnemius, which has approximately two thirds the cross-sectional size of the soleus. The gastrocnemius is primarily a fast-twitch aerobic type 1 muscle, whereas the soleus is predominated with slow-twitch type 2 fibers. The time of

Figure 6.22. The ankle is the primary power output for normal walking. Stance phase of the ankle is best broken into ankle rockers. First rocker is from foot contact to foot flat and is controlled by an eccentric contraction of the tibialis anterior. Second rocker is the time in which the foot is flat on the ground and the tibia is rolling forward on the fixed foot, a motion that is mainly controlled by an eccentric gastrocsoleus contraction. Third rocker occurs from heel rise until toe-off and is controlled by a concentric contraction of the gastrocsoleus. During this ankle rocker period, the normal period of gait defined in the context of the whole gait cycle also occurs. The ankle motion, ankle moments, and power curves also demonstrate the ankle rocker phases.

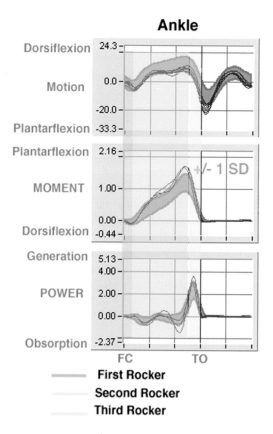

contraction in the gait cycle between the gastrocnemius and soleus is very similar,[1] and for practical clinical conditions, especially in children with CP, they can be considered to be contracting at the same time. The secondary plantar flexors are the tibialis posterior, the flexor digitorum longus, the flexor hallicus longus, and the peroneus longus and brevis. All these muscles are predominantly active during terminal stance phase and preswing. The only muscle with consistent activity during weight acceptance is the tibialis posterior. All together, these muscles only generate approximately 10% of the force of the soleus. The main function of these muscles is to stabilize the foot segment.

Foot Segment

The foot segment is a very complex structure that depends heavily on muscle force to maintain its function as a stable ground contact segment. The function of the subtalar joint is to allow the foot to be stable when the ground surface is uneven. The subtalar joint has very complex motions. The motion through the subtalar joint is linked to midfoot motion, especially the calcaneocuboid joint and the talonavicular joints. The importance of these joints for normal gait is to provide stability to the foot. This stability is controlled by muscles, with the tibialis anterior and the peroneus longus working in opposing directions, and the peroneus brevis and the tibialis posterior working in opposing directions. These muscles are primarily responsible for providing mediolateral stability. The long toe flexors and extensors can significantly increase the length of the foot segment by stiffening the toes so they also become a stable part of the foot segment.

Knee

The knee joint connects the thigh and shank segments, and its primary role is allowing the limb to shorten and lengthen. This function greatly improves the efficiency of gait. If the limb is given no ability to change its length, the vertical movement of the center of gravity would be approximately 9.5 cm compared with 0.5 cm in normal functioning gait. This decreased vertical oscillation represents an energy savings of approximately 50%.[1] The primary knee extensors are the vastus muscles and the rectus femoris. The primary knee flexors are the hamstring group including semimembranosus, semitendinosus, biceps femoris, and gracilis. The secondary knee flexors are the gastrocnemius and the sartorius. The only single joint knee flexor is the short head of the biceps; however, all the vastus muscles are single joint knee extenders.

At initial contact, the knee is slightly flexed approximately 5°. With the knee in almost full extension, the step length is maximized; however, with slight flexion, the knee is ready to absorb the shock of the impending weight transfer. At foot contact, the vastus muscles and the hamstring muscles all tend to be contracting in an isometric contraction to stabilize the knee joint. During weight acceptance, the knee flexes approximately 10° to 15°, allowing the HAT segment to move forward over the supporting foot without having to raise the HAT segment. In middle stance phase, the knee gradually goes into extension again to maintain the height as the mass moves forward on the planted foot. The movement in middle stance phase tends to be largely passive, controlled only by the eccentric gastrocsoleus contraction. This phase of knee extension is controlled by the calf muscles throughout the influence of the knee extension–ankle plantar flexion couple (Figure 6.23). The moment and power produced in the knee in stance phase is minimal, with early extension moment and a later stance phase flexion moment predominating (Figure 6.24). In late stance phase, the knee starts rapid knee flexion,

Figure 6.23. Knee control in normal gait is mainly controlled by the gastrocsoleus through its control of the plantar flexion–knee extension couple; this means the ground reaction force can be controlled by the degree of ankle dorsiflexion during gait to increase or decrease the knee extension. The efficient function of the plantar flexion–knee extension couple requires that the foot be aligned with the knee axis, and the foot has to be able to generate a stable moment arm. If the foot is externally rotated relative to the knee joint axis, the extension moment arm shortens and the knee valgus moment arm lengthens. Therefore, the gastrocsoleus is less effective in controlling the knee joint in flexion-extension, and it places an increased valgus stress on the knee.

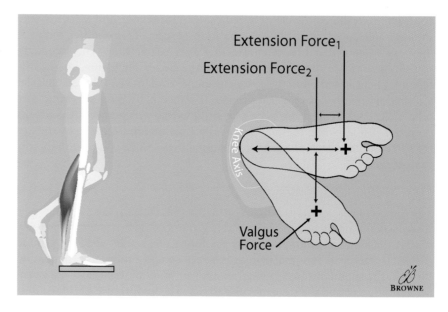

coordinated with the ankle starting plantar flexion and the heel rising off the ground. This knee flexion is passively produced by momentum of the forward movement of the hip joint, the vertical vector of the plantar flexors push-off burst, and the initiation of the hip flexor power burst. All hamstring muscles are quiet during this aspect of toe-off, except for some mild variable contraction of the gracilis and the sartorius, and sometimes with the short head of the biceps. These muscles are the only ones that normally can provide active knee flexion in late stance phase, which is a period of time when the hip is flexing as well. As the knee flexion velocity increases, the rectus femoris starts contracting in preswing phase, with most activity at toe-off and the first 20% of swing phase. The rectus has an eccentric contraction to slow the velocity of knee flexion and transfer this momentum into hip flexion. At the time of peak knee flexion, the rectus muscle turns off and the knee extension begins as a passive motion of gravity working on the elevated foot and shank segment, as well as the momentum of active hip flexion. Enough knee flexion has to occur so the limb is shortened so that the foot will not strike the ground as it swings under the body segment. In terminal swing phase, the passive knee extension is increasing rapidly and the velocity of the knee extension has to be decelerated by an eccentric contraction of the semitendinosus, semimembranosus, and biceps femoris, which also act as hip extensors. These hamstring muscles now transfer force from the forward swinging foot and shank segment into hip extension. The hamstring muscles guide the hip and knee into proper alignment for initial contact. It is at this period of time where control of hip and knee flexion by the hamstring muscles is crucial in the control of step length.

There are some other secondary muscles functioning at the knee, such as the fascia latae and the biceps femoris, which assist with rotational control and valgus stability. The semimembranosus and the semitendinosus with the gracilis may assist in controlling internal rotation of the tibia and varus instability. However, most of these forces are controlled by the ligamentous restraints in the knee joint.

Hip

The hip joint is the only joint with significant motion in all three planes during gait. The hip is also a principal power output joint along with the ankle

A

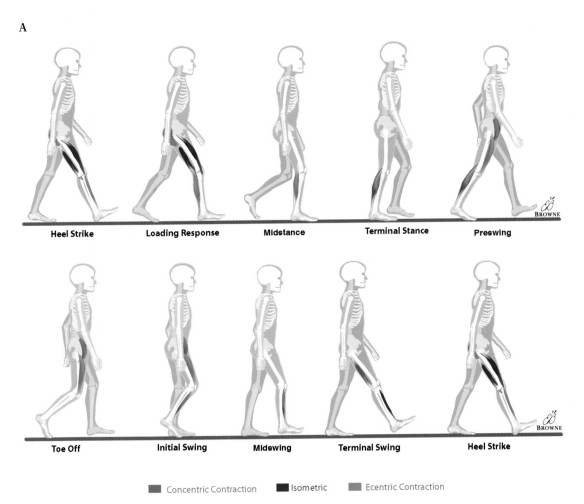

Heel Strike   Loading Response   Midstance   Terminal Stance   Preswing

Toe Off   Initial Swing   Midswing   Terminal Swing   Heel Strike

■ Concentric Contraction   ■ Isometric   ■ Ecentric Contraction

B

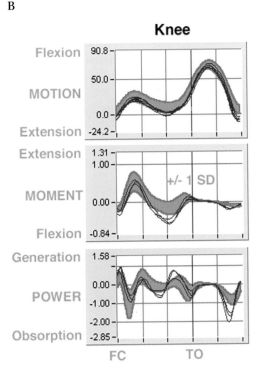

Figure 6.24. Complete control of the knee includes stabilizing function of the hamstrings and quadriceps, especially at foot contact, which is provided by isometric contraction, a hip extensor that uses momentum to extend the hip and knee at the same time. In midstance and terminal stance phase, the gastrocsoleus is the primary controller of the knee position. In swing phase, the rectus initially controls knee flexion through an eccentric contraction and the hamstrings use an eccentric contraction to decelerate the forward swing of the foot, thereby limiting knee extension (A). These motions are well demonstrated on the knee kinematics along with the normal moments and power absorption at the knee. Significantly more power is absorbed at the knee than is generated, demonstrating the fact that the knee's primary function is to provide stability and change the limb's length between stance and swing phase (B).

in normal walking. The position of hip flexion at initial contact significantly contributes to step length along with knee extension. At initial contact, the hip starts into extension under the influence of strong gluteus maximus contraction. Additionally, all of the hamstring muscles plus the adductors are active at initial contact and remain active during weight acceptance phase. This forceful hip extension provides a large hip extension moment in early stance phase and a power output to lift the forward falling of the body. Also, at initial contact and in weight acceptance, the abductor muscles are active to contract and hold the center of gravity in the midline. There is an initial hip adduction motion in weight acceptance followed in midstance and terminal stance with gradual abduction. In mid- and terminal stance, the hip abductors and extensor muscles are relatively quiet, with the fascia latae being consistently active. Middle stance is a time of low-level muscle activation as momentum provides primary stability with only minimal control by the fascia latae. During terminal stance and preswing, the adductor muscles become active and act as hip flexors and adductors. In terminal stance, the hip flexion is again initiated, which can occur passively as an effect of the momentum of the body moving forward off the planted foot and the forceful contraction of the ankle plantar flexors. This force provides transfer of momentum from knee flexion into hip flexion by the rectus as the rectus activates to decrease the acceleration and control the magnitude of knee flexion (Figure 6.25). The other alternative is a concentric contraction of the primary hip flexors, which include the iliacus and psoas muscles. Also, the secondary hip flexors, including the gracilis, adductor longus, and brevis, may be active.

During swing phase, there is gradual hip adduction correlated with hip flexion. In general, the hip flexors adduct and internally rotate and the primary extensor muscles abduct and externally rotate the hip (Figure 6.26). The control of the rotation is not well understood. Early stance phase is a major time of power generation at the hip, second only to the late stance push-off power burst of the gastrocsoleus at the ankle to provide the force, which propels the body forward.

This power is primarily generated from the gluteus maximus extending the hip as momentum is driving the forward-falling body. During midstance, there is little power absorption or generation; however, in terminal stance and preswing, the power burst occurs secondary to the active force output to generate forward motion of the leg through hip flexion. In middle swing, there is very little muscle activity; however, by terminal swing, the hip extensors, especially the hamstrings and gluteal muscles, are again becoming active to decelerate the forward swing of the shank and foot, and transfer that force into hip extension.

Pelvis

The pelvis moves through space in a motion akin to swimming, with a combination of pelvic anterior and posterior tilt, pelvic obliquity, and pelvic rotation (Figure 6.27). The pelvis articulates superiorly at the lumbosacral junction in the gait model discussed here. The motion of the pelvis in current clinical calculation algorithms is considered to move relative to the room coordinate system and not relative to the lumbosacral junction. All other motions distal to the pelvis are relative to the immediate proximal segment. The pelvis is a very confusing segment because it is articulated by three other segments, two thighs and the HAT segment. This means that the pelvis has a segment cycle of a stride and not a step, as each of the limbs has. Motion of the pelvis may be presented as a right step and a left step motion cycle; however, this is presenting the same data only in a different order and is quite different than the data presented for instance at the knee joint for right and

A

Hip

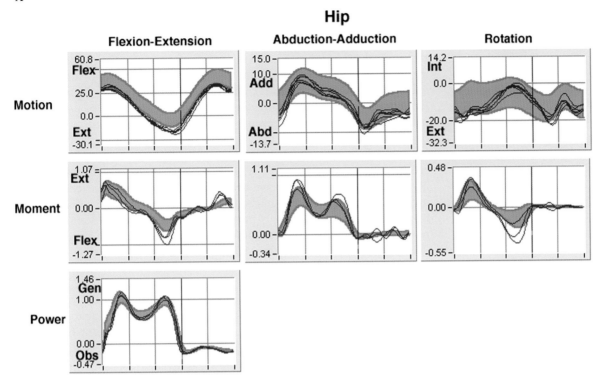

Motion   Flexion-Extension   Abduction-Adduction   Rotation

Moment

Power

B

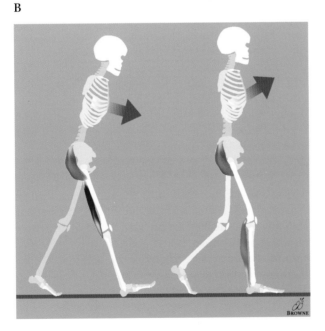

Figure 6.25. Because the hip has free three-dimensional motion, it requires muscle control in each of these dimensions (A). The muscle that controls sagittal plane motion at foot contact and weight acceptance is primarily the gluteus maximus, which provides concentric contraction (B). This muscle activity is the secondary power generator for motion, and when the gastrocsoleus becomes inactivated, such as in the use of very high heeled shoes, the gluteus maximus becomes the primary power generator. Hip flexion in terminal stance phase is produced by the gastrocsoleus and the hip flexors. Deceleration of hip flexion in terminal swing phase is controlled by the eccentric contraction of the hamstrings.

left steps. Another way to present motion data of the pelvis is to present it as half-cycle data from right heel strike to left heel strike and from left heel strike to right heel strike. This presentation presents two different data sets and allows an assessment of the symmetry of pelvic motion. Again, the difference between these two graphic presentation modes should be understood when looking at the data. This same problem of how to present motion relative to the gait cycle also applies to the trunk segment and the head segment.

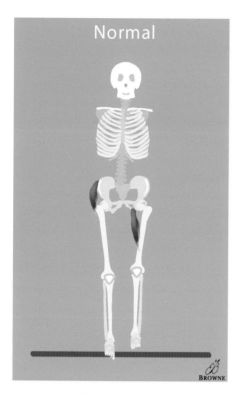

Figure 6.26. Coronal plane motion is controlled by an isometric contraction of the gluteus medius in early stance phase and by adductor contraction in initial swing phase.

Pelvic motion at initial contact on the right is rotated right side forward, then slowly rotates into maximum left side forward at left heel contact, and then back again to full right side forward at right heel contact. Therefore, pelvic motion has one rotation cycle during each stride with the normal total rotation being less than 10°, and this rotation increases with increased walking velocity. Pelvic tilt follows the swing limb, meaning that the posterior pelvic tilt is maximum at foot contact, then as the opposite limb starts hip flexion, the pelvis follows into anterior pelvic tilt, followed by posterior tilt maximum again at toe-off on the opposite side. Pelvic tilt therefore goes through two rotation cycles with each stride concurrent with the swing limb. Normal total range of pelvic tilt is less than 5°, but also increases with increasing speed of walking. Pelvic obliquity is neutral at initial contact. During weight acceptance, the pelvis drops on the opposite side, reaching a maximum pelvic drop in early midstance, then the pelvis starts elevation back toward the neutral position by initial contact on the contralateral side. The pelvic obliquity makes one rotation cycle in each stride with a range of motion of less than 5° (see Figure 6.27).

HAT Segment

The HAT segment is very complicated and the interactions are not well worked out. Motion of the HAT segment tends to be similar to the pelvic segment (Figure 6.28). The trunk muscles serve an important function of maintaining the trunk stable much in the same way the ankle is stabilized by muscles connecting at the foot. These trunk muscles include the abdominal muscles and the paraspinal muscles used for general postural control. The motion of the arms can have a significant impact on the stability and position of the center of gravity in the HAT segment. The arms swing reciprocally with the swinging leg, meaning when the right leg is in forward swing, the left arm is swinging forward (Figure 6.29). If there is a major problem that limits motion in the upper extremity, the contralateral lower extremity will demonstrate the mechanical impact during gait. Also, the head is a separate segment within the HAT segment, which can be positioned so as to impact the center of mass. However, the head postures are more likely to be used for balance and receiving sensory feedback than for altering the center of mass of the HAT segment.

A Simplified Understanding of Normal Gait

The foregoing description of the function of all the segments and joints during gait has been greatly simplified compared with current full understanding. The mechanical understanding of the whole body will simplify this structure even more, but it provides a framework to apply a mechanical clinical understanding to pathologic gait that can be helpful in formulating treatment options.

Simplified Joint Functions

The body is seen as a cargo segment setting on the motor train. The motor train element is made up of linked, rigid segments. The foot is the segment in contact with the ground and its main function is to make a stable, solid connection with the ground and have mechanical lever arm length in the plane of forward motion and at right angles to the ankle and knee joints. The ankle joint is the primary motor output of energy and power for forward motion of gait. Also, the ankle is the primary stabilizer for postural stability. The calf is a straight, rigid segment between the knee and ankle joints. The knee is a hinge joint whose main function is to allow the limb to lengthen and shorten, and the knee needs to be a stable connection between the shank

A

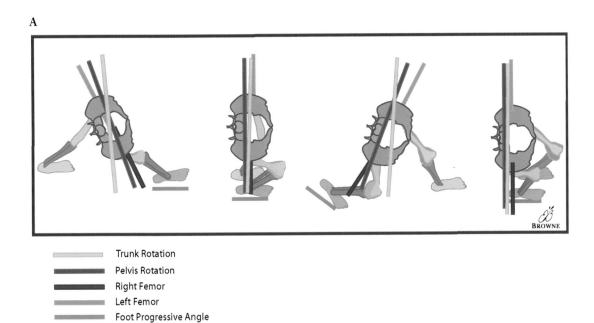

	Trunk Rotation
	Pelvis Rotation
	Right Femor
	Left Femor
	Foot Progressive Angle

B

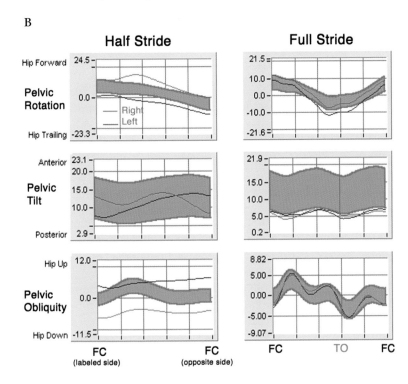

Figure 6.27. The most significant motion of the pelvis is in the transverse plane, although there is motion in both the sagittal and coronal planes as well (A). Transverse plane control of the limb starts with the foot fixed on the floor; however, as toe-off occurs, some internal rotation occurs that has to be accommodated at the pelvis and hip. The cycle of the pelvis does not have a right and left cycle because it is one unit without an articulation in the middle. The cycle is half as long as the stride in the limbs; therefore, we prefer to look at right and left half cycles (B); this allows a comparison of right to left symmetry rather than plotting the same data twice, only out of phase, which is what occurs with full cycle plotting.

and thigh segments. The knee joint axis and ankle joint axis should be parallel and at right angles to the forward line of progression. The thigh is a straight, rigid segment with torsional alignment allowing the knee to have its axis at a right angle to the forward line of progression. The hip allows motion in three dimensions. The hip is the secondary or alternate source of power output for forward mobility. At initial contact, hip flexion combined with knee extension define the step length. The hip also has to keep the pelvis and HAT segment stable with minimal motion. The role of the pelvis is to have enough motion to accommodate the hips so as to decrease the motion of the center of mass of the HAT segment.

Trunk Motion - Full cycle plots

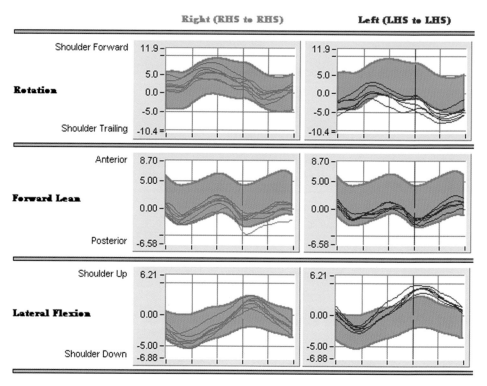

Figure 6.28. Movement of the trunk as defined by the top of the shoulders and chest follows the motion of the upper extremity and is opposite of the pelvis; thus, the trunk rotates forward during ipsilateral stance and contralateral swing phase (Figure 6.27A), just the opposite of the pelvis, that rotates forward with the swing limb. Motions in the other planes are also out of phase with the pelvis. This opposite direction motion of the trunk and pelvis works to decrease the total motion of the center of mass and therefore decreases work required for walking.

Simplified Cycle Functions

Using these very simplified rules of gait, this mechanical understanding can be combined into a full description of the gait cycle. At initial contact, the heel strikes with the knee being almost extended and the hip flexed. The pelvis is rotated forward and tilted posteriorly. During weight acceptance, the foot comes to foot flat with solid contact with the ground. For weight acceptance, the leg initially shortens with knee flexion and ankle dorsiflexion, and hip flexion occurs to slow the forward fall of the HAT segment. This forward fall is primarily controlled by the hip extensors. The knee is stabilized by the hamstrings and the vastus muscles. The shock absorption function also occurs with knee flexion, allowing the leg to shorten, and the energy is absorbed through the eccentric contraction of the gastrocsoleus, vasti, and hamstring muscles. In middle stance, only the gastrocsoleus has a low level of eccentric contraction with momentum carrying the body forward. In terminal stance, the gastrocnemius and soleus contract with a concentric contraction to produce plantar flexion, causing heel rise and increasing knee flexion, which allows the leg to shorten to accommodate for the rapidly increasing plantar flexion. Hip flexion also starts under the impact of this gastrocsoleus push-off contraction. Hip adductors contract to aid hip flexion and adduction in terminal stance. In preswing, the knee is rapidly shortened under the control of the eccentrically contracting rectus muscle. Initial swing phase is marked by the knee shortening to allow the foot to swing through. Also, at preswing and in initial swing, hip flexor power is increased to produce power causing forward swing of the limb at the hip joint. In midswing, there is little muscle activity as most of the motion is produced by momentum. In terminal swing phase, the hamstring muscles start eccentric contraction to decelerate the knee extension and hip flexion to provide stability

A

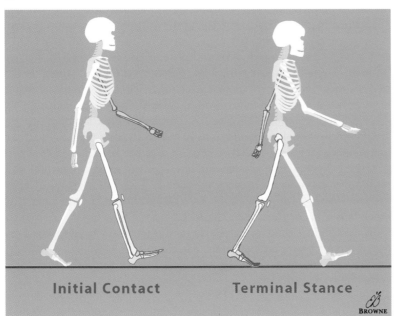

Initial Contact   Terminal Stance

BROWNE

Figure 6.29. The upper extremities also move in the opposite direction of the ipsilateral lower extremity. This out-of-phase swinging again balances the trunk and helps to preserve energy during ambulation (A). More specifically, the hip motion and the shoulder motion tend to be exact inverse motions that can easily be appreciated by plotting shoulder and hip flexion extension side by side (B).

B

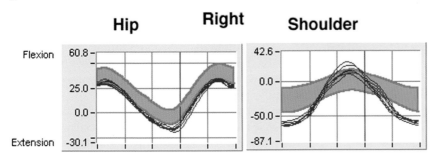

during initial contact. Hip extensors and hip abductors also activate in terminal swing and are active at initial contact.

In a very simplified version, one now sees that the foot is solidly planted, then accepts the weight of mass with as much absorption of shock as possible. The limb then shortens by knee flexion to allow the HAT segment to roll over the top, and in late stance, an energy burst produced by the gastrocsoleus is put into the system to keep it rolling forward. Weight is again transferred and the leg is shortened to allow it to swing through and be placed for the next cycle.

Abnormal Gait Adaptations

Pathologic problems can occur in any of the subsystems or mechanical components of the whole neuromuscular system that is required to make walking possible. When a problem arises in one part of this system, compensations are made in relatively consistent patterns. Usually, these compensations help resolve the deficiency at the heart of the pathology; however, sometimes the compensations can become a source of the pathology as well. The great complexity in the system makes finding verifiable reasons for compensations very difficult, and most of the explanations are based only on close observations of patients and trying to understand the results of the observed changes. It is even more difficult to try to understand the neuroanatomic anatomy and alterations that give rise to specific patterns of gait. Because there currently is not a good neuroanatomic explanation of how the central program generator works, understanding its response to pathologic insults is even more difficult. Therefore, these pathologic changes will be explained on the basis of dynamic motor control theory, which provides understanding of why patterns develop as the system is pulled toward chaotic attractors. For a full description of dynamic motor control, refer to the section on motor control. This method of making predictions based on dynamic motor control theory is similar to techniques used to predict weather patterns. However, in this situation, the impact of growth and development upon a neuromotor system with abnormal control is being predicted. With this theoretical approach, the predictions improve with increased information and the predictions are much better in the short term than long term. Short-term and smaller interventions are easier and more reliable to predict than long-term outcomes and the results of larger interventions. Therefore, the goal is to obtain as much information about each of the neurologic subsystems and the mechanical components as is possible.

Balance

Balance is an absolute requirement for safe ambulation. There are children with relatively good ability to make steps and to hold onto a walker but who have no protective response to falls. These children do not even realize they are falling and fall with a pattern often described as a falling tree. Children with this falling tree pattern, or children who consistently fall over backward, cannot be independent ambulators even with a walking aid unless it is fully supported with a design similar to a gait trainer.

As many young children start walking, problems with balance emerge. Some investigators believe that balance is the primary subsystem that precludes walking in a normal 8-month-old baby. When the baby's balancing system matures, he is ready to become a toddler. This pattern also seems to persist in many young children with diplegia who continue long term with a toddler pattern gait. If the balance system is limited in its ability to keep the body stable in an upright position, the secondary response is to cruise along stable objects or to hold onto objects that can be pushed, such as push toys or walkers. If children are able to walk without holding on, balance feedback is enhanced by keeping the arms in the high guard or medium guard positions. This arm-up position allows using the arm position to alter the center of gravity in the HAT segment and works with the same mechanical principle as the long pole that is used by high-wire walkers at the circus. Another adaptation for poor balance is to use momentum in such a way that children can walk when they are going at a certain minimal speed, but when this velocity decreases or they try to stop, they fall over or have to hold onto a stable object. This adaptive response to poor balance is similar to that which is normally used when riding a bicycle.

Poor balance can be assessed by a decrease in the gross motor function measure and high variability in step length and cadence. Also, there is increased shoulder range of motion and increased elbow flexion reflecting the high guard arm position. Children with severe ataxia often have high variability of hip, knee, and ankle motion patterns on the kinematics. Poor stability, primarily due to foot positioning problems such as toe walking, planovalgus, or equinovarus, also magnifies the central balance problems.

The Impact of Growth and Development

The balance system usually matures rapidly in the first 3 years of life, often making substantial observable gains every 6 months. Significant gains continue in the second 3 years, but usually in a less dramatic fashion. Slow improvements often continue into middle childhood, reaching full balance maturity at 8 to 10 years of age. Usually, during the adolescent growth spurt, balance appears to be deteriorating; however, this is only the appearance of the adolescent clumsy stage that most normal teenagers endure. By several years after the completion of growth, balance will return to a similar level of middle childhood; however, because these children are much heavier and taller, falls are more painful and they may not run along, fall, and then get up again with the same vigor with which they did at age 7 years. Also, for teenagers who are 17 years old, it is not socially acceptable to be repeatedly falling, especially in public.

Interventions

The primary interventions for addressing balance deficiencies are therapy-based techniques that will stimulate children's balance systems. These activities include walking on an edge, walking slowly, and doing activities on one foot, such as hopping. These activities have to be closely matched to the children's immediate abilities. It is important that children be provided with an appropriate aid for walking, usually a walker for young children, and then switched to forearm crutches in middle childhood. Also, crutches or canes used in therapy can stimulate balance, even if these devices are not functional for day-to-day ambulation. It is important to provide as stable a base of support as possible, which is usually accomplished by adding foot orthotics to young children. The orthotic should hold the foot plantigrade and correct planovalgus foot deformities. The first orthotic should be a solid ankle AFO to stabilize the ankle and foot so that children can focus on control of the hips and knees. Stable shoes with good, flat soles should also be used.

Motor Control

Motor control is the primary central program generator function that directs the muscles to contract at the appropriate time. Motor control function is complex and difficult to comprehend, especially considering that only one muscle, the gastrocnemius, has approximately 2000 motor units. Each of these motor units has to be contracted considering the position of the knee and ankle, the velocity of the contraction, the specific fiber type, and the time of the gait cycle. Adding this complexity to the balance system explains why the largest part of the central nervous system is taken up with controlling the peripheral motor system. When this system has a pathologic defect, it tries to maintain control, but generally at a level of less detail. A simple example of this effect occurs in the upper extremity of a hemiplegic hand in which individual fine motor control of finger flexion is lost; however, the child maintains gross grasp finger flexion in which all the fingers and thumb flex at the same time. Sometimes, this even extends to mirror movements on the other side so when the fingers flex on the less-involved side, the fingers also flex on the more-involved hand.

As motor control is decreased, many changes occur. The changes of motor control are definitely drawn to patterns that appear to be attractors for specific limitations. A pattern of simpler movements, often based on mass movement similar to the mirror motion described in the hand, is the most common alteration. Athetosis, dystonia, chorea, and ballismus are other movement patterns. A full discussion of these patterns occurs in the chapter on motor control (Chapter 3). The tendency toward mass movement initiates significant secondary adaptive changes. This pattern of decreased motor control often has increased muscle tone, which stiffens the system to make control easier. The increased tone also tends to cause muscle fiber shortening, which decreases the joint range of motion, again decreasing variable options available for motor control. Often, the motor control that is available seems to focus on the major joints and gross function at the expense of small joints and small motions. This means the motor control system is able to control motion of the hip, knee, and ankle, but may not be able to control foot position, leading to a higher rate of foot deformities. The system also does better with single-joint muscles than with multiple-joint muscles. Again, there is much less complexity in controlling a muscle that only affects one joint than with a muscle that affects two or three joints simultaneously. An example is the quadriceps muscles, where the rectus often has problems with motor control; the vastus seldom has problems related to motor control. Because many of the multiple-joint muscles work as body stabilizers or provide body stiffening, in the face of decreasing motor control these muscles tend to contract too much and add significant stiffness to the system.

Assessing motor control requires several measures, but a decrease in the fourth dimension in the GMFM is a good indicator of motor control problems. Also, in the physical examination, the individual muscle motor control gives a measure of the function of the central program generator, and the presence of mass movement or the confusion tests indicates increasing motor control problems. The confusion test is positive when children can dorsiflex only in concurrence with hip and knee flexion. The assessment of athetosis usually demonstrates high variability around a single cluster, especially in trunk motion and upper extremity motion. The movement pattern of dystonia often presents with variability around two or three clusters. Often, there is the appearance of motion being drawn to two separate attractors.

The Impact of Growth and Development

Motor control is variable in its development. By the time children are 6 to 7 months old, the central program generator already consistently makes stepping motions if the children are placed on the floor and held so they do not fall. The fine motor control of the feet and the upper extremity come on slowly, following a pattern similar to balance development. The first 3 years have the most rapid development, then very significant development continues over the subsequent three years. By middle childhood, motor development reaches its maturity; however, new motor skills can be learned throughout life.

Athetosis is often present first as poor balance, then the movements start in the second and third years. By age 3 to 5 years, the pattern is well set and seems to change little. Dystonia, when it is mild, may be seen first in the 3- to 5-year-old age range and is often stable during middle childhood. Although there have been no published data, our experience with children has been that the dystonia tends to get worse around adolescence. This increased severity does not seem to recede as the individuals enter young adulthood.

Interventions

Intervention for motor control pathology is similar to balance in that the first intervention should be therapy using a teaching model similar to teaching children to be dancers or ice skaters. This therapy involves cognitive understanding and repetitive performance of a task to be learned. This therapy has to be within the context of the children's physical abilities, meaning that some children have too much damage to the central program generator to learn to walk and no amount of teaching will get them walking. Also, because of the tendency to focus on major joint control over small joint control, providing stability of the small joints, especially the foot with the use of orthotics, is an important aspect of the first stage. This initial stabilization can be followed later by surgical stabilization of the foot if indicated. Assessing when the adaptive mechanisms have become a pathology in themselves, and addressing these pathologic adaptations, are important parts of the treatment. For example, the stiffness imparted by an overactive rectus femoris may be needed in some children, but in others, it is a definite impairment in its own right. Children who walk very slowly with a walker as household ambulators only, have scores on the fourth dimension of the GMFM of 35%, and have significant toe drag, will likely gain more from the stiffness imparted by the rectus than if this stiffness were removed. Many of these children will recruit the vastus to again provide the knee stiffness because of their need for support in stance. On the other hand, children who are independent ambulators at 8 years of age, but are consistently dragging their feet because the rectus is active too long in swing phase, will respond very well to having the impairment of the knee stiffness removed. When planning treatment, the level of motor control has to be considered in the decision making to determine if the apparent problem is adding to or further impairing children's overall function.

Interventions for athetoid gait patterns are mainly directed at stabilizing joints, such as the feet if the problem is instability. Surgery or other active interventions are seldom of much help in individuals with athetosis unless they have associated spasticity that is causing secondary problems. The spasticity is beneficial in athetosis as a means of placing a shock absorber or brake on the movement disorder. With dystonia, joint stabilization is the only viable option to improve gait. For both athetosis and dystonia, finding the correct walking aid with functioning arm support often requires a great deal of trial and error.

Motor Power

Gait requires energy output that has to be expended by the muscles to create motion. This motion requires the cardiovascular system to bring the energy to the muscles. Weakness can come from problems in any of the energy production pathways. When the problem of decreased energy available is expressed as muscle weakness, an almost normal gait pattern may be preserved through the use of increased motor control to improve efficiency. This is what occurs in children with primary muscle disease, such as muscular dystrophy. These individuals have an extremely energy-efficient gait when oxygen consumption is measured.[37] These same children, though, have very limited ability to walk. Children with CP may also have weakness due to small muscle size from spasticity and decreased energy delivery secondary to poor conditioning, but they can seldom make up for these deficiencies with increased motor control. Instead, it is much more common for children with CP to have increased energy cost of walking as a way of compensating for poor motor control and poor balance. Adding stiffness through increasing spasticity and co-contraction of the muscles increases the energy costs of walking; however, these changes provide a functional benefit of lowering the demands on the balance and motor control subsystems. This combination of muscle weakness and cardiovascular conditioning often coalesces to form a milieu in which individual children are drawn to either primary wheelchair ambulators or community ambulators with assistive devices (Case 6.3). Young adults who primarily ambulate with wheelchairs in the community will lose cardiovascular endurance to the point where community ambulation is no longer possible because of weakness. Therefore, forcing these individuals into wheelchairs further exacerbates the loss of endurance. Individuals who primarily walk will stay well conditioned and usually continue walking. In intermediate ambulators, there also seems to be a psychologic factor that feeds into the process. If individuals have a strong drive to walk, they will continue walking, but if the drive to not walk is stronger, it will soon be reinforced with poor endurance from not walking. Motor power is measured in individual muscles using the motor strength scale from the physical examination. Overall oxygen consumption is measured during walking, and this is combined with the heart rate response as the best measure of children's cardiovascular condition and the energy efficiency of walking.

Impact of Growth and Development

The strength of children's muscles relative to their body weight is greatest in young children, and this strength ratio decreases gradually as they grow into middle childhood. There is rapid decrease in the strength ratio during adolescence. Also, as children with spasticity grow, muscles have less growth than would normally occur, therefore leaving these children even weaker. Cardiovascular endurance does not usually become an issue until the preadolescent or adolescent stage. Children in early and middle childhood tend to want to be out of the wheelchair and be as active as their physical ability allows. Then, a combination of factors come together to push these children into either primary wheelchair ambulation or primary ambulation without a wheelchair in the community. The factors that occur just before and during adolescence include the children's weight, physical ability, psychologic drive, family structure, amount of expected community ambulation, and the physical environment of the community.

Interventions

The primary interventions are to maintain cardiovascular conditioning, especially at the adolescent stage, through some activity that the children enjoy. This plan works best if children start at an early age. For example, a child who learns to swim at age 5 or 6 years and continues to swim during middle childhood tends to be more comfortable with this activity and will therefore improve his physical conditioning through swimming. If an attempt is made to teach children to swim at age 15 years for physical conditioning, they will often be very resistant because of the difficulty of becoming comfortable in the water. Also, working on strengthening exercises for children with spasticity does no harm and actually has been documented to provide some benefit.[14]

Musculoskeletal Subsystem: Specific Joint Problems

As was noted in the description of normal gait, the musculoskeletal subsystems function as a series of mechanical components linked by joints. Each of these segment components and the connecting joints has a specific role in gait. As problems occur with gait, these mechanical subsystems are the place where the adjustments occur. Again, there can be adaptive adjustments that accommodate for the problem at a different location, or the problem may be primary and the source of the problem requiring the adaptation elsewhere. Sorting out this impact is very important when planning treatment because secondary adaptations need no treatment, as they will resolve when the primary problem is addressed. However, there are situations where an adaptive secondary change over time can become part of the primary problem. An example of such a problem is the combination of toe walking with hemiplegia in young children. The mechanical system prefers to be symmetric, and in young children who have great strength for their body weight, if forced to toe walk on one side, will usually prefer to toe walk on both sides (Case 6.4). If children have a pure hemiplegic pattern and the unaffected ankle has full range of motion, an orthotic is needed only on the affected side. This orthotic will stop the toe walking on the opposite side as well. If the toe walking has been ignored in older children and they have been walking on their toes for 4 to 6 years, the unaffected side, even if there is no neurologic pathology, will have become contracted; therefore, they cannot walk feet flat comfortably. The adaptive deformity has now become a primary impairment in its own right and if surgical treatment is planned, the unaffected leg must be addressed as well.

Foot and Ankle

The foot has the role of being a stable segment aligned with the forward line of progression and providing a moment arm connected to the floor. The ankle provides the primary energy output for mobility and provides motor output for postural control, as well as being part of the shock absorption function during weight acceptance.

The Foot as a Stable, Stiff Segment

The primary role of the foot segment is to provide a stable, stiff connection to the ground during stance phase. The primary problems occurring at the foot are foot deformities that preclude a stable base of support. These deformities are mainly planovalgus, and less commonly, varus deformity. Another problem is the loss of stiffness of the foot segment, which occurs because of increased range of motion in the midfoot allowing for midfoot dorsiflexion, also called midfoot break. This combination of foot pathology leads to less stability of the foot as a stiff segment and further leads to less stable support with the ground by focusing the pressure into a smaller contact area (Case 6.5). The primary cause of foot deformities is poor motor control, which is added to by the mechanics forcing this deformity into progression. The degree of dysfunction caused by the foot deformity is best assessed with a pedobarograph, where only pressure on the medial midfoot would suggest a very severe foot deformity with poor mechanical function. Also, an assessment of the ankle moment often demonstrates low plantar flexion moment in late stance, but a high or normal plantar flexion moment in early stance. A foot that has lost its stiffness also cannot provide support against which the gastrocnemius muscle can work to provide push-off power.

Secondary Adaptations

When a foot is unstable, balancing and motor control subsystems are stressed and one response is to increase the stiffness at the proximal joint through increased tone and increased motor co-contraction, especially at the knee. The vastus muscles, as primary knee extenders, are usually activated to assist with maintaining upright posture with the knee in flexion as part of the crouched gait pattern. These secondary changes, especially in adolescents with greatly increased body mass, add to the pathomechanics causing a foot deformity to become more severe. Most often, the foot is the initial primary cause of the crouched gait pattern (Case 6.5).

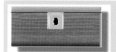
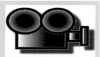

Case 6.4   Charvin

Charvin, a 5-year-old girl, presented with the parents' complaint of toe walking. On physical examination she was noted to have Ashworth grade 2 tone in the left gastrocnemius, −5° of ankle dorsiflexion with both knees extended and knee flexion, and 3+ ankle reflex. The right ankle had 10° of dorsiflexion with knee extension, 15° with knee flexion, normal muscle tone, and normal reflexes. Examination of the remaining lower extremities was normal, and the left upper extremity had no increased tone, but seemed clumsier with rapid movements. Observation of her gait demonstrated a child with excellent balance, normal upper extremity arm swing, and bilateral toe strike with persistent bilateral toe walking. A diagnosis of hemiplegia was made and she had a full gait analysis, which demonstrated normal timing of the left tibialis anterior muscle (Figure C6.4.1). A diagnosis of

type 2 left-side hemiplegia was made, although she had significant toe walking on the right as well. This toe walking was felt to be compensatory for the left ankle equinus. An open Z-lengthening of the tendon Achilles was performed, and she walked with a flat foot strike. Over the next 10 years, she continued to have intermittent toe walking related to rapid growth spurts, and persisted with premature heel rise on the left. By the time she reached full maturity at age 15 years, she desired a final correction, and she had a gastrocnemius lengthening that improved her premature heel rise and high early ankle plantar flexion moment on the left side. In addition to having decreased early dorsiflexion peak and premature plantar flexion, which improved bilaterally, she was able to slightly improve her push-off power generation on both sides (Figure C6.4.2).

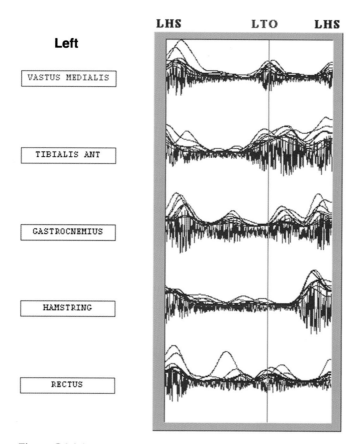

Figure C6.4.1

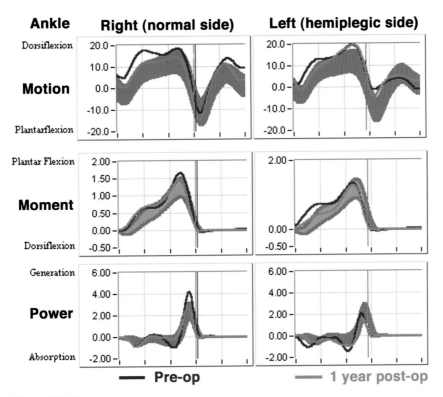

Figure C6.4.2

Treatment

In young children, the primary treatment of the unstable feet is the use of custom-molded foot orthotics, usually starting with solid ankle AFOs; then, if the deformities are not too severe, the AFOs can be articulated. However, if the foot deformity is severe, articulated orthotics do not work well because motion tends to occur in the subtalar joint. At some point, many of these children need surgical stabilization of the foot. There are many surgical options that are discussed fully in the chapter on the foot and ankle.

The Foot as a Functional Moment Arm in Contact with the Ground Reaction Force

The other major function of the foot, in addition to being a stable, stiff segment, is to be a moment arm upon which the ground reaction force can act; this means the foot has to have an alignment that is in line with the forward line of progression and at right angles to the ankle and knee joint axes. Torsional malalignment of the foot does not allow the power output at the ankle to have a moment arm on which to work. This torsional malalignment may have its primary etiology as part of the foot deformity. The plano-valgus deformity may cause an external rotation of the foot relative to the ankle joint axis and the equinovarus causes internal rotation of the foot relative to the ankle joint axis. The torsional malalignment may also be due to tibial torsion, femoral anteversion, or pelvic rotation (Case 6.6). The alignment of the foot is best assessed by the foot progression angle on the kinematic evaluation. The source of the rotational malalignment is best determined by tibial torsion and femoral rotation measures on the kinematic evaluation compared with the physical examination. On the physical examination, femoral rotation with hip extension is assessed. Tibial torsion is

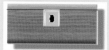

Case 6.5   Joshua

Joshua, a boy with asymmetric diplegia, walked with a posterior walker. By age 6 years, he was walking independently, although very asymmetrically, with extreme knee stiffness on the left. At that time he had a rectus transfer on the left, and he continued to do well until age 15 years. As he was going through his adolescent growth, he gradually developed more right foot planovalgus and external rotation, and complained of having increased knee pain with ambulation. He was placed in a ground reaction AFO but, because of poor moment arm due to the external rotation, this was of little help. The knee pain was believed to be due to high joint reaction force external valgus moment at the knee and high shear stress in the knee. The foot pressure demonstrated a moderate right planovalgus foot deformity with an external foot progression angle of 35°, although a weightbearing radiograph of the foot was nearly normal (Figure C6.5.1). He also had 45° of external thigh–foot angle on physical examination. Based on these data, the crouch and knee pain were thought to result from a combination of planoval-

gus and external tibial torsion. Also, a radiograph of his knee demonstrated mild increased knee valgus measuring 12°. The planovalgus was corrected with a lateral column lengthening and the tibial torsion with an osteotomy of the tibia (Figure C6.5.2). It was elected to leave the knee valgus because this was on the border of normal and due to secondary forces from the leg below. One year after the surgery, he was walking without knee pain and no orthotics; however, he still had a mild degree of knee valgus but with improved crouch (Figure C6.5.3). The right foot demonstrates a mild residual valgus deformity; however, the left foot is slightly overcorrected into varus (Figures C6.5.4, C6.3.5). The right gastrocsoleus is still somewhat incompetent based on the prolonged heel contact or late heel rise on the right (Figure C6.5.4). To completely correct this deformity, a high tibial varus osteotomy would have been required. This demonstrates the typical occurrence of these deformities as an adolescent goes through the final growth, often with problems occurring at several levels, which combine to cause a severe problem.

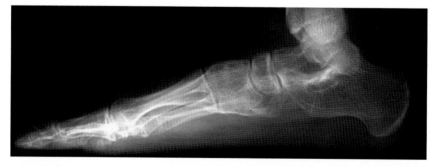

Figure C6.5.1

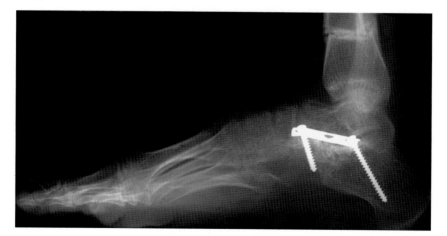

Figure C6.5.2

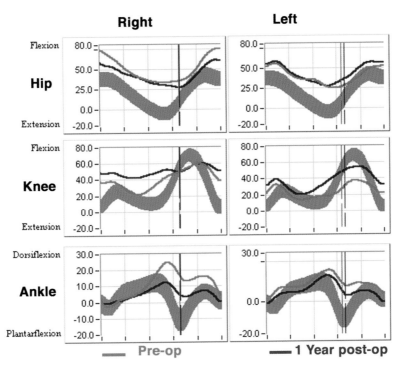

Figure C6.5.3

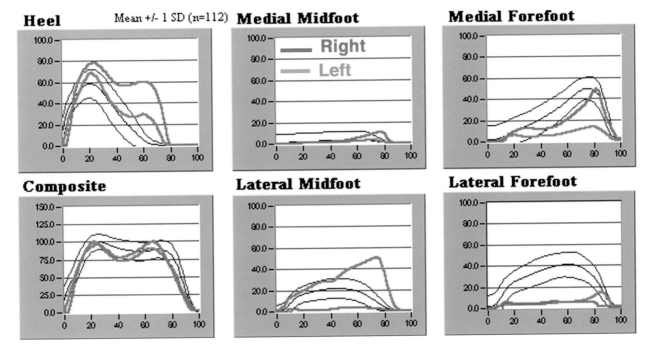

Figure C6.5.4

Left   **Right**

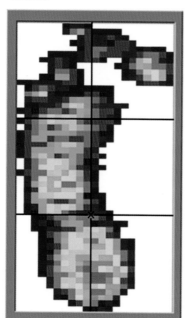
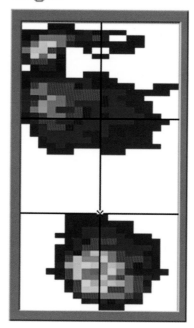

Figure C6.5.5

measured with a transmalleolar axis-to-thigh angle. In general, a normal foot progression angle is 0° to 20° external. Most individuals with CP do well until the angle is more than 10° internal or 30° external. The foot progression angle, which is more than 30° external, will rapidly start to have a negative effect on the moment arm, as an effective length of the moment arm rapidly shortens. This number is due to the length of the moment arm being the length of the foot times the cosine of the rotation angle (Figure 6.30). Therefore, changes of the first 20° to 30° cause minimal change in the affected moment arm.

Secondary Adaptations

As the moment arm becomes less effective, the plantar flexion moment generated by the ankle decreases. As with foot deformities, the same secondary effects of increased stiffness and increased co-contractions occur. There may also be a residual moment, which tends to cause the deformity to get worse. In a foot with severe external rotation, the moment arm in the direction of forward motion has decreased greatly. However, the moment arm generating an external rotation moment has increased and now may be a mechanical factor to increase the deformity, either by increasing the foot deformity, or by causing increased external tibial torsion as children grow. This external rotation moment arm may also cause external rotation subluxation by rotating the tibia through the knee joint. There is an increase in the varus-valgus moment arm as well, but this seldom seems to cause mechanical or growth problems, probably because the force is somewhat reduced with the increased co-contraction required for walking, which is common in this combination of deformities. Many children have a combination of external rotation and planovalgus foot deformity, which makes a double-dose insult to the moment arm function of the foot. This insult is a principal cause of severe crouched gait and has been termed lever arm disease by Gage[3] (see

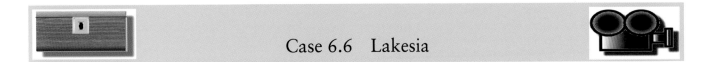

Case 6.6   Lakesia

Lakesia, a 15-year-old girl with a diagnosis of spastic diplegia, was in a regular high school and was a varsity swimmer on the high school swim team. She had also been playing lacrosse as a recreational sport. Over the past 2 years, she had grown rapidly and gained weight. During that time she gradually started to develop more knee pain, worse on the left than the right, to the point that she had trouble walking around her school and she

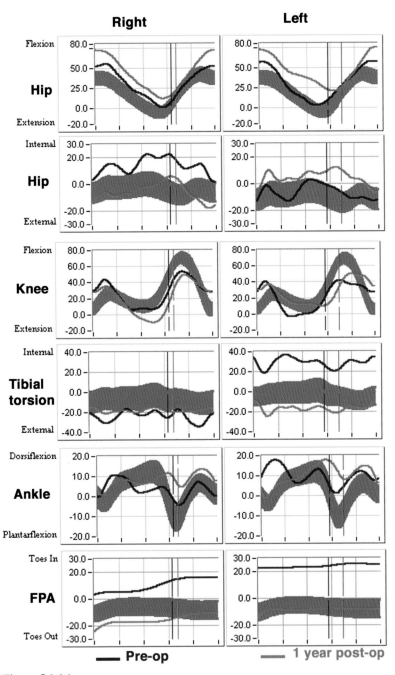

Figure C6.6.1

could not run to play lacrosse. Her family doctor told her to buy and use a wheelchair. Her gait involved a significant amount of trunk lurching with mild crouching, stiff knee gait, and internal rotation of the knees. On physical examination, both knees had mild diffuse tenderness, with no effusion, mechanical instability, click, or joint line tenderness. Hip motion demonstrated 80° of internal rotation, 10° of external rotation, full knee flexion and extension with popliteal angles of 70°, and transmalleolar-to-thigh axis of 30° external on the left and 20° on the right. Both feet demonstrated a planovalgus deformity and both feet had significant bunions. Radiographs of the knees were normal. She was initially evaluated in the sports clinic where a diagnosis of intraarticular pathology was made, and she was scheduled for knee arthroscopy, where an inflamed plica was found and excised. Following a 6-month rehabilitation program, she still continued with the same pain, and she was now using the wheelchair

for all ambulation except for household ambulation. An evaluation in the gait laboratory found significant internal rotation of the hips, external tibial torsion on the right, and internal tibial torsion on the left with the planovalgus feet, increased knee flexion at foot contact, and decreased knee flexion in swing phase (Figures C6.6.1, C6.6.2). Because there was minimal EMG activity in the rectus in swing phase (Figure C6.6.3), a trial of Botox to the left rectus also demonstrated no change in the motion of the left knee in swing phase. It was thought that the decreased knee flexion in swing was due to the poor push-off and poor mechanical advantage on the hip flexors at push-off. She was immediately referred to physical therapy and taught crutch walking to try to get her out of the wheelchair. She was then reconstructed with bilateral femoral derotation osteotomies, left tibial rotation, bilateral lateral column lengthenings, bunion corrections, and hamstring lengthenings. One year following surgery, she

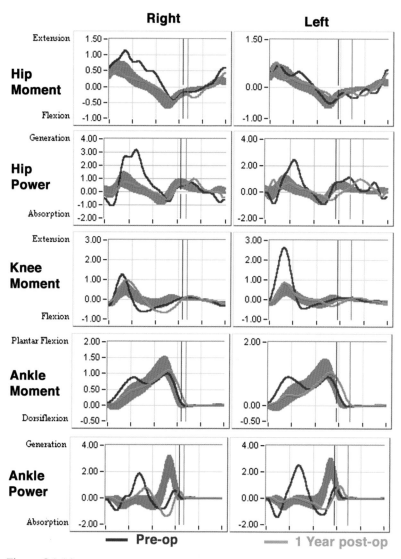

Figure C6.6.2

was pain free, was again swimming on the varsity swim team, and was no longer using the wheelchair for any community mobility, except for very long walks such as at airports or amusement parks. In all community ambulation, she used the Lofstrand crutches, which she preferred over the wheelchair.

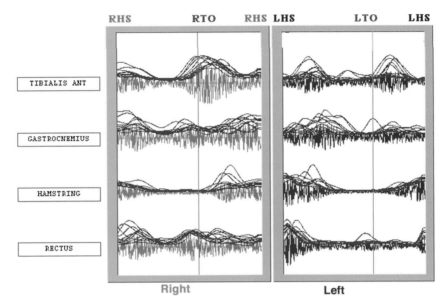

Figure C6.6.3

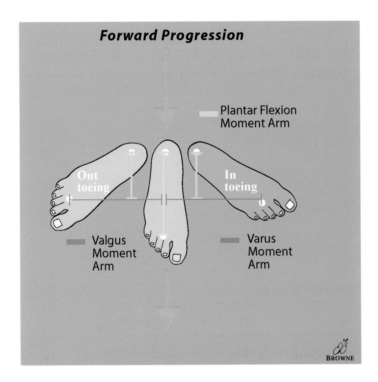

Figure 6.30). The lever arm is another name for a moment arm, and the importance of this concept to the etiology of crouched gait is often missed. Failing to understand the importance of the moment arm in the crouched gait pattern is like spending time sewing a skin wound on the leg of a child with an injury while failing to see the underlying fracture. All orthopaedists

Figure 6.30. The torsional alignment of the foot, knee, and the forward line of progression of the body is very important. If the foot is not stable or lined up with the knee axis, the plantar flexion–knee extension couple cannot function, and the child drops into a crouched gait pattern. As the foot rotates relative to the knee axis, the moment arm of the foot decreases. The length of the moment arm is determined by the cosine of the angle of rotation. This means that there is very little effect on the first 20° to 30° of external or internal rotation; however, over 30°, the moment arms rapidly lose length, and the moment arm falls very fast when there is more than 45° of external rotation.

know that the open fracture is really much more significant than the skin wound, and likewise, the lever arm dysfunction at the foot is much more significant as a contribution to crouched gait in most children than the knee flexion, which is readily apparent (Case 6.5).

Treatment

Malrotation of a foot progression angle can be treated with a foot orthotic if a major portion of the malrotation comes from the foot deformity. If the malrotation is secondary to torsional deformity more proximally, the only treatment option is surgical correction of the malrotation. In some children, the rotation is present in two or three locations and a decision has to be made if all or several need to be corrected. A relatively common example is severe planovalgus feet with external tibial torsion and increased femoral anteversion. In this situation, based on the physical examination and kinematic measurements, a judgment of how many of the deformities need to be corrected has to be made. These data have to be combined with an intraoperative assessment. For example, after the planovalgus foot deformity has been surgically corrected, the foot-to-thigh angle should be checked. If the foot-to-thigh angle is more than 25° to 30° externally, tibial osteotomy is definitely needed, but if the foot-to-thigh angle is between 10° internal and 10° external, no tibial osteotomy is needed. The midpoint ranges have to include consideration of children's level of function with more accurate correction attempted in children with better functional ability. In situations in which there is internal tibial torsion and femoral anteversion, the decision about doing one or both levels may be especially difficult. Correcting significant equinus also causes the foot to go from internal rotation to external rotation. Therefore, when making the decision on the need for rotational correction, the final determination should be made after surgical correction of the equinus (Figure 6.31). One rule that should almost always be applied is do not create compensatory deformities, or in other words, do NOT externally rotate the tibia past neutral to compensate for femoral anteversion. This compensation often leads to progressive deformity of external tibial torsion.

Figure 6.31. As the foot develops more equinus, it also tends to go into internal rotation of the foot relative to the tibia. When the severe equinus is corrected, as the foot goes into dorsiflexion it also goes into external rotation relative to the tibia. When correcting severe equinus, this secondary rotational change always has to be considered, so one should not be surprised that the individual now has severe external tibial torsion after tendon Achilles lengthening.

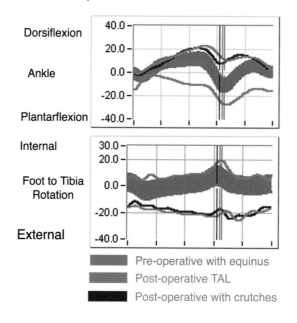

The Ankle as a Power Output Joint

The ankle is the principal power output joint and is an important part of being a shock absorber along with the knee. Ankle position at initial contact is very important in the shock absorption function. If initial foot contact is with toe strike, the foot and gastrocnemius may absorb some energy; however, if the position is foot flat, there is often a very hard strike, with the floor having to absorb the energy of initial contact. Children walking with this pattern can often be heard walking down hallways because of the loud sound and vibrations set up in the floor. The lack of shock absorption is measured on the vertical ground reaction vector of the ground reaction force. The loading response may show a magnitude of 1.5 to 2 times body weight when normal children's loading force should be between 1.1 to 1.2 times body weight (Figure 6.32). The loss of shock absorption also occurs in children in whom there is an incompetent gastrocsoleus, a situation where they strike only on the heel but have little ability to absorb the load except through the heel pad. This situation is primarily seen in children whose Achilles tendon has been transected by tenotomy. During weight acceptance, the position of the ankle joint is determined by the gastrocsoleus muscle. If the muscle is contracted and unable to allow 15° to 20° of dorsiflexion by eccentric contraction, a premature heel rise will occur. If the eccentric contraction initiates a concentric contraction, a premature plantar flexion will occur in midstance phase, causing a midstance phase rise in the center of gravity, called a vault. A major burst of power generation will be associated with the vault (see Figure 6.32). The premature gastrocnemius and soleus contraction may also cause the heel to rise, but with increased knee flexion. The center of gravity does not rise; however, the child's crouch increases. The second possible response to increased plantar flexion in midstance is knee extension, producing back-kneeing. The reasons for these three attractors for knee response to overactivity of the gastrocnemius in midstance is discussed in the knee section.

The primary reason for the gastrocnemius and soleus having a premature contraction in midstance phase may be a contracture of the gastrocnemius, which most commonly does not allow the muscle sufficient excursion for the required 20° of dorsiflexion. The treatment of this contracture is lengthening of the muscle–tendon unit, usually by gastrocnemius lengthening only. Appropriate gastrocnemius lengthening can restore some push-off power and normalize the ankle moment.[39, 40] Another primary cause of premature gastrocnemius contraction may be related to decreased motor control, making independent control of eccentric contractions difficult. These difficulties may be correlated with increased tone and increased sensitivity in the tendon stretch reflex, which together initiate a concentric contraction at the foot contact. This concentric contraction continues through weight acceptance and midstance and is best treated with an AFO that blocks plantar flexion but allows dorsiflexion.

As the gait cycle moves to late stance, the time for the power burst of the gastrocnemius occurs. If the transition from midstance to terminal stance has the ankle in plantar flexion, the mechanical advantage of the moment arm of the foot will be compromised. If the ankle is in 0° to 10° of plantar flexion, this may not be a significant compromise; however, if the ankle is in 45° of plantar flexion as terminal stance is entered, there is very little ability to generate a push-off power burst. The amount of the power burst also depends on the amount of stretch and muscle fiber length relative to the rest length or, in other words, it depends upon the muscle's position on the length–tension curve. If the muscle is already almost completely shortened

A   B

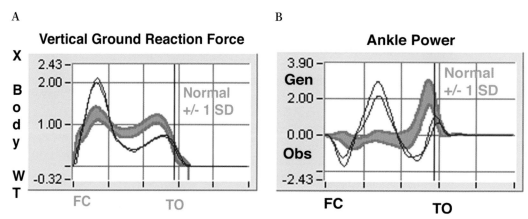

Figure 6.32. At initial contact and loading phase, the stance limb functions as a shock absorber. When the limb is not shortening through the knee, there is a very high impact force as the weight is shifted on the loading limb; this is seen best on the vertical vector of the ground reaction force (A). If the ankle then also develops a premature plantar flexion in midstance called a vault, power that lifts the center of mass vertically is generated (B).

through a contraction, little additional power can be generated. Power output that is required for the push-off power burst can be generated only with a concentric contraction, in which the muscle actually shortens. The poor prepositioning of the ankle joint in terminal stance often precludes significant push-off power generation (see Figure 6.32). The secondary adaptations for the decreased ankle push-off power generation require that the hip extensors become the primary power generators for forward motion of gait. This proximal migration of power generation is often combined with increased pelvic rotation. This change increases the total energy of walking, but is a good trade-off when motor control is not sufficient to manage the more distal ankle power generation. This same process is invoked in the role of fashion by the use of high-heeled shoes. The high-heeled shoes prevent the prepositioning of the ankle in slight dorsiflexion during terminal stance, therefore precluding the push-off power from the gastrocsoleus. This forces power generation to the hip extensors, which also increases the amount of pelvic rotation.

Treatment of the plantar flexion prepositioning of the ankle at the start of terminal stance can include the use of orthotics. Although the orthotic can block the midstance problems of vault, back-kneeing, or increased crouch, it will not preposition the foot to allow push-off power burst because it prevents active plantar flexion. An articulated AFO may preserve some push off power; however, it is greatly reduced from normal. The use of a leaf-spring orthosis is another option; however, the stiffness required to prevent the midstance phase plantar flexion almost always prevents the terminal stance phase plantar flexion burst as well. In many patients, the gastrocnemius is much more of a problem than the soleus. The gastrocnemius covers three joints and tends to develop a more severe contracture more quickly. Based on the physical examination, the degree of contracture between the gastrocnemius and the soleus can be separated based on the degree of dorsiflexion of the ankle with the knee flexed versus extended. This examination records the excursion of the soleus compared with dorsiflexion of the ankle with the knee extended, which reflects the excursion of the gastrocnemius. Usually, lengthening only the gastrocnemius will greatly improve the premature contraction problem in middle stance, and in some situations, allows improved push-off power development by improved prepositioning of the ankle. It is very important to avoid overlengthening because the ankle generally functions better in mild equinus than hyperdorsiflexion, a position where it can generate no plantar flexion. Many children who had their Achilles tendons transected require lifelong use of AFOs to stabilize their ankle joints.

C

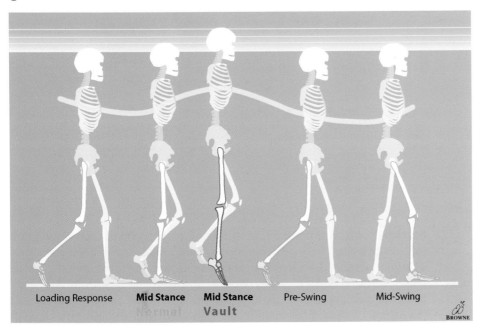

D

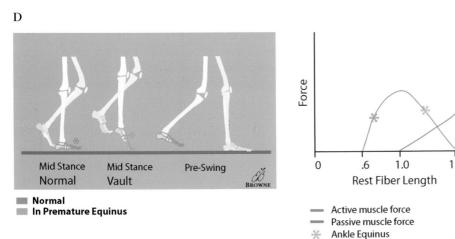

Figure 6.32 (continued). From the peak of the vault, the body falls forward into terminal stance (C); however, the ankle is usually still in equinus, thereby decreasing the ability for the ankle to generate power from additional push-off. This occurs because the muscle tends to be positioned on the wrong side of the length–tension curve to have maximum ability to generate power, and the remaining range of motion is limited (D).

Ankle Dorsiflexion in Swing Phase

Dorsiflexion in swing phase has two roles. First, in early swing phase, dorsiflexion helps to shorten the limb and allows swing through. Second, in terminal swing phase, dorsiflexion is part of prepositioning the limb for initial contact. Most children with CP have active dorsiflexor power produced by the tibialis anterior. If the EMG of the tibialis anterior is phasic in its activity, but very little dorsiflexion is produced, the cause is usually co-contraction with the gastrocnemius and soleus, or the tibialis anterior is attempting to contract against a contracted gastrocnemius muscle. In the presence of a phasic contracting tibialis anterior muscle, the ability for it to produce dorsiflexion will be enhanced with gastrocnemius lengthening. If the plantar flexion contracture was severe, the tibialis anterior may be overstretched and will require using an orthotic for some time to contract and function in its proper length (Figure 6.33). Some children with incompetent Achilles tendons

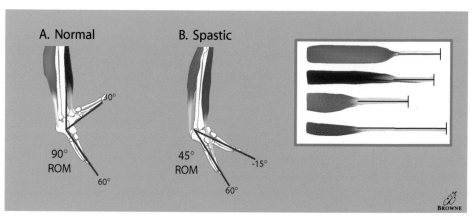

Figure 6.33. A problem of equinus contracture that gets most of the attention is the shortened gastrocsoleus which limits the active range of motion. This active range of motion can be changed by lengthening the tendon Achilles; however, the second problem is that the tibialis anterior has developed an overlengthened tendon and it too is functioning in the equinus position. After lengthening the tendon Achilles, the tibialis anterior is now much too long; therefore, it is not functioning as an antagonist muscle in the same range in which the gastrocsoleus is working. Time is required for the tibialis anterior to shorten.

develop dorsiflexion contractures because there is no gastrocnemius strength to overcome the tibialis anterior power. Some children with inadequate dorsiflexion combined with a stiff knee have severe toe drag in early swing phase. The dorsiflexion is a secondary cause of toe drag with the stiff knee being the primary cause. Often, this order is confused and the equinus gets the primary blame. For example, an individual with complete paralysis of the tibialis anterior and a drop foot but otherwise a normal functioning extremity, will never drag his toes. He will instead develop hyperflexion of the hip and knee to allow clearing of the foot. The only time an equinus foot position will cause toe drag is when it is associated with a knee that has decreased knee flexion in early swing phase. Many children with toe drag have dorsiflexion of the ankle and still drag their toes. This dorsiflexion also explains why children wearing orthotics that prevent plantar flexion still have toe drag. This again shows that the toe drag actually was due to the knee and not the plantar flexion. The treatment of decreased dorsiflexion power preventing active dorsiflexion is a very light, flexible leaf-spring AFO. These AFOs will control dorsiflexion and still allow some plantar flexion to occur. These AFOs are useful only when the gastrocnemius and the soleus have relatively normal tone and muscle length.

Knee

The primary function of the knee is to allow limb length adjustment and to provide stability in stance phase. At initial contact, the knee should have slight flexion so it can participate with the ankle in absorbing the shock of weight transfer. If the knee is completely extended, it does not easily have smooth flexion and therefore will not provide good shock absorption. The degree of knee flexion is modulated mainly by the hamstrings, and in children with CP, full knee extension at initial contact usually is the result of overlengthening of the hamstrings. Full knee extension at initial contact is also seen in children with hypotonia and ataxia.

Increased knee flexion at foot contact is much more common. This increased flexion helps shock absorption; however, this is often associated with plantar flexion and toe strike, which places an immediate strong external extension moment on the knee that the hamstrings have to resist. During weight acceptance, there tend to be two patterns of knee motion; one is immediate extension from initial contact position and the other is increased knee flexion, which may occur because of eccentric gastrocsoleus contraction, weak gastrocnemius, or a poor moment arm of the foot. The amount of knee flexion during weight acceptance should be 10° to 20° if it is normally controlled by the gastrocnemius and soleus eccentric contraction. If the degree of knee flexion is more than 20°, it is likely due to weakness of the gastrocsoleus or an insufficient moment arm at the foot.

As the gait cycle proceeds to midstance, if there was knee flexion during weight acceptance, knee extension should now begin. If the knee flexion continues into midstance, then a crouched gait pattern is present (Case 6.7). The primary causes of increased knee flexion in midstance are knee flexion contractures, hamstring contractures, a deficient foot moment arm, and gastrocsoleus weakness (Figure 6.34). A secondary etiology may be significant hip flexion contracture, which can limit knee extension in midstance. Often, there are several causes of increased knee flexion in midstance and all primary and secondary causes should be identified. This identification involves considering the actual magnitude of the flexion by evaluating the knee extension in midstance on the kinematic evaluation, the ankle moment in midstance, and the knee moment in midstance. If the ankle moment is normal or below normal, and the knee flexion is not increased, then the ankle weakness and foot moment arm are the most likely causes. If the kinematics show the knee extending to the limits of the fixed knee flexion contracture measured on physical examination, then the knee joint contracture is a likely cause. If the ankle has a high plantar flexion moment and the knee has a high flexion moment, it is likely a combination of contracture of the gastrocnemius and the hamstrings. If the hip extension peak occurs early, is decreased, and the physical examination shows a significant hip flexion contracture, then hip flexion contracture may also be contributing to the midstance phase knee flexion deformity. If children use ambulatory aids such as crutches and the hamstring muscles are not really contracted, there is a tendency for them to fall into back-kneeing, both when the gastrocsoleus is overactive, and when it is too weak. If children are independent ambulators or have overactive hamstrings, they will be strongly drawn to a crouched gait pattern. If children are very strong and have high tone, they will be drawn to keep the knees stiff and vault in midstance phase. This vault action raises the body and increases the energy cost of walking; however, it has the benefit of allowing the contralateral leg to clear the floor during swing. Also, by raising the body in midstance, the body can then fall forward in terminal stance so forward momentum can be used at initial contact and the contralateral limb can use the gluteus to lift the body back up again (Figure 6.35).

The back-kneeing position in midstance phase is an especially difficult problem to address. This position has been shown to follow three patterns, with one pattern having predominantly overactive gastrocsoleus muscles, the second having the HAT segment center of gravity move anterior to the knee often in the face of a weak gastrocnemius, and the third having the HAT center of gravity moving posterior to the hip but anterior to the knee.[41] Treatment for all back-kneeing is to make sure the gastrocnemius has enough length to allow dorsiflexion with knee extension. If dorsiflexion with knee extension is possible, children should be placed in an orthosis that allows 3° to 5° of dorsiflexion while limiting plantar flexion to minus 5°. This orthosis can usually be an articulated AFO. If there is a pattern in which the ground reaction force is moving either significantly in front or behind the knee in the face of a weak gastrocsoleus, a solid ankle AFO should be used to assist the gastrocsoleus in ankle control. Back-kneeing that is especially difficult to control is that which is present in children who use walkers or crutches, because the center of mass of the HAT segment can be so far forward that when they are placed in AFOs, the toes of the shoes and AFOs will just rise with all the weight being borne on the heel. This persistent back-kneeing in spite of appropriate orthotics in children with assistive devices may cause progressive back-kneeing because of increasing knee hyperextension and the development

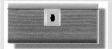

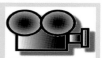

Case 6.7   Michael

Michael, a 5-year-old boy, was evaluated 1 year after he walked independently without the use of his walker. His parents complained that he fell a lot and had trouble stopping without falling at the end of a walk. Michael appeared to be age-appropriate cognitively and had significant spasticity in the lower extremities. He also had some increased tone in the upper extremities and poor hand coordination. His gait demonstrated toe walking with mild knee flexion in stance phase and significant internal rotation of the hips. After a full evaluation, he underwent a reconstruction with bilateral femoral derotation osteotomies, distal hamstring lengthening, and gastrocnemius lengthening. In his rehabilitation, gait training focused on ambulation with crutches, which he learned to manage well. By age 10 years, he was in a regular school and walked with Lofstrand crutches (Figure C6.7.1). He then fell and sustained a femur fracture, which was treated in his community hospital by placing him in a hip spica cast for 3 months. Following this, he could barely walk short, in-home distances with a walker (Figure 6.7.1). Shortly before the fracture accident, his parents went through an acrimonious divorce. Following removal from the cast, he was placed in a wheelchair and there was

little or no effort to try to rehabilitate him. Over the next 3 years, his father, who was very enthused about the boy's ambulatory ability, successfully petitioned the court to get custody from the mother, who felt ambulation was hopeless. This change in homes greatly lifted the boy's spirits, and in spite of not being able to stand to transfer himself by age 14 years, he was enthused about trying to get back to walking. By this time he had severe crouch stance posture, severe planovalgus feet, knee flexion contractures, and hamstring contractures (Figures C6.7.2, C6.7.3). At this time, Michael was doing well academically in a regular school. He underwent bilateral planovalgus correction with triple arthrodesis (Figure C6.7.4), gastrocnemius lengthening, posterior knee capsulotomies, and hamstring lengthening. By 6 months postoperatively, he could again walk in the house for short distances using a walker and ground reaction AFOs. By 9 months postoperatively, he made further progress with increased walking endurance, and by 2 years after surgery, he was again doing community ambulation and had worked back toward crutch use. The problems that caused Michael to stop walking were all reversible, including social home environment, his depression and lack of motivation, and the physical deformities. The key to having clinical confidence in getting him out of the wheelchair was having documentation in the videos or other gait analysis of his

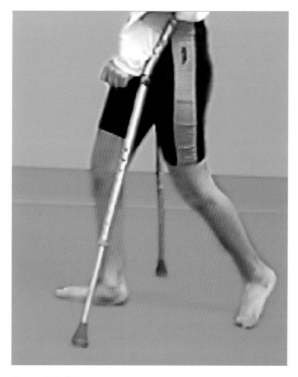

Figure C6.7.1

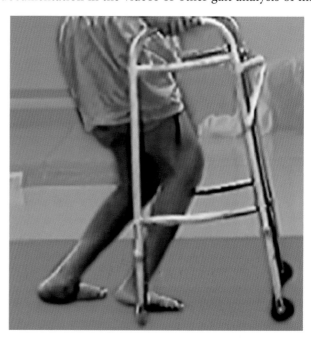

Figure C6.7.2

prior walking ability, and then making sure that all the factors were addressed before the physical deformities were corrected. The success of getting Michael walking again was probably as much a result of the change in home environment as it was the medical care.

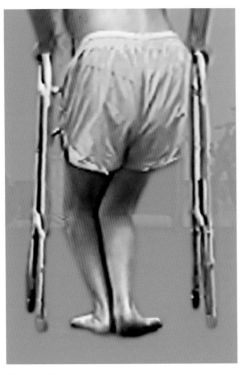

Figure C6.7.3

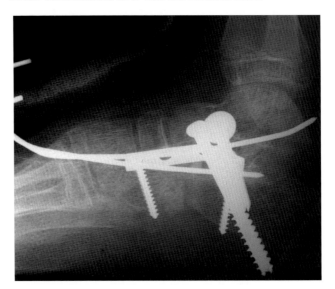

Figure C6.7.4

of pain. The only treatment for this kind of progressive back-kneeing is through the use of a knee-ankle-foot-orthosis (KAFO) with extension blocking hinges at the knee.

As the gait cycle progresses to terminal stance, the knee should start to flex as part of the process to accommodate the plantar flexion from the ankle joint and to start the process of shortening the limb for swing through. If flexion is delayed or decreased, it may be due to a lack of push-off power burst from the ankle, a lack of hip flexor power, too much contraction of the rectus, or co-contraction between the hamstrings and the vastus muscles. As the joint moves to early swing phase, the peak of flexion should be occurring in initial swing in the first 20% to 30% of swing phase. The stiff knee gait syndrome may be present if there is a decreased magnitude of knee flexion, meaning less than 55° to 65° of peak flexion, or the flexion occurs in midswing phase. This syndrome is the principal cause of toe drag. The primary cause of this stiff knee gait syndrome in children with CP is a rectus muscle that is contracting out of phase or with too much force. Secondary causes of decreased knee flexion in swing phase are the low push-off power bursts from the gastrocsoleus, decreased hip flexor power, and a knee joint axis that is severely out of line with the forward line of progression. To diagnose the overactive rectus as the primary cause requires an EMG of the rectus, which is active for a prolonged period in swing phase, the time of maximum swing phase knee flexion is late, and the magnitude of maximum swing phase knee flexion is decreased. Additional data to reinforce the rectus muscle as the cause of the stiff knee are provided by the physical examination showing a contracted rectus muscle with a very positive Ely test and a rectus that is spastic. A poor push-off power burst at the ankle and little or no hip flexion power generation at toe-off suggests that some of the problem is coming from these sources.

Figure 6.34. The hamstrings effect on knee flexion in stance or crouched gait results from the hamstrings muscle ability to generate the same magnitude of force at three different points on the length–tension curve based on the level of contracture. At normal fiber length, the muscle still has the ability to generate more force with increased contraction. With a moderate contracture, there is decreased force generation as the muscle further lengthens and, with a severe contracture, there is rapid increase in force due to passive increase in tension from the connective tissue (A). In addition to the impact of the contracture on the hamstrings force-generating ability, the ability to generate joint moment depends on the position of the hip and knee joint. The hamstrings may be at the same length and generate the same force; however, if the hip and knee are flexed, as in a crouched gait, there is a large moment arm at the knee generating much more knee flexion force than when the knee is near full extension (B). Therefore, the end-to-end length of the muscle in crouch may be the same as in upright stance, but this does not mean the hamstring contracture is not a problem. One must consider the contracture effect on the length–tension relationship, and as this drives the knee into flexion, the crouch is a self-propagating position because more knee flexion increases the hamstrings mechanical advantage through an increasing knee moment arm.

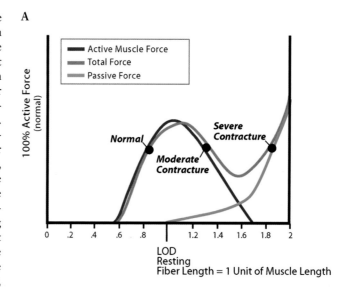

When the stiff knee syndrome is due to an overactive rectus, the required treatment is to remove the rectus from its insertion on the patella (Case 6.8). This removal requires transferring the rectus to some other muscle, with the sartorius and the gracilis being the most common sites. The specific site of the transfer does not matter[42]; however, it has to be transferred and not only released from the quadriceps tendon.[43, 44] If the tendon is released only, it will probably reattach to the underlying tendon and go back to doing its old job again. The primary goal of this transfer is to remove the action of the rectus from knee extension but preserve its function as a hip flexor. Usually, the contraction pattern is appropriate for hip flexion, and if it is to have an effect on the knee, it should work as a knee flexor. Good results with increased knee flexion in swing phase and an earlier peak knee flexion have

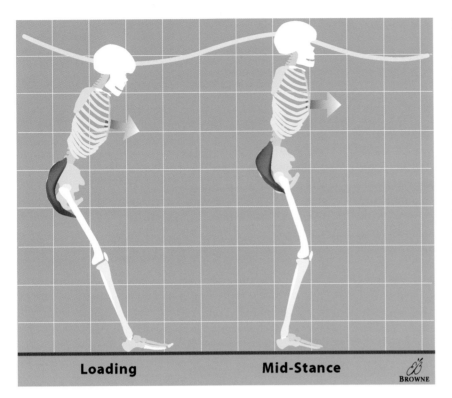

Loading **Mid-Stance**

Figure 6.35. The gluteus maximus, primarily and along with the other hip extensors, are the secondary muscles generating forward motion. This function is accomplished by the muscle having a strong contraction at foot contact and early stance, in which the forward falling HAT segment and center of mass are decelerated and lifted. The strong contraction between momentum of the forward falling body and the fixed foot uses the lifting of the body by a concentric contraction. When the gastrocsoleus is inactivated by an equinus contracture or by the use of very high heeled shoes, the hip extensors become the primary power output muscles generating power for walking.

been well documented by several studies.[42–44] The distal transfer is better than the proximal release[45] and works best when there is good walking velocity and swing phase EMG activity of the rectus but not constantly on rectus EMG activity.[46]

During terminal swing phase, the knee should be extending in preparation for initial contact. This extension is controlled by eccentric contraction of the hamstring muscles. The impact of the hamstring insufficiency to allow the knee to fully extend has already been noted. A much more common problem is overactivity of the hamstrings with early initiation on the EMG. Often, the primary problem is a contracture of the hamstrings and overactivity of the hamstrings muscle; however, the secondary cause is decreased momentum from slow hip flexion. This increased knee flexion at the end of swing phase causes short step lengths (Figure 6.36).

Treatment of diminished knee extension in terminal swing phase is primarily directed at the hamstrings, where surgical lengthening is the main treatment option. The function of the hamstrings is extremely complex, and the benefit of hamstring lengthening to improving knee extension at initial contact is less consistent.[47] Most reports showing positive results of hamstring lengthening come from the pregait analysis literature and have no dynamic data; however, they suggest that the popliteal angle remains improved after 2 to 4 years.[48, 49] There are reports showing improvement in stance knee extension, loss of knee flexion in swing phase, and mild increased lumbar lordosis after hamstring lengthening.[50, 51] There have been many modeling studies showing that the hamstring length is often not significantly shortened when measured from origin to insertion in the crouched gait midstance posture.[32, 33] These findings fail to consider that these patients also have greatly decreased muscle fiber length as demonstrated by high popliteal angles. These modeling origin to insertion measurements miss the significant impact of the change of muscle power based on the position the muscle falls on the

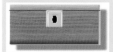
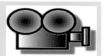

Case 6.8   Josie

Josie, a 16-year-old girl, presented with the complaint of frequent tripping and wearing out the front of her shoes very quickly. She has never had surgery, attends high school where she is an average student, and desires treatment for her complaints. On physical examination she had good hip motion, and full knee range of motion with popliteal angles of 45° bilaterally. An Ely test was positive at 60°, the rectus had 1+ spasticity on the Ashworth scale. Ankle dorsiflexion with the knee extended was 5°. Kinematics showed knee extension in stance to the normal range but only 35° peak flexion in swing phase. The ankle kinematic showed early ankle plantar flexion. The ankle moment had a significant early plantar flexion moment. The ankle power showed a midstance genera-

tion burst indicating a significant vault. An EMG of the rectus showed constant swing phase rectus activity, but no significant stance activity. Bilateral rectus transfers were performed, and she had significant increase in swing phase knee flexion immediately after surgery (Figure C6.8.1). This improvement was maintained 3 years later, along with excellent improvement in symptoms. She now reports much less tripping and never wears out the toes of her shoes. Although patients with isolated stiff knee gait are rare, this demonstrates the excellent benefit of rectus transfer when the indications are correct. Often, the cause of swing phase knee stiffness is not so isolated but also includes poor hip flexor power and poor ankle push-off.

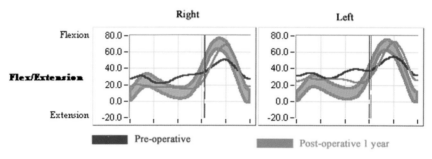

Figure C6.8.1

length–tension curve and the impact of the change of the moment arm based on joint position (see Figure 6.34). With the knee flexed 60°, the moment arm for knee flexion by the hamstrings is much greater than when the knee is extended. This same change in moment arm also occurs at the hip; however, the length the moment arm changes is less significant at the hip. There are also three separate muscles, the semimembranosus, semitendinosus, and long head of the biceps, which make up the primary hamstrings, and each of these muscles has a different fiber length but very similar origin and insertion sites. As all the variables involved with hamstring contraction are added to the force generated, which depends on the velocity of the contraction, the complexity of the control of the force impact on the hip and knee from the hamstrings is demonstrated. These variables include three muscles, each with different fiber lengths, approximately 1500 motor units in each muscle, and variable moment arms at two points for each muscle. With this great level of complexity, it is easy to see why these muscles are not commonly well controlled in children with motor control problems. This complexity can also explain why the outcome of lengthening is not very predictable. However, based on clinical experience, severely short hamstrings do not work well even if the simplistic modeling suggests that the origin-to-insertion length of the hamstrings in the midstance part of the gait cycle is long enough.

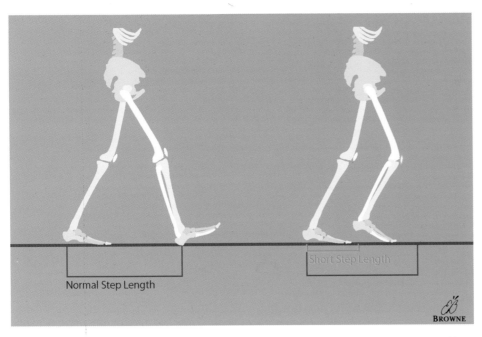

Normal Step Length

Short Step Length

BROWNE

Figure 6.36. An important function of the knee is to develop extension at foot contact. Lack of knee extension at foot contact can be a significant a cause of short step lengths.

Hip

Sagittal Plane

The major role of the hip joint is to allow progression of the limb under the body and provide three degrees of motion between the limb and the body. The hip joint is also the secondary power output source. In the sagittal plane, the hip is typically flexed at initial contact, which is seldom a problem even if the flexion is slightly exaggerated. At weight acceptance the hip is starting to extend as the body is moving forward over the fixed limb. The ankle and knee should be acting as shock absorbers. If the ankle and knee are held stiff, the hip extension may be slowed. The hip extenders are very active in weight acceptance as the body falls forward and is dropping with momentum. The main hip extenders are the gluteus maximus and the gluteus medius along with the hamstrings, which forcefully contract and output power, effectively lifting the body up again. If the hip extensors are weak, some compensation may occur by shifting even more proximally and using the spine extensors or the paraspinal muscles to create increased lumbar lordosis. Weak hip extensors are assessed by physical examination and by the weight acceptance hip extension moment and power generation in early stance phase. Another sign of hip extensor weakness is an early crossover of the hip moment from extension in early stance to flexion in terminal stance. This crossover should occur between mid- and late stance and not during weight acceptance. Treatment of weak hip extensors should include a strengthening program. For severe weakness, an ambulatory aid, either a crutch or a walker that allows the arms to assist the hip extensors in lifting the forward fall of the body during weight acceptance, should be prescribed.

In midstance phase, the hip continues to extend as the weightbearing limb moves behind the body. Hip flexion contractures are contractures of the hip flexors, primarily the psoas, which cause the extension to be limited. This limitation requires secondary adaptation of increasing anterior pelvic tilt and preventing full knee extension (Figure 6.37). Hip flexion contraction may be measured by several different physical examination methods, but it is most important to have a sense of what the normal range is for the method used.

Figure 6.37. The primary hip flexors assist with increasing hip flexion acceleration in preswing and into early swing phase. If these muscles are not functioning because of weakness or contracture, the abdominal muscles can provide an adaptive mechanism by increasing pelvic tilt motion to augment inadequate hip flexion.

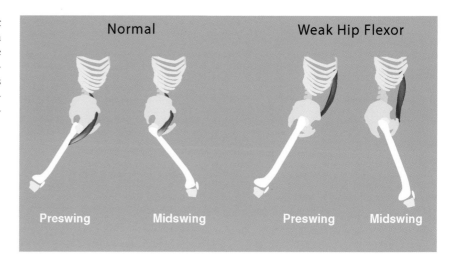

Hip extension in the kinematic measurement in midstance should come nearly to neutral; however, the normal range for the specific marker placement should be considered. Treatment of hip extension deficiency includes stretching exercises of the hip flexors or lengthening the psoas through a myofascial lengthening of the common iliopsoas tendon. Lengthening of the psoas has not been shown to consistently decrease anterior pelvic tilt[52]; however, one report found that it did better in younger children.[53] Modeling studies suggest that the iliopsoas may be shortened more relative to normal in crouched gait than the hamstrings.[32] Occasionally, a contracture of the rectus femoris or the fascia latae can contribute to the hip flexion contracture. Contractures of the rectus femoris and the fascia latae should be evident on physical examination.

In terminal stance phase, the hip again starts to flex, and much of the power for this hip flexion in normal gait comes from the gastrocsoleus push-off burst. However, in most children with CP, this gastrocsoleus burst is deficient and the direct hip flexors are the primary power output source to move the limb forward. This burst is also the main source of power that causes knee flexion. The primary hip flexor muscles are first the iliopsoas, followed slightly later in the cycle by the adductors, primarily the adductor brevis and the gracilis. Inactivity or weakness of the hip flexors is demonstrated by delayed hip flexion on the kinematic measurement and by absent hip flexion moment or late crossover from the extension to flexion moment in late stance phase. The compensations for a weak hip flexor are increased pelvic movement, usually a posterior pelvic tilt in terminal stance and a slow velocity of walking, especially caused by decreased cadence. Treatment of hip flexor weakness is first to avoid excessive surgical lengthening of the psoas and adductors. Strengthening exercises are the only option for adding strength to these muscles if weakness is the major problem. The use of assistive devices, such as walkers or crutches, will not help with the problem of hip flexor weakness and often makes it worse. The weakness of the hip flexors in terminal stance is magnified by crutch use because crutch users generally lean forward, increasing their hip flexion and causing the need for even more hip flexion in swing phase. The forward lean also tends to put less prestretch on the hip flexors, making them even less effective as power generators. Having the muscle at the optimum position on the length–tension curve is an important way to increase the muscle's functional strength, but crutch use tends to do the opposite with hip flexors. Another common disability from weak hip flexors is the inability to step up on a curb or a stair step. Problems stepping into vehicles or bathtubs are also common complaints.

In initial swing, the hip flexor continues to be active as the force for initiating the forward swing of the swing phase limb. The hip flexor is also the force that produces the knee flexion. Problems of terminal stance are continued with the same implications in initial swing. In midswing, there is seldom much direct impact, except for the common problem in CP of premature initiation of hamstring contractions, which tends to limit hip flexion and knee extension at a time when momentum is needed going into terminal swing. In terminal swing, the excessive activity of the hamstrings is again the most common problem. The effects of this activity are most dramatic at the knee, but the hamstrings contraction, if it is very excessive, may also limit hip flexion in terminal swing. Compensation occurs at the pelvis, where a posterior pelvic tilt may occur as a compensation for excessive hamstrings force in terminal swing. If the hamstrings or vastus muscles are very weak, the gluteus maximus and medius may substitute by a forceful contraction in terminal swing, which causes the knee to fully extend. This contraction places the knee in a fully extended preposition for initial contact (Figure 6.38). This is a position of maximum inherent stability for initial contact and weight acceptance, but it allows poor shock absorption at the knee.

Coronal Plane Hip Pathology

The coronal plane motion of the hip is used to keep the center of mass of the body in midline and allow the feet to be under the body close to the midline. At initial contact, the hip is abducted slightly, which decreases in midstance and then increases again at toe-off. During swing, the process is repeated. If there is a contraction of the adductor at initial contact, there will be less hip flexion and the foot will be positioned across the midline, where it tends to impede the forward line of progress during swing phase of the contralateral limb. This pattern, in which the foot is positioned across the midline, causes the scissoring gait pattern. In the scissoring gait pattern, the swing phase foot gets trapped behind a foot that has been placed too medially. If the adductor contraction or overactivity is unilateral, the uncontracted hip can abduct, compensating along with pelvic obliquity. This pelvic obliquity will then cause a limb length discrepancy, which has to be compensated for. The primary assessment of coronal plane hip pathology is based on physical examination measurement of hip abduction with the hip extended and the measurement of hip abduction on the kinematic evaluation. The hip should abduct slightly at initial contact. Then, there may be several degrees of abduction in midstance phase and swing phase. The main treatment for overactive or contracted adductors usually requires surgical lengthening. A contracted adductor is not a common problem in children who are functional ambulators. Some children who are marginal ambulators and often require gait trainers consistently have increased adduction such that the feet are always crossed and they cannot step. Some of these children have adduction because of poor motor control, in which a total flexor response to initiate stepping is used (Case 6.9). This flexor response includes hip flexion, adduction, knee flexion, and ankle plantar flexion. Even if the adductor is lengthened, for some of these children the motion continues unless all the adductors are removed, which will only cause a new problem. Unilateral increased hip adduction can also be a secondary response to limb length

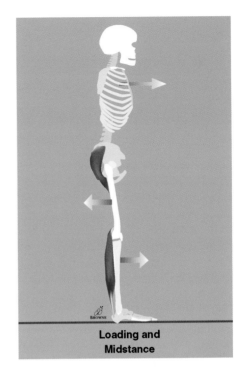

Loading and Midstance

Figure 6.38. The hip extensors also provide important function in controlling knee position. During stance, this is provided in coordination with the gastrocsoleus in which knee extension is produced as a result of hip extension. Momentum is moving the body forward over the fixed stance phase foot, allowing the hip and gastrocsoleus to control knee stability. In swing phase, the deceleration of the hip flexion by the hip extensors can allow the knee to swing into full extension if the hamstrings are not activated.

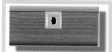

Case 6.9   Jacob

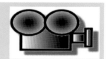

Jacob, a 10-year-old boy, was brought in by his father with the main complaint that he could not walk because his feet crossed over each other when he stood and tried to walk. His father was most concerned about the boy's spasticity, which he felt was limiting his ability to walk and was making bathing, dressing, and transferring more difficult. On physical examination, Jacob was not able to sit unsupported. He could self-feed with a spoon (if the food was sticky like mashed potatoes), had no speech, and was in a special education classroom for children with severe cognitive limitations. The physical examination demonstrated Ashworth grade 1 and 2 spasticity throughout most muscles in the lower extremity and the upper extremity. He had no ability to do individually isolated joint movement in the lower extremity. The hip demonstrated a symmetric 30° of abduction, popliteal angles were 40°, hip internal rotation was 50°, and ex-

ternal rotation was 30°. Jacob was cooperative in trying to stand and take steps when being held from the back. He had a gait trainer, which he enjoyed. Based on this assessment, Jacob was believed to have significant spasticity; however, this was not felt to be the main cause of the scissoring. The scissoring was due to poor motor control and poor motor planning. It was not thought that he would benefit from further surgical lengthening of the adductor because these were not contracted, and part of the cause of the scissoring was his poor coordination in the use of hip flexors to advance the limb. A baclofen trial was given, but he could not stand with the decreased spasticity after the baclofen injection, and his parents felt the benefit of the decreased spasticity during custodial care would not make up for his functional loss of not being able to stand.

inequality. In children with CP, this inequality can be a physically short limb, but is more commonly a functional limb shortening due to asymmetric hip, knee, or ankle flexion. Treatment of the limb length inequality will treat the hip adduction. Asymmetric adduction on one hip and abduction on the opposite hip may also be caused by fixed pelvic obliquity emanating from spinal deformities.

Increased hip abduction leads to a wide-based gait, which is cosmetically unappealing and is very functionally disabling if the children are functional ambulators. The wide-base position forces excessive side-to-side movement of the body to keep the center of mass over the weightbearing limb. If children have increased abduction with a wide-based gait but have no abduction contracture on physical examination, the cause of the wide-based gait is weakness of the adductor muscles. Usually, the cause is incompetent adductors secondary to excessive adductor lengthening, or the addition of an obturator neurectomy to an adductor lengthening (Case 6.10). The best treatment of this problem is to prevent it from happening by not doing this type of surgery on a functional ambulator. However, if presented with the problem, working on strengthening the remaining adductor strength and allowing the children to grow often slowly corrects the problems. There are no other treatments available. The wide-based gait may also be due to an abduction contracture, usually of the gluteus medius or fascia latae. The etiology of wide-based gait due to a contracture requires identifying the source of the contracture, and the kinematic measure should show increased abduction, especially in midstance phase. Once the specific source of the abduction contracture is identified, the treatment is surgical lengthening of the contracted muscle. Fixed contractures of the hip joint may also cause the same effect as muscle contractures. Sometimes, this contracture requires a

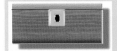

Case 6.10   Sean

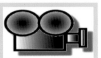

Sean, a 5-year-old boy with quadriplegia, had an adductor lengthening and distal hamstring lengthening to treat spastic hip disease at age 3 years. By age 5 years, he walked efficiently with a walker; however, his parents were concerned about his wide-based gait and foot drag. On physical examination, he was not able to get into the walker without assistance, but had functional gait once he was in the walker. His hip abduction was 50° on each side, full hip flexion and extension was present, the popliteal angle was 40°, and he had grade 2 spasticity in the rectus, with a positive Ely test at 40°. Kinematic evaluation showed increased hip abduction and decreased knee flex-

ion in swing phase with EMGs of the rectus, which were very active in swing phase. His hip radiographs were completely normal. His gait was characterized by a wide-based gait with foot drag and knee stiffness in swing phase. Based on these data, Sean had bilateral rectus transfers because the knee stiffness was believed to be adding to the tendency to have a wide-based gait. He was initiating a circumduction maneuver because of adductor weakness to assist with foot clearance. After the rectus transfers, his base of support narrowed and knee flexion increased nicely. His foot drag also decreased.

---

radiographic evaluation of the joint to determine if the source is the muscle only or a combination of the muscle and the joint.

Transverse Plane Deformity

Transverse plane deformity in children is common and is often confused with coronal plane deformity. The difference between scissoring, which is excessive hip adduction, and hip internal rotation gait is often missed. Scissoring is a completely different motion requiring a different treatment (Figure 6.39). Hip rotation is defined as a rotation of the knee joint axis relative to the center of hip motion in the pelvis. In normal gait, this rotation around the mechanical axis of the femur allows the feet to stay in the midline and allows the pelvis to turn on top of the femur, which are both motions that work to decrease movement of the HAT segment and therefore conserve energy. At initial contact, the normal hip has slight external rotation of approximately 10°, then it slowly internally rotates, reaching a maximum at terminal stance or initial swing phase. If the hip is positioned in internal rotation at initial contact, then during stance phase as the knee flexes, there is an obligatory hip adduction and the knee may impact the opposite limb (Case 6.9). If the internal rotation is present during midstance, such as in a crouched gait pattern, the knees often rub during swing phase of the contralateral limb. Internal rotation positioning in terminal swing also causes the knee to cross the midline, a problem that continues into initial swing. Another primary effect of this internal rotation is placing the knee axis out of line with the forward line of motion. This position causes significant alteration in mechanical efficiency of the push-off power that the ankles generate. Secondary adaptation to the internal rotation of the hip includes decreased knee flexion in weight acceptance in swing phase, decreased ankle push-off power burst, and requires the use of more hip power. If the internal rotation is unilateral, the pelvis may rotate posteriorly on the side of the internal hip rotation, then the contralateral hip compensates with external rotation. The amount of internal rotation is assessed by physical examination with children prone and the hips extended (Case 6.11).

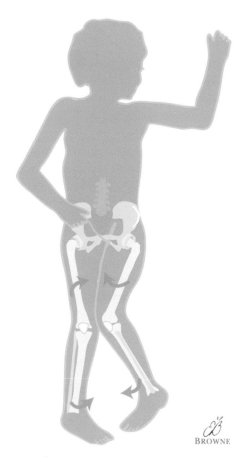

BROWNE

Figure 6.39. Crossing over of the knees is often called scissoring gait. However, it is better to use the term scissoring gait only when it is caused by true hip hyperadduction. Most of the time, crossing over of the knees is due to internal rotation of the hips, often secondary to increased femoral anteversion and not caused by primary increased hip adduction.

The kinematic measure should show external rotation through almost all of the gait cycle. There are two problems with the kinematic measure of which clinicians must always be aware. First, the measure is very dependent on defining the axis of the knee joint by the person placing the marker. An error of 5° to 10° in defining the knee joint axis is to be expected. The second major issue is all clinical gait software programs currently use rotation as the last Euler angle to derotate. This means that often the measured degree of rotation is less than clinicians perceive, probably because they are mentally derotating the hip first. This is not an error in the kinematics or the clinicians' assessments but is related only to the method of expressing the position. Clinically, the hip rotation may be more significant than the kinematic measure suggests.

The principal cause of the increased internal rotation is increased femoral anteversion. A secondary cause may be a contracture of the internal rotators. A third cause may be motor control problems as mentioned with increased scissoring, which are often seen in marginal ambulators. For children who previously had surgery on the hip and in whom there is a question as to the specific cause of the internal rotation, measurement of the femoral anteversion with ultrasound or CT scan should be considered. Children in middle childhood or older who are functional ambulators tend to do poorly with internal rotation that is greater than 10° during terminal stance phase. From middle childhood on, there is little apparent spontaneous correction of the internal rotation. Children who are very functional ambulators and have any internal rotation during stance phase are easily cosmetically observed as having internal rotation. Some children with 0° to 15° of internal rotation of the hip in stance phase seem to have very few measurable mechanical problems; however, parents often notice that they trip more frequently, which may be due to decreased knee flexion to avoid knees crossing over the midline. These increased problems that require sophisticated motor control probably cause children with CP to be more clumsy. Also, during running when there is increased knee flexion, a heel whip will appear if children have persistent internal rotation. This heel whip clearly adds to children's poor coordination during running. Treatment of increased internal rotation is a derotation femoral osteotomy, which will improve the foot progression angle.[54] If the source of the internal rotation is felt to be a contracture of the internal rotators of the hip, the most usual cause is the anterior fibers of the gluteus medius and the gluteus minimus.[55]

Excessive external rotation of the hip during gait is rarely a primary problem of gait in children with CP. Usually, this external rotation is associated with hypotonia and may be part of a progressive anterior hip subluxation syndrome (Case 6.12). Typically, these children start losing functional ambulatory ability as the hip increases its external rotation at the same time the anterior subluxation is increasing. The treatment is to correct the hip joint pathology. The second situation where external rotation may be seen is secondary to excessive external rotation of the femur for treatment of femoral anteversion. The rule of thumb should be that a little external rotation is better than a little internal rotation, with the goal being 0° to 20° of external rotation. However, too much external rotation, meaning greater than 20°, is worse than a little internal rotation of 0° to 10°. The goal should be to have 0° to 10° of femoral anteversion, and the kinematic measure should show 5° to 20° of external rotation of the femur during stance. Femurs with excessive external rotation may need to be turned back into internal rotation again. Imaging studies should be obtained to fully assess the deformity before undertaking repeat surgery because external rotation contractures

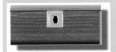 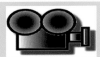

Tonya, an 11-year-old girl with a diagnosis of spastic diplegia, complained of increased difficulty in walking due to clumsiness and pain from her knees knocking together. This problem had become much more symptomatic over the past year. Tonya had normal cognitive function, and no other medical problems. On physical examination, she had 70° of hip internal rotation and −10° external hip rotation. Hip abduction was 20°, popliteal angles were 60°, and the feet were normal. Her gait demonstrated a foot flat gait pattern with mild knee flexion in stance, decreased knee flexion in swing, severe in-

ternally rotated knees with heel whip, and mild increased lumbar lordosis. Kinematics showed hip internal rotation of 20° in stance phase. The EMG of the rectus showed mild increased activity in swing phase and that hamstring activity was normal (Figure C6.11.1). Based on the EMG activity, the main problem was believed to result from femoral anteversion, and she had femoral derotation osteotomies bilaterally. This procedure resolved all her complaints and substantially improved her knee motion and hip extension.

Rectus EMG recording   Skin electrodes

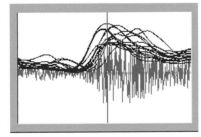 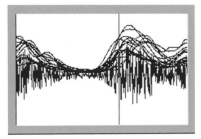

Right   Left

Figure C6.11.1

can occasionally occur. These external rotation contractures usually involve the posterior half of the gluteus medius and the short external rotators of the hip joint.

Pelvis

Pelvic motion is viewed as motion of the pelvis in the space of the room coordinate system. Observational gait analysis of pelvic motion is difficult because this body segment does not have clear borders and it is socially difficult to have children undressed at the pelvic level. Therefore, trying to see the pelvis move is somewhat like watching the neighbor's television through a window covered with a curtain. Pathologic motion of the pelvis occurs either with excessive motion or asymmetric motion. Excessive pelvic motion is defined as more than 10° on the kinematic measure in any of the three directions and is usually due to increased tone, which has stiffened the hip joint and limits hip motion (Table 6.9). Often, treatment is not needed as this is a functional way of increasing mobility that has only a slightly increased energy cost. This increased pelvic rotation may cause heel whip during running, therefore making running more difficult. The only available treatment is to decrease muscle tone by rhizotomy or intrathecal baclofen, both of which cause or bring out muscle weakness. Often, the weakness is more impairing to the gait function than the stiffness.

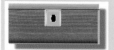

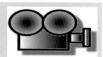

Case 6.12   Hameen

Hameen, a 10-year-old boy with hypotonia and mental retardation, had increased difficulty in ambulation. He used to walk everywhere using a posterior walker, but now his mother stated that he refused to walk except for very short distances. She did not perceive that he had any pain. Nine months before this presentation, he had a femoral osteotomy for a subluxating hip at another hospital. Following this osteotomy, his gait had not improved, although he was walking almost as well as he was before that surgery. His health had otherwise not changed, except his mother felt his external rotation of the feet, especially on the left side, was getting worse. On physical examination he was noted to have generalized hypotonia, hip abduction was 60°, full flexion and extension, hip external rotation to more than 90°, and an internal rotation to 60°. The left hip had a click with rotation. Anterior palpation suggested that the femoral head was subluxating anteriorly. A radiograph was obtained that showed a mild lateral displacement of the femoral head with a healed femoral osteotomy (Figure C6.12.1), and the CT scan showed that it was slightly anterior (Figure C6.12.2). He was observed walking with a posterior walker and severe external rotation of the left hip. The cause of his decreased walking tolerance was thought to be the anterior hip subluxation, and he had a Pemberton pelvic osteotomy without a varus femoral osteotomy because the soft tissue was believed to have enough laxity (Figure C6.12.3). By 1 year after the surgery, he had returned to his usual walking tolerance, and by 6 years after surgery, he was a fully independent community ambulator with a stable hip (Figure C6.12.4). Although he continued to have external foot progression on the left and bilateral back-knee, he was without symptoms (Figure C6.12.5).

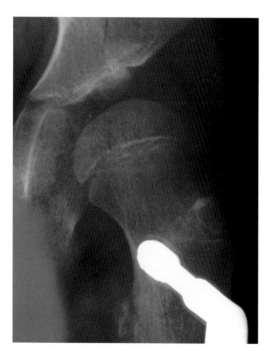

Figure C6.12.1

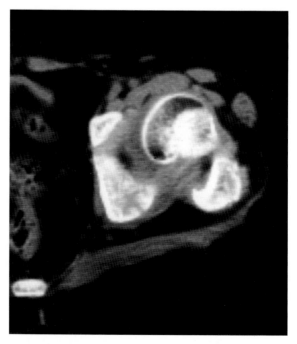

Figure C6.12.2

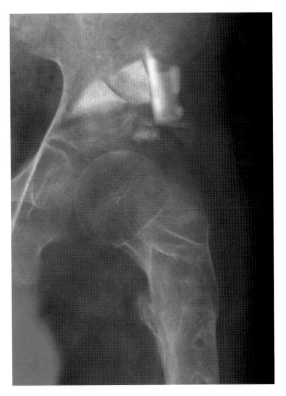

Figure C6.12.3

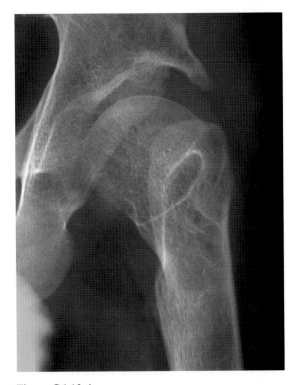

Figure C6.12.4

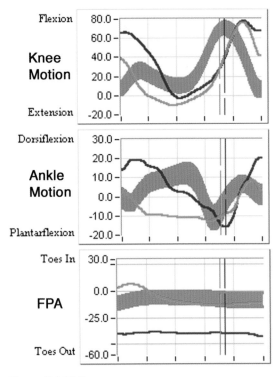

Figure C6.12.5

Table 6.9. Segment and joint compensations.

Problem	As the primary etiology	Compensatory effect for
Pelvis		
Increased anterior tilt	As part of lumbar lordosis that is compensated by increased hip flexion	Compensating for a hip flexion contracture or hip extensor weakness
Increased tilt motion		Hip stiffness or hip weakness
Asymmetric pelvic rotation	Hemiplegia type motor control	Asymmetric femoral rotation with the pelvis posterior on the internally rotated side
Increased rotation		Decreased push-off from gastrocsoleus, hip stiffness, hip flexor weakness
Asymmetric pelvic obliquity	Lumbar scoliosis	Hip abduction or adduction contracture, limb length discrepancy, ankle plantar flexion contracture
Increased drop on swing side		Abductor muscle weakness
Hip		
Decreased flexion in swing	Hip joint stiffness or extension muscle contractures (hamstrings or gluteus)	Weak push-off power burst from the ankle plantar flexors
Decreased flexion	Hip flexor weakness	
Decreased extension stance	Hip flexor contracture, joint stiffness	Lack of knee extension
Increased abduction	Weak adductor muscle, joint or abductor contractures	Adduction contracture of the opposite hip, ataxia
Increased adduction (scissoring)	Adductor contracture	Poor motor control
Increased internal rotation	Increased femoral anteversion, contracture of internal rotators	Asymmetric pelvic rotation, external tibial torsion
Increased external rotation	External rotation contracture, retroversion of femur	Asymmetric pelvic rotation often due to opposite hip internal rotation, internal tibial torsion
Knee		
Increased flexion at foot contact	Knee flexion contracture, premature hamstring activity, hamstring contracture, toe strike due to ankle equinus, weak push-off, or hip flexor	
Decreased knee flexion at foot contact	Weak hamstrings	Quadriceps weakness, hypotonia
Lack of weight acceptance knee flexion	Knee stiffness	Ankle plantar flexor contractures
Decreased midstance flexion (back-knee)	Contracture or overactivity of gastrocsoleus, or weak gastrocsoleus	Poor motor control, hamstrings that are too weak compared with the gastrocsoleus
Increased midstance flexion (crouch)	Knee joint contracture, hamstring contracture, lever arm disease (planovalgus feet)	Lack of plantar flexion, balance problems, severe abnormal foot progression angle, hip flexion contracture, ankle equinus
Lack knee flexion swing (stiff knee gait)	Overactivity of the rectus muscle, knee stiffness, quadriceps contracture	Poor push-off power from the gastrocsoleus, poor hip flexor power
Foot		
Equinus at foot contact	Gastrocnemius and/or soleus contracture, weak dorsiflexors	Severe knee flexion contracture
Lack of first rocker	Gastrocnemius and/or soleus contracture or muscle overactivity, ankle stiffness, weakness of dorsiflexors	
Premature second rocker	Lack of first rocker, spastic or contracted gastrocnemius or soleus	Lack of knee extension in midstance
High early plantar flexion moment	Spastic or contracted gastrocnemius or soleus	
Decreased late stance plantar flexion moment	Contracture of gastrocsoleus, or weak gastrocsoleus	
Decreased push-off power	Lack of plantar flexion in third rocker	Lever arm disease, planovalgus, severe torsional malalignment
Internal or external foot progression	Tibial or femoral torsion, planovalgus, or varus feet	Severe muscle weakness or poor balance, and is used to stabilize posture

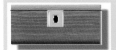
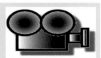

Case 6.13   Christopher

Christopher, a 6-year-old boy, presented with a diagnosis of CP and a peculiar gait pattern. His parents were concerned that he tripped a lot and they wanted to improve the appearance of his walking. He had normal speech and was cognitively age appropriate. He had no other medical problems, and his parents felt that he had had very little change in his gait in the past year. On physical examination he had significant spasticity in his left upper extremity, with internal rotation at the shoulder, elbow flexion, and wrist flexion. He could use gross grasp of the fingers. He was using the hand as a helper hand without prompting. He had full hip flexion and extension, and abduction was 15° on the left and 28° on the right. Internal rotation of the hip was 80° on the left and 50° on the right. External rotation was 5° on the left and 30° on the right. Knee popliteal angles were 55° on the left and 40° on the right. Ankle dorsiflexion with extended knee was −7° on the left and 0° on the right. Dorsiflexion with the knee flexed was 0° on the left and 8° on the right. His gait demonstrated severe pelvic rotation with the left side being posterior 45° to 65° throughout the whole cycle. The left knee appeared to be internally rotated relative to the pelvis. The right foot was internally rotated and the left foot was neutral. Both knees were in hyperextension in midstance, with increased knee flexion at foot contact. The upper extremity was held in elbow flexion and internal rotation of the shoulder. Christopher's pelvic rotation seemed mostly caused by asymmetric hip rotation with the left hip being internally rotated; therefore, a left femoral derotation osteotomy was performed to correct this. The deformity was probably being exaggerated because of his hemiplegic motor control problems. Lengthening of the adductor on the left also helped to allow the limb to externally rotate and abduct. Lengthening the tendon Achilles on the left and the gastrocnemius on the right helped the knee extension in midstance. Following these procedures, the pelvic rotation improved significantly; however, he developed a planovalgus foot, partly due to a split transfer of the tibialis posterior tendon, which should not have been done. Several other operative procedures for other problems were required during his growth period; however, the pelvic rotation remained corrected until he reached full maturity.

Pelvic Rotation
Asymmetric pelvic rotation may be primarily caused by motor control, or as a secondary adaptation for asymmetric hip rotation. Children with very asymmetric neurologic involvement, especially severe hemiplegic patterns, often lead with the most functional side of the body. Leading with the functional side of the body seems to be a motor control attractor, probably because it is easier to control the impaired limb in the trailing position. If the asymmetry is only 10° to 20°, trailing of the involved side is not very cosmetically apparent and usually needs no treatment. Most rotations greater than 20° are cosmetically apparent and cause functional problems, such as increased tripping and poor coordination, especially in highly functional ambulators. If the rotation is severe, sometimes reaching 45° to 60°, children are walking sideways, which is ineffective and very cosmetically noticeable (Case 6.13). Severe rotation is often a combination of asymmetric hip motion and motor control, which should be addressed by making all efforts to correct hip asymmetries and even slightly overcorrecting these asymmetries. Many children have pelvic rotation asymmetry due to asymmetric hip rotation or adduction. Physical examination should focus on hip rotation with hips extended and with hip abduction. The hip on the side of the pelvis that is rotated posteriorly should have more internal rotation or have less passive external rotation. Typically, this hip has increased adduction and often flexion contracture as well. The treatment is to do a unilateral hip derotation

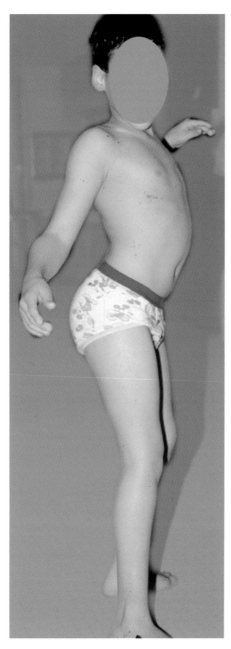

Figure 6.40. Some children who are independent ambulators have significant hamstring contractures requiring lengthening of the hamstrings. They should be carefully examined to be sure that there are not significant hip flexor contractures. This boy, 1 year after hamstring lengthening, has developed severe hyperlordosis primarily because the hip flexors were not lengthened. There are children, however, who naturally take on this posture and, when they are examined, do not have a hip flexion contracture.

and adductor lengthening if the adductor is contracted, meaning there is less than 20° of hip abduction with the knee extended. Excessive adductor lengthening should not be done; a percutaneous adductor longus tenotomy only is often sufficient.

Pelvic Tilt

Anterior pelvic tilt may have increased magnitude, be asymmetric, or be increased in either direction. Increased magnitude of pelvic motion is very common and is related to increased tone in the lower extremities. Also, the increased magnitude serves as another proximal power input joint as a way of propelling the swing limb forward. This increased stiffness and use of pelvic tilt is also present with hip flexion contractures, specifically the iliopsoas, and has been called the double bump pelvic motion. This term is somewhat misleading because it suggests a new pathologic movement pattern of the pelvis, which is not true. This pelvic motion is only a magnification of the normal movement. Again, in many patients, this pelvic motion serves a useful secondary adaptation to help with swing phase in a limb with increased stiffness or decreased power output. If children are very functional with good ankle push-off power generation, it is possible to decrease this pelvic motion through lengthening the hamstrings and the psoas, which increases the hip joint range of motion. If the hip is the main source of power output, these lengthenings run the risk of shifting the length–tension curve such that the weakness of the hip muscles will be magnified and the pelvic tilt range may increase even more to compensate.

Increase in anterior pelvic tilt primarily occurs due to increased hip flexion contractures, or secondarily occurs due to increased lumbar lordosis. The normal upper range for anterior pelvic tilt is 15° to 20°, although this varies somewhat with different marker placement algorithms. An increase to 25° is common in children with CP. Weakness of the hip extensors and increased force in the hip flexors are the primary causes of increased anterior pelvic tilt. Primary lumbar lordosis is another cause, and it may be difficult to separate primary lumbar lordosis from lumbar lordosis as a secondary response to increased anterior pelvic tilt due to increased hip flexion forces. Increased pelvic tilt and lumbar lordosis are strong attractors in motor control, possibly because they increase stability and lock the lumbar spine, thereby producing more mechanical stiffening. Iliopsoas lengthening should be performed if lumbar lordosis is flexible, hip flexor contracture is present, hamstring lengthening is needed to improve knee kinematics, and these individuals are independent ambulators. If a child does not meet all these criteria, iliopsoas lengthening may have more side effects than benefits. If the lordosis is stiff, muscle surgery will not affect anterior pelvic tilt. If the iliopsoas is not contracted, psoas lengthening will only weaken effective hip flexion. However, if hamstring lengthening is performed and the contracted hip flexor is not lengthened, the anterior pelvic tilt will almost definitely get worse. These individuals often develop the jump position with forward lean of the trunk on the anterior tilted pelvis. Over time, the compensation is obtained by having increased lordosis (Figure 6.40). For individuals who use walkers or crutches, hip flexor lengthening will increase apparent weakness due to increased anterior pelvic tilt from always leaning forward.

Increased posterior tilt is usually defined as abnormal if there is any posterior tilt past neutral. The principle cause of posterior pelvic tilt is a contracture of the hamstrings. The posterior pelvic tilt has to be correlated by physical examination. The posterior tilt may be due to gluteus contractures; however, we have never seen this in children with CP. Treatment is lengthening of the hamstrings if they are contracted. A secondary cause of posterior pelvic tilt is lumbar kyphosis or, more commonly, total spinal kyphosis. Correction of the kyphosis will correct the posterior pelvic tilt.

Pelvic Obliquity

Most causes of abnormal pelvic obliquity are due to asymmetric contractures of the hip adductors or abductors or weakness of one of the muscle groups. This pelvic obliquity may be secondary to apparent or real limb length discrepancy, or it may be secondary to fixed scoliosis. Pelvic obliquity may be asymmetric when one side has strong muscles and hip hiking on the swing side is used to help with clearance.

The Trendelenburg gait, often discussed by writers concerned with hip pathology, is really only a magnification of normal movement pattern, much like the double bump anterior pelvic motion. This gait is a response to mild weakness in the abductors as the hip on the swing side drops more to pretension the abductor muscle until it finds the strength to resist. Increased movement of the center of mass of the HAT segment over the weightbearing limb is usually combined with this, thereby decreasing the force needed to resist the drop of the pelvis. This pattern may also suggest mechanical instability of the hip joint, such as hip subluxation,[56] and hip radiographs should be obtained. With severe weakness of the abductor muscles, the center of mass of the HAT segment will move completely over the weightbearing limb, usually with elevation of the pelvis on the swing side. This movement is called a hip lurch, in which the trunk muscles can also be used to control the drop of the pelvis on the swing limb side (Figure 6.41). Treatment of Trendelenburg gait is by strengthening of the abductor muscles when possible. Treatment of the lurch gait pattern is by strongly encouraging patients to use forearm crutches, which will decrease both the energy of walking and the force on the joints in the lower extremities, especially the knee joint. Some of these movement patterns may also occur secondary to pain in the hip joint. Therefore, a good history should be available with the gait analysis.

Figure 6.41. Obliquity of the pelvis can change in different ways to accommodate muscle weakness, hip pain, or motor coordination problems. In normal gait, the abductors are used to maintain the pelvis with only minimal motion. As the muscles develop mild weakness, the pelvis may drop on the swing limb side in a motion commonly called Trendelenburg gait. There is little movement of the center of mass in this gait pattern. As the weakness or pain becomes more severe, the pelvis raises on the swing limb side as the center of mass moves laterally over the stance phase limb, causing a gait pattern commonly called a lurch. As the muscle weakness becomes more severe, the pelvis may drop on the swing limb side as the center of mass moves laterally over the stance limb.

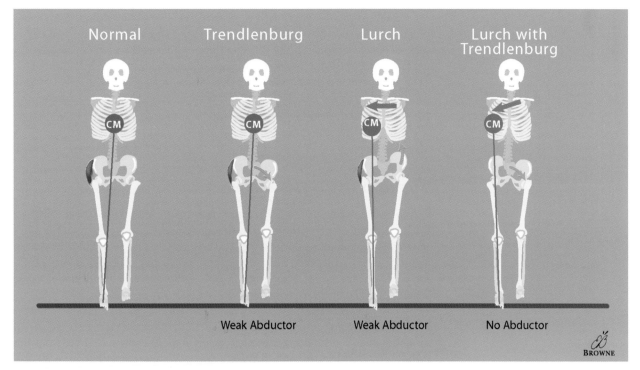

Figure 6.42. The motor control system can adjust the trunk alignment and the position of the center of mass or center of gravity (COG) so either the ground reaction force goes directly through the hip joint, therefore requiring little hip muscle power posterior to the hip in which the hip flexors are the main active muscles, or anterior to the hip joint, requiring mainly hip extensor use. It is often hard to understand why the motor control system chooses one pattern over the other in children with CP.

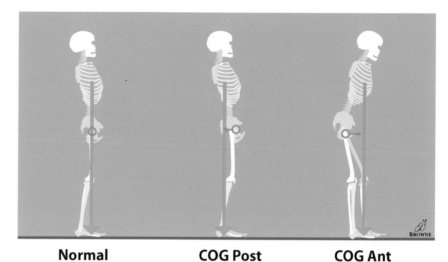

Normal   **COG Post**   **COG Ant**

HAT Segment

The real function of gait is to move the HAT segment in space. This segment, however, is not only passive cargo. By the use of trunk muscles, neck muscles, and arm movements, the HAT segment can position its center of mass to assist in gait. In normal gait, the HAT segment primarily involves passive motion, which will cause the center of mass to have the least movement away from the line of progression. Through the motor control system, the center of mass can be positioned in front of the hip joint to allow the hip extensors to be more effective as power generators, or it can be positioned behind the hip joint so the weak hip extensors are not stressed and the anterior hip capsule or hip flexors are the primary supports of the mass (Figure 6.42). As was discussed with lurching, the trunk muscles can output force and provide power for movement in children (see Figure 6.41). The contribution of active power generation of the HAT segment is not well understood. Typically, the trunk is rotated posteriorly on the involved side of individuals with hemiplegia. Often, the arms are in the high to medium guard positions with elbow and shoulder flexion in individuals with poor balance. Treatment specific for asymmetries of trunk motion or increased magnitude is primarily directed at determining the need for assistive devices. Individuals with 20° to 30° of trunk motion side to side usually do better with walking aids such as crutches, especially for long-distance walking.

Cerebral Palsy Gait Patterns, Treatments, and Outcomes

Ambulatory children with CP require treatment of the whole motor system, not consideration of a problem in only one segment or subsystem of the gait's pattern. The goal is to understand all the primary and secondary problems as much as possible, then address all these problems in one operative event. Dr. Mercer Rang popularized the concept of avoiding the birthday syndrome for surgery. The birthday syndrome was a common approach in the 1960s and 1970s. In this treatment approach, children would typically have an Achilles tendon lengthening one year, hamstring lengthening the next year, adductor and iliopsoas lengthening the year after, then they would need another Achilles tendon lengthening. This process would go on with yearly surgery throughout children's growth years. With tools for gait evaluation, few children should need to have more than two surgical experiences during their childhood years to treat problems related to gait. The surgery can be arranged for children and families so it occurs when the families can best manage the time commitment and children are least impacted with respect to school. As the pathologies for each joint, movement segment, and motor subsystem are combined into the whole functioning musculoskeletal system, patterns of involvement have to be defined. Children's anatomically involved pattern of CP needs to be determined first, meaning separating out hemiplegia from diplegia from quadriplegia. In this overall pattern, children whose primary problems are ataxia or movement disorders also have to be considered. These problems do not fit neatly into the hemiplegia and diplegia pattern of involvement. Within each of these patterns, there has to be a further sub-categorization to reach an understanding of the most common patterns.

Hemiplegia

Almost all children with hemiplegic pattern CP walk. Typically, these children are very functional ambulators, and their major orthopaedic problems are related to improving gait pattern and upper extremity position. A few children, usually with severe mental retardation, do not become functional ambulators. Often, nonambulation is related to poor function in the upper extremity, which makes the use of an assistive device difficult. There have been several attempts to classify patterns of hemiplegic gait,[57, 58] but the classification of Winters et al.[58] is easy to remember and has the most direct implications for treatment (Figure 6.43). This classification divides hemiplegic

Figure 6.43. The best classification of hemiplegia is that of Winters et al.,[58] in which type 1 is due to a weak or paralyzed ankle dorsiflexor causing a drop foot. Type 2 has equinus foot position due to a contracture of the gastrocnemius or gastrocsoleus preventing dorsiflexion. Type 3 has spastic or contracted hamstrings or quadriceps muscles in addition to type 2 ankle. Type 4 has spastic or weak hip muscles in addition to type 3 deformity. Almost all patients are relatively easy to classify into one or the other type, which is then helpful for planning treatment. Transverse rotational plane malalignments do not fit into this classification and should be seen as an additional problem.

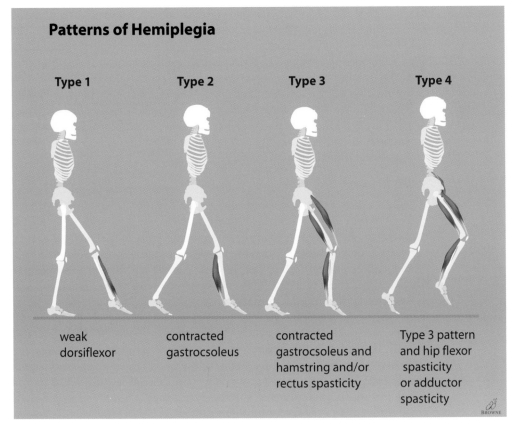

Patterns of Hemiplegia

Type 1 — weak dorsiflexor

Type 2 — contracted gastrocsoleus

Type 3 — contracted gastrocsoleus and hamstring and/or rectus spasticity

Type 4 — Type 3 pattern and hip flexor spasticity or adductor spasticity

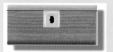

Case 6.14   Tania

Tania, an 18-year-old girl, had hemiplegia as result of a traumatic brain injury sustained at age 8 years. Her main complaint was that she could not lift her foot. Physical examination of her right ankle demonstrated an active toe extensor, and some apparent activity of the tibialis anterior on withdrawal stimulus of a pin stick on the sole. Ankle dorsiflexion was 10° with knee flexion and 20° with knee extension. Ankle kinematics showed no active dorsiflexion in swing phase and no EMG activity of the tibialis anterior (Figure C6.14.1). Observation of her gait demonstrated an extended hallux in swing phase, but no apparent dorsiflexion was in swing phase. Knee and hip motion appeared to be normal. She was ordered a leaf-spring AFO that worked well when it was worn.

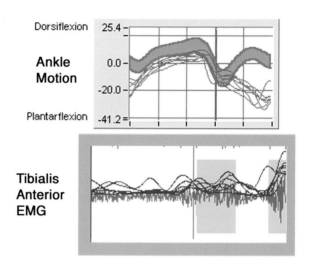

Figure C6.14.1

gait into four patterns. Type 1 has ankle plantar flexion in swing phase with an inactive or very weak tibialis anterior, which is the cause of the plantar flexion. Type 2 has an equinus gait pattern but with spastic or contracted plantar flexors, which overpower an active dorsiflexor. Type 3 includes the ankle position of type 2, further adding abnormal function of the knee joint. Type 4 includes all problems of type 3 with the addition of abnormal function of the hip joint muscles. The separation of these types is usually easy through a combination of physical examination, EMG, kinematic evaluation, and kinetic data. As with all biological groups, however, there are intermediate patients. This system does not consider transverse plane deformities; however, most children with significant residual internal femoral torsion are types 3 or 4, and tibial torsion occurs with types 2, 3, or 4.

Type 1

In children with hemiplegic pattern CP, type 1 is the least common pattern of involvement. Type 1 occurs more with adult stroke or with a peripheral nerve injury. If this type is identified in a child with CP, the physical examination will demonstrate full passive dorsiflexion; however, no active dorsiflexion can be demonstrated. The kinematic examination will show plantar flexion at initial contact and no dorsiflexion in swing phase. The EMG will demonstrate a tibialis anterior that is silent or nearly silent. The primary treatment for type 1 hemiplegia is a relatively flexible leaf-spring AFO (Case 6.14). In very rare situations where the tibialis posterior has normal tone and normal phasic firing, the tibialis posterior can be transferred through the interosseous membrane to the dorsum of the foot. However, this transfer is mainly used with peripheral nerve palsy. With central lesions, relearning is difficult as this is an out-of-phase transfer, and transfer of the spastic tibialis posterior leads to very severe foot deformities.

Type 2

The most common subtype of hemiplegia is type 2, making up approximately 75% of all children with hemiplegia. Typically, children learn to walk independently between 15 and 20 months of age, either with toe walking or foot flat with a planovalgus. The early treatment is to provide the children support through the use of an orthotic, usually starting with a solid ankle AFO, then following with an articulated AFO for the second orthotic. If a child has a very spastic gastrocsoleus, botulinum toxin injection for two or three cycles can help parents apply the AFO and make AFO wear more comfortable for the child. Usually, by 4 to 7 years of age, the gastrocsoleus contracture has become so severe that brace wear is no longer possible. On physical examination, children often demonstrate a contracture of both the gastrocnemius and soleus. The kinematic examination will show equinus throughout the gait cycle, and knee flexion at foot contact may be increased as children preposition the knee to avoid high external extension moments from the ground reaction force during weight acceptance. Often, these children will be toe walking on the unaffected side as well, and a careful assessment is required to make sure that this is compensatory toe walking and not mild spastic response in a limb that was erroneously thought to be normal. The physical examination and kinematic evaluation are most useful for this assessment. The unaffected ankle should have adequate dorsiflexion measuring 5° to 10° with knee extension. The ankle moment should show normal late stance phase plantar flexion moment or a variable moment, one or two of which may look almost normal. The affected ankle will also be more consistently abnormal with high early plantar flexion moments. If children have been allowed to walk on the toes until late middle childhood, their unaffected ankles will often develop plantar flexion contractures from persistent toe walking. The physical examination will show a reduced ankle range of motion, and the ankle moment will still show the same variability with much better power generation than the affected ankle. The step length of the affected side is usually longer and the stance phase time of the normal limb is longer. These changes occur because the affected leg has a normal swing phase but is more unstable in stance phase. If the normal ankle is contracted it will need a gastrocnemius lengthening or the normal ankle will become a driving force toward toe walking after correction of the contracture on the primarily involved side (Case 6.15).

Outcome of Tendon Lengthening

The need for postoperative orthotic use varies, but braces are not routinely needed. If children do not gain foot flat at initial contact by 3 to 6 months after surgery, an AFO should be used, usually an AFO that allows dorsiflexion to encourage the tibialis anterior to gain function. This AFO can be either an articulated AFO or a half-height wrap-around AFO with an anterior ankle strap. With appropriate early treatment, most children with type 2 hemiplegic pattern CP can be free of an orthosis by early grade school. Some children will develop an equinus contracture again in late childhood or adolescence. If an adolescent is willing to tolerate the orthosis, another round of Botox injections and orthotic wear can delay surgery until he is near the completion of growth. Approximately 25% of type 2 hemiplegics will need a second gastrocnemius or tendon Achilles lengthening in adolescence. Adolescents or young adults with type 2 hemiplegia should seldom need to wear an orthosis after this last lengthening. Long toe flexor spasticity may also be present, but this seldom needs surgical treatment.

In early childhood, the feet are often in a planovalgus position; however, as children gain increased tone, gastrocnemius and soleus equinus develops.

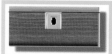

Case 6.15   Christian

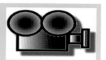

Christian, a boy with hemiplegia, started walking at 17 months of age. He used a solid ankle AFO until he was 2.5 years old. He then used articulating AFOs until he was 4 years old, when he complained that the orthotics caused him pain. After multiple attempts to make the orthotics comfortable, he was allowed to walk without orthotics for 1 year until age 5 years, when he had a full analysis. The physical examination demonstrated that he had popliteal angles of 35° bilaterally, and ankle dorsiflexion on the right was only −25° with both knee flexion and extension. On the left, he had ankle dorsiflexion to 20° with knee flexion, but only 5° with knee extension. The observation of his gait showed that he was toe walking bilaterally, although higher on the right than the left. It was recommended that he have an open Z-lengthening of the tendon Achilles. Postoperatively, he used an articulated AFO for 1 year, and following this, he developed good active dorsiflexion with a plantigrade foot position (Figure C6.15.1).

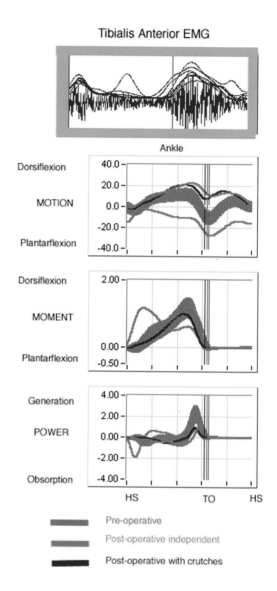

Figure C6.15.1

Almost always, this equinus causes the planovalgus to correct and sometimes even overcorrect. Children with type 2 hemiplegia develop planovalgus that needs treatment only on rare occasions. Surgical treatment should not be considered until 8 to 10 years of age because this planovalgus frequently resolves spontaneously. The predominant problem for children with type 2 hemiplegia is equinovarus, usually due to a spastic or overactive tibialis posterior. In occasional children, equinovarus is due to a spastic tibialis anterior. The diagnosis as to the cause of the varus between these two tendons requires a combination of physical examination and EMG data. The physical examination will often demonstrate increased tone in the muscle most responsible. The EMG should show a tibialis anterior that is active during preswing and initial swing phase, and again in terminal swing at initial contact. Significant activity during midstance is abnormal. The tibialis posterior may be active throughout stance phase, more so in terminal stance, and should be silent in swing phase.[59] Most commonly, the tibialis posterior is constantly active on EMG and spastic on physical examination, although there are cases where it is only active in swing phase. If the subtalar motion is supple, allowing full correction of the varus, a split transfer of the tibialis posterior to the peroneus brevis on the lateral side is performed. If the tibialis anterior is most affected, it is split transferred to the cuboid or to a slip of the peroneus longus. If both tendons are abnormal, both can have a split transfer performed at the same time. If the subtalar joint is not allowing overcorrection into some valgus, a calcaneal osteotomy may be required, although this is rare in type 2 hemiplegia.

Rotational Deformities

Transverse plane torsional deformities are not common in type 2 hemiplegia and are usually mild, similar to torsional deformities in normal children. Because the torsional deformities are mild, surgical treatment should not be considered until late middle childhood or adolescence. Limb length discrepancy is usually approximately 1 cm shorter on the involved side, which is anatomically perfect. Shoe lifts should not be given, as they will only require children to make an adaptation, which increases the difficulty of swinging the leg through. This degree of shortness causes no short-term or long-term problems.

Treatment of the spasticity, which is limited to the plantar flexors in type 2 hemiplegia, is only by local measures such as tendon lengthening, Botox, and/or bracing. There is no role for dorsal rhizotomy or intrathecal baclofen because the local treatments are effective and much simpler. Because both the gastrocnemius and soleus seem to contract together in many of these children, it is reasonable to consider nighttime orthotic wear to try to stretch the soleus and perhaps the gastrocnemius. A nighttime orthosis is usually attempted when contractures are present; however, most children object to this orthosis because they are unable to fall asleep and therefore, in practice, this seldom works.

Type 3

Children with type 3 involvement have all the concerns and problems of the children with type 2 involvement. Children with type 3 hemiplegia tend to start walking slightly later than with type 2, usually at 18 to 24 months of age. They almost all start walking on the toes of both feet but usually will not need assistive devices to start walking. The diagnosis of type 3 hemiplegia requires establishing evidence that the knee is involved in the pathology as well. On physical examination, there may be increased tone in the hamstrings or rectus muscles and increased hamstring contracture, usually at least 20° and often 30° to 40° more than the unaffected side. Knee flexion at initial contact will be high, more than 25°. In midstance, the knee flexion continues to be increased. All type 3 patterns have abnormal hamstring activity. On the EMG, this activity is usually premature onset in swing phase and prolonged activity in stance phase. The presence of a fixed knee flexion contracture of more than 5° is also evidence of hamstring involvement. The step length is usually shorter than the normal side and the stance time is variable, sometimes longer and sometimes shorter depending on the stability of stance phase (Case 6.16). Treatment of the hamstring contractures and overactivity may

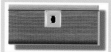 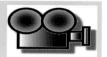

Case 6.16   Kwame

Kwame, an 18-month-old boy, was initially seen with a complaint that he was late in learning to walk. He was reported to have been premature by 8 weeks, but had been healthy since discharge from the hospital. On physical examination he had increased tone through the lower and upper extremities, but it seemed worse on the left side. He was placed in an AFO and, over the next 6 months, he started walking. By age 5 years, he was developing significant internal rotation of the femur and having a stiff knee gait as well as significant toe walking bilaterally. At this time, the physical examination showed that he had hip abduction of 25° on the left and 45° on the right, and internal rotation on the left of 75° and on the right of 60°. The popliteal angle on the left was 68° compared with 50° on the right. The left ankle dorsiflexion with the knee extended was −20°, while on the right it was 4°. The knee flexed ankle dorsiflexion on the left was −8°, while on the right it was 11°. The kinematics demonstrated low nor-mal knee flexion in swing phase, increased knee flexion at foot contact, bilateral early ankle dorsiflexion in stance phase, with less total dorsiflexion on the left side. Internal rotation of the left femur was also noted (Figure C6.16.1). The EMG showed much less clear activity patterns on the left with the rectus having high variability and the hamstring having very early initiation on the left. The right side looked normal (Figure C6.16.2). Except for the internal rotation of the hip, the primary pathology seemed to be in the left knee and ankle; therefore, this is a type 3 hemiplegia. Based on this, the femur was derotated, hamstring lengthened, distal rectus transferred to the sartorius, and a tendon Achilles lengthening was performed (Figure C6.16.3). He did well for 4 years, but then he again developed a significant ankle equinus requiring a second tendon Achilles and distal hamstring lengthening. As he entered puberty, he was doing well with a nearly symmetric gait pattern.

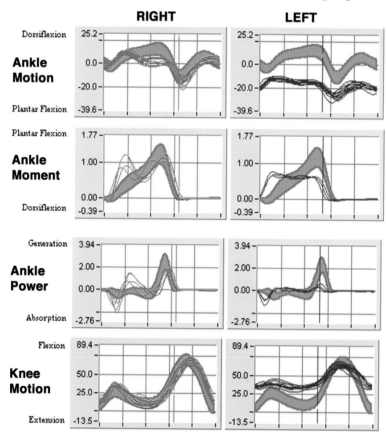

Figure C6.16.1

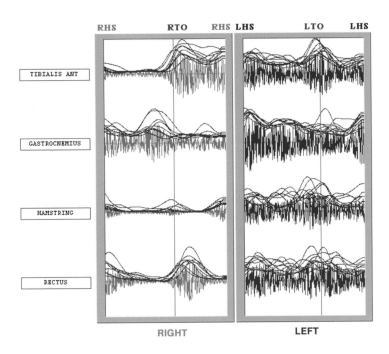

Figure C6.16.2

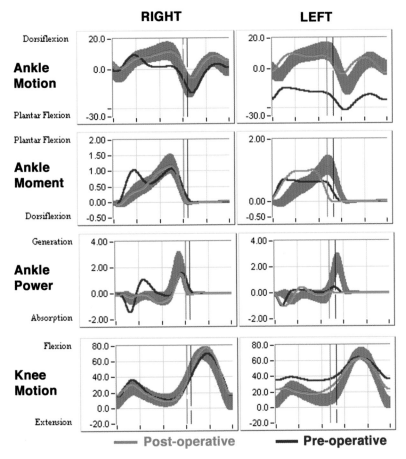

Figure C6.16.3

be with botulinum toxin injections for several cycles in young children, along with gastrocnemius injections. When the hamstring contracture is causing progressive knee flexion contracture, surgical lengthening should be performed. If the gastrocsoleus contractures need to be addressed, the hamstrings should also be lengthened at the same time, or knee flexion in midstance will draw these children to either toe walk again or stand with a crouched gait on the affected side, which also draws the unaffected side into a crouched gait pattern with increased knee flexion in stance.

Stiff Knee Gait

Some children with type 3 hemiplegia have involvement of the rectus. This involvement will be noted by the parents as a complaint of toe dragging, frequent tripping, and rapid shoe wear, especially on the anterior aspect of the shoes. The physical examination may or may not demonstrate increased rectus tone and a positive Ely test. The kinematic evaluation will show swing phase peak knee flexion to be less than the normal, usually less than 50°, and the peak is often late, close to midswing. For children with late or low knee flexion in swing, when the EMG activity of the rectus muscle in swing phase is increased and evidence of complaints of toe dragging is present, then a distal transfer of the rectus is indicated. This transfer is almost always performed with hamstring lengthening and gastrocnemius or tendon Achilles lengthening. Similar to type 2 hemiplegia, approximately 25% of the children will need two tendon lengthenings, one at age 4 to 7 years, and a second at adolescence. A few children will need three lengthenings. These tend to be children who needed the first lengthening very early, sometimes as early as the third year of life. The goal of delaying the first tendon lengthening is to try to avoid the second or third tendon lengthening, although there is no physical documentation that this strategy is effective.

Rotational Deformities

Transverse plane deformities are more common with type 3 hemiplegic involvement. If tibial torsion or femoral anteversion are causing increased tripping or are very cosmetically objectionable by 5 to 7 years of age, surgical correction can be considered. If children have a very asymmetric pelvic rotation as an adaptation for unilateral femoral anteversion, correction should be considered as early as age 5 to 7 years. Because the functional impairment is greater, the limb length discrepancy tends to be slightly greater than for type 2 hemiplegia, often between 1 and 2 cm at maturity. For most children, this limb length discrepancy works perfectly well to help with foot clearance during swing phase in a limb that does not have as good ability to shorten during preswing and initial swing phase. A shoe lift should not be used, and radiographic monitoring of limb length is needed only with a discrepancy of over 1.5 cm. If the knee flexion contracture is more than 10°, additional shortening will occur. To prevent further leg shortening, knee flexion contracture prevention is important. Like type 2 hemiplegia, there is no role for the global treatment of spasticity in type 3 hemiplegia.

Type 4

Type 4 hemiplegia is the third most common pattern; however, it is relatively rare, probably making up less than 5% of all children with hemiplegia. It is relatively common to find type 4 hemiplegia that overlaps with asymmetric diplegia or mild quadriplegia, and it is uncommon to find a child with type 4 hemiplegia who is completely normal on the contralateral side. Children with type 4 involvement usually walk later, between the ages of 2 and 3 years. Many children will use a walker during the learning period of walking. The walker usually needs to be fitted with an arm platform on the involved side. The diagnosis of type 4 hemiplegia is made by the presence of increased tone in the adductor or hip flexor muscles and by evidence on the kinematic examination of decreased hip extension in midstance. Both the stance time and the step length will be shortened as the limb neither can swing normally nor is very stable in stance phase. All the problems and considerations of type 2 and type 3 have to now be added into the treatment of type 4. In addition, concern for overactivity and contracture of the adductors and hip flexors has to be considered as well. It is important to recognize that children with type 4 hemiplegia can develop spastic hip disease, so they have to be monitored by physical examination and radiographs for hip dysplasia.

From the perspective of children's gait, the decisions about surgery are usually based mostly on the function at the level of the ankle and knee. Based on the evaluation of these joints, surgery of the hip has to be considered as an additional procedure. Adductor lengthening is only needed occasionally. If the abduction is greater than 20° on physical examination and abduction is present at foot contact, surgery is seldom indicated. Iliopsoas lengthening is indicated if hamstring lengthening is to be done, a hip flexion contracture of more than 20° is present, anterior pelvic tilt is more than 25°, and there is less than 10° of hip flexion at maximum extension in mid- or terminal stance. Usually, these lengthenings are needed only once; however, additional lengthenings, especially hamstring and gastrocnemius lengthenings, are very commonly needed. Probably 75% to 90% of children with type 4 hemiplegia need at least two lengthening procedures and approximately 25% may need a third lengthening procedure. Treatment of the distal problems follows the pattern of type 2 and type 3; however, the muscle tone and contractures tend to be worse.

Rotation Deformities

Transverse plane deformities, especially increased femoral anteversion, are common in type 4 hemiplegia. Usually, this is added to the neurologic tendency for pelvic rotation with the affected side rotated posteriorly. In occasional children, this pelvic rotation may be so severe that they present with almost sideways walking. This sideways walking pattern can also be described as crab walking. This gait pattern is very ineffective and should be addressed at the young age of 5 to 7 years. Femoral derotation, which will then allow the pelvis to rotate anteriorly on the affected side, is required, and children will have a more symmetric gait pattern. Femoral derotation should be considered if the pelvic rotation is more than 15° to 20° on the involved side and the physical examination shows an asymmetric femoral rotation with more internal rotation on the affected side. Femoral derotation can be combined with all the other soft-tissue lengthenings that may be needed. Children with type 4 hemiplegia may develop foot deformities similar to diplegia in which the planovalgus improves into middle childhood, but then gets worse again in adolescence.

Limb Length Discrepancy

Limb length discrepancy should be an active concern because many of these children have 2 to 2.5 cm of shortness on the affected side. The functional impact of the limb shortness is increased with the tendency for knee and hip flexion deformities to add more functional shortening to the real shortening. Also, this leg length discrepancy may be further complicated by adductor contractures that may limit hip abduction allowing the pelvis to drop on the affected side, which further magnifies the limb length inequality. If the limb length cannot be functionally accommodated, the use of a shoe lift is recommended for type 4 hemiplegia. This group also merits close radiographic monitoring of limb length with the goal in some children of doing a distal femoral epiphyseodesis to arrest growth on the non-involved side. The goal in type 4 hemiplegia is to have the affected limb length equal to 1 cm longer than the non-involved side because of the functional impact of the inability to accommodate for joint positions during stance phase, which take precedence over swing phase dysfunction (Case 6.17). There is benefit to having a longer affected limb only in definite type 4 hemiplegia. In all other types, which make up more than 95% of hemiplegia, the affected limb should be approximately 1 cm shorter for maximum function (Figure 6.44).

In some children with type 4 hemiplegia, the use of intrathecal baclofen can be considered for treating severe spasticity even though it is unilateral. We have not used intrathecal baclofen in this population and there are no reports specifically addressing its use. However, the local treatment of the degree of spasticity present in many children with type 4 hemiplegia is not very effective.

In severe type 4 hemiplegia, an assistive device is needed long term for ambulation. These children usually require a platform walker unless they can walk with one crutch or cane. The most functional device is found by trial and error in physical therapy. In the children who have many ambulatory problems, wheelchairs are needed. Because of the presence of one normal arm, a double-rim one-arm-drive chair should be considered.

Diplegia

Diplegic pattern involvement has a wide spectrum, blending with the quadriplegic pattern at the more neurologically severe end of bilateral involvement and blending with the hemiplegic pattern on the more severely asymmetric end of the spectrum. Attempts to classify diplegic gait patterns usually end with parameters directly related to age, such as limb length,[60] or indirectly related to age, such as jump position versus crouch[61] (Figure 6.45). There is no easy and relatively separable severity grouping such as is defined for hemiplegia. There are definitely children with mild diplegia and children with severe diplegia, but these groups seem to be opposite ends of a standard distribution curve with a mean being moderate involvement. Severity of involvement tends to increase from distal to proximal similar to hemiplegia; however, there are few children with diplegia with only ankle involvement. Most children with diplegia have some hip, knee, and ankle involvement. The method for planning treatment that is easy to remember and relates directly to the treatment plan is based on the age of children rather than on the individual severity. Therefore, young children, middle childhood aged children, and adolescents to young adults will be the age groups, and within each age group, mild, moderate, and severe involvement is considered.

Diplegia in Young Children (the Prancing Toe Walker)

Mild Involvement

Children with mild diplegia may start walking between 18 and 24 months of age. Usually, these children initiate independent ambulation by toe walking with extended hips and knees. Typically, the spasticity in the gastrocnemius and hamstrings is mild, and there may even be a question of these children being idiopathic toe walkers or mild diplegic pattern CP. The toe walking is easy to control with an AFO, and as children gain motor control and balance, some will start to walk foot flat without an AFO. However, other children will become more spastic, occasionally with severe spasticity requiring Botox injections just to tolerate brace wear. If these children are

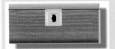

Case 6.17   Jeremy

When Jeremy was 9 years old, his parents complained that he tripped over his right leg and could not run. Jeremy had moderate mental retardation and no other history of medical problems. The left side was normal on physical examination, but on the right side he had weakness, especially at the hip abductors and extensors. He had no spasticity of the gastrocnemius, but increased tone in the hamstrings with a popliteal angle of 50° on the right and 30° on the left. Ankle dorsiflexion on the right was 15° with knee flexion and 5° with knee extension. Hip abduction was limited to 10° on the right, full flexion was present, and a 2.5-cm shortness was noted on the right side (Figure C6.17.1). Jeremy was put in an AFO and given a 1.5-cm shoe lift, which improved the tripping symptoms. An adductor and hamstring lengthening was performed, and the leg length was monitored with annual scanograms. Because this was believed to represent a type 4 hemiplegia without much compensation attempted by toe walking, a femoral epiphyseodesis was planned when his remaining growth would leave the right leg approximately equal to 1 cm long. At age 12.5 years, the epiphyseodesis was performed (Figure C6.17.2) and by age 16 years, he was left with several millimeters of increased lengthening on the right side (Figure C6.17.3). He was weaned off of the shoe lift and out of the AFO. At the completion of growth, he walked without assistance. This is the typical limb length problem of type 4 hemiplegia, which should be managed to gain equal limb lengthening to slightly overlengthening on the involved side. With the other types of hemiplegia, the goal is to leave the child with a 1- to 2-cm shortness on the involved side, which will help with limb clearance and accommodate for the tendency for premature heel rise from gastrocnemius spasticity or contracture.

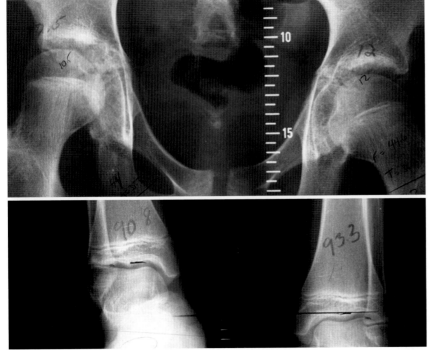

Figure C6.17.1

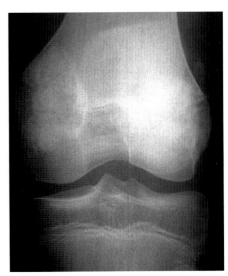

Figure C6.17.2

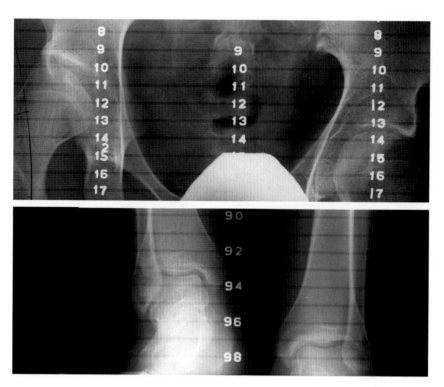

Figure C6.17.3

still toe walking without an AFO by 5 to 7 years of age, surgical tendon lengthening should be considered. If the ankle dorsiflexion with knee extension is less than 5°, and the maximum dorsiflexion in stance phase is occurring during weight acceptance instead of terminal stance, gastrocnemius lengthening is indicated. If there is a high early plantar flexion moment with a big power absorption and poor push-off power generation, gastrocnemius lengthening is also indicated. If the initial contact knee flexion is increased above 20° and the popliteal angle is increased, then hamstring lengthening should also be considered. It is expected that children with mild diplegia will need only one surgical procedure to maximize gait. Most children with mild diplegia do not have transverse plane deformities; however, if they do, the correction can be made at the same time, between the ages of 5 and 7 years (Case 6.18).

Moderate Degree of Involvement

Most children with diplegia would be defined as moderate. If balance is adequate, most moderate children walk independently between the ages of 24 and 36 months. If balance is a problem, walker use will continue to be required, starting with crutch training around 4 to 5 years of age. Functional community ambulation with crutches should not be expected until age 5 years and sometimes will not occur until children are 8 to 10 years old. In the first year of independent ambulation, these children will walk with the arms in the high guard position, walk fast up on the toes, and when they want to stop, they will run to find fixed objects like a wall or fall to the floor. Most children walk with knee stiffness, extended hips and knees, and with increased rotation of the pelvis. Some children have transverse plane deformities with increased femoral anteversion being most common, but they also may have tibial torsion. Many children at this age with moderate diplegia

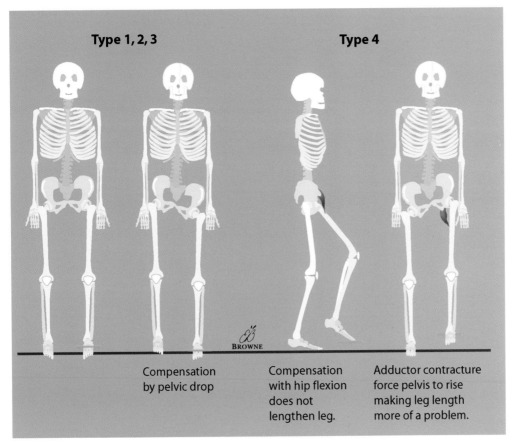

Type 1, 2, 3   **Type 4**

Compensation   Compensation   Adductor contracture
by pelvic drop   with hip flexion   force pelvis to rise
                       does not   making leg length
                       lengthen leg.   more of a problem.

walk with ankle equinus and varus. Surgical treatment is planned for between 5 and 7 years of age after children have had 6 to 12 months of no
improvement in ambulatory speed, walking endurance, or improvement in
balance. The primary treatment at this age is aggressive physical therapy
using the teaching modalities and repetitive practice to improve balance
and motor control. Passive stretching may be taught to caretakers as well as
performed by therapists. Localized treatment with Botox may be beneficial
if there are specific focal problems such as gastrocnemius, spasticity, or hamstring spasticity that are causing impediments to progress in gait learning
(Case 6.19).

Severe Involvement

The most severe end of the diplegic pattern are children who have very
significant asymmetry, who start walking with a walker at 2 to 3 years of age
and, if they come to independent ambulation, do so only after 4 or 5 years of
age, usually following surgery. These children are high, early toe walkers in
their bare feet. They may be able to get feet flat, often with significant planovalgus. Many of the toe walkers have varus foot position associated with
equinus. Transverse plane deformities are common, with both tibial torsion
and femoral anteversion. Spasticity tends to include the hip, knee, and ankle
almost equally. These children have to be closely monitored for spastic hip
disease, which will occur in a significant number and requires early adductor lengthening. Often, these children are best treated with solid AFOs until
they are 4 or 5 years of age. Physical therapy is the mainstay of treatment,
with the focus being the same as with children with moderate involvement.

Figure 6.44. In hemiplegic types 1 to 3, it is
better to have a mild shortness of the affected
limb. Naturally, this ends up being between
1 and 2 cm, which helps limb clearance in
swing. However, in type 4, there is a tendency to have increased hip adduction and
flexion contractures that greatly magnify any
other leg shortness. Also, hip extension and
abduction are major mechanisms for accommodating leg length shortness, and when this
is deficient in type 4 hemiplegia, the limb
shortness becomes an impairment in its own
right. Therefore, careful attention should be
paid to limb length in type 4 with a goal usually of having symmetric limb lengths. An
occasional patient may even function better
with a longer limb on the affected side.

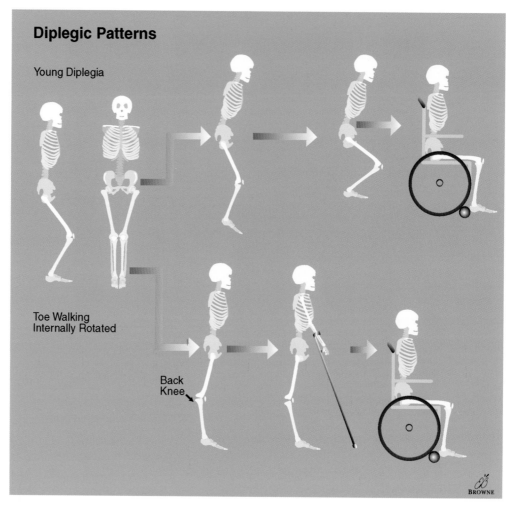

Figure 6.45. The patterns of diplegia are more difficult to define than those of hemiplegia. It is better to divide the stages or ages rather than pattern of involvement. Children younger than 5 years old tend to toe walk with equinus knee stiffness and often internal rotation of the hips. By middle childhood, they often develop a crouched gait pattern which, if left untreated, gets rapidly worse during the adolescent growth period. This problem may drive a child into a wheelchair if it is untreated and severe. Some children in middle childhood start to back-knee, and this may become worse in adolescence to the point where it causes severe knee pain if it is not addressed again, causing the child to end up in a wheelchair.

These children seldom have significant benefit from Botox because of the diffuse widespread involvement of the increased spasticity.

Surgical Treatment of the Prancing Toe Walker

Surgical treatment planning is usually focused at the interface between early childhood and middle childhood. By 4 or 5 years of age, children are reaching a plateau in neurologic development and the rate of learning motor and balance skills is plateauing as well. Socially, children are preparing to enter kindergarten or first grade if they have adequate cognitive skills. For cognitively high functioning children, the goal should be to have the gait impairment surgically corrected and rehabilitation completed before entering first grade. Entering first grade is a significant transition point for many children as they change from primary gross motor skills orientation to primary fine motor skills and cognitive skills learning. This transition period should include decreasing physical therapy and transitioning to normal age-appropriate athletic activities that individual children's functional levels and community ambulatory abilities allow. For example, having a child play soccer 2 days a week with a team would be better than spending that time in physical therapy doing medically oriented therapy, especially for a child who is an independent ambulator.

As children reach a gait functional plateau, usually between 5 to 7 years of age but sometimes as early as 4 years of age, a full analysis and evaluation

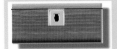

Case 6.18   Cherisse

Cherisse, an 18-month-old girl with increased stiffness in the legs, was seen for slow walking development. Although there was no history of birth problems, she had a workup with a brain MRI that was normal, and a diagnosis of diplegic CP was made. She was placed in an AFO and her mother was encouraged to have her move using heavy push toys. By age 2 years, she was walking independently and by age 3 years, she was walking on her toes, going faster but falling a lot. She was wearing an articulated AFO and was in physical therapy where she had good continued improvement up to age 4 years. Therefore, she was continued for another year in the same program. By age 5 years, both her mother and therapist who were working with her felt that there had been little additional progress in the past 6 months. At this time, her physical examination demonstrated a popliteal angle of 50°, knee extended ankle dorsiflexion of 5°, and bilateral and knee flexed ankle dorsiflexion of 15°. Internal rotation of the hips was 70° with external rotation of 20°. Other ranges of motion were normal. Kinematics demonstrated increased knee flexion at foot contact, premature ankle dorsiflexion, and internal rotation of the hips (Figure C6.18.1). The gastrocnemius had 2+ spasticity and the hamstrings and hip adductors had 1+ spasticity. Her mother was given the option to have either a dorsal rhizotomy or orthopaedic surgery, and she chose to do the orthopaedic procedures. Cherisse had bilateral hamstring lengthening, gastrocnemius lengthening, and femoral derotation osteotomy. One year after surgery, her gait had improved with better knee motion and correction of the internal rotation. This improvement was maintained 4 years later. It is expected that this girl will likely not need more surgery and that she will be an excellent ambulator as an adult.

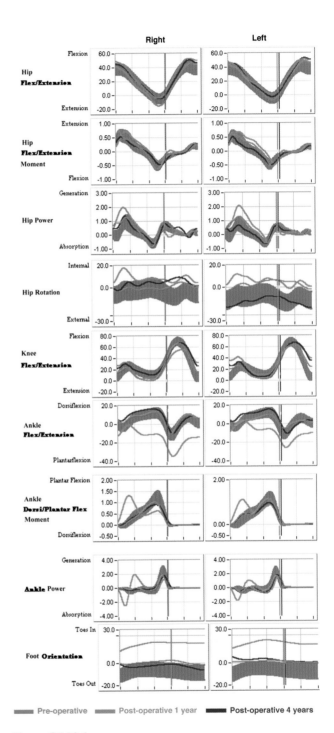

Figure C6.18.1

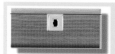

Case 6.19   Daymond

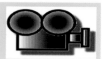

Daymond, a 2-year-old boy, presented with a history of prematurity and slow motor development. At that time, he was just starting to hold on to and push some toys. He was placed in solid ankle AFOs and, after 1 year of physical therapy, he was able to walk slowly in the posterior walker, but could not get into the walker by himself. By age 4 years, through continued therapy, he learned to get up into a standing position and increased his walking speed. He was also switched to articulating AFOs. By age 5 years, he was walking well with the walker, and in therapy, he was working on balance development with the use of quad canes, which were nonfunctional for ambulation outside the therapy environment. By age 6 years, he was practicing with Lofstrand crutches and by age 8 years, he was starting to practice walking independently. He was finding more stability and walking more with back-kneeing and ankle dorsiflexion even though he did not have equinous contractures (Figure C6.19.1). It was clear at this time, however, that he would be a permanent crutch user as age 8 years is a common plateau point, and he had been receiving intensive therapy, which means significant additional improvement cannot be expected. He had no significant structural limitations that could be corrected, and most of his ambulation problems were related to poor balance with the arms in the high guard position. Over the next 4 years, he continued to work on his balance, but as he entered puberty, it was clear that he would never be able to walk independent of the crutches except for very short times in home areas.

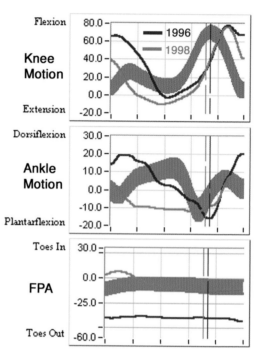

Figure C6.19.1

of their gait function is performed. A surgical plan is made and the actual surgery planned to least disturb families' normal activities. First, a decision has to be made if a tone reduction procedure is indicated or if the treatment is to be all musculoskeletal based. If children are independent ambulators and the physical examination demonstrates increased tone throughout the lower extremities and minimal fixed muscle contractures, the kinematics demonstrate decreased range of motion at the hip, knee, and ankle, and there are no transverse plane deformities, these children are considered excellent candidates for a tone reduction procedure. Children who meet all these criteria are very rarely seen, so there are almost always relative contraindications. At this time, the reported data from rhizotomy in this age group suggests that ambulatory ability is not improved much over physical therapy alone.[62] Dorsal rhizotomy decreases spasticity and the joint range of motion increases, especially at the hip and knee.[63–65] Muscle contractures do not resolve, and there is no impact on transverse plane deformities.[66] There are very few data comparing direct musculoskeletal surgery with dorsal rhizotomy, with the only report suggesting a better chance of independent ambulation following muscle surgery than dorsal rhizotomy.[67] Based on these reports and our own experience, we no longer recommend dorsal rhizotomy to any child; however, it is still used in some centers. The use of intrathecal baclofen for this population has not been reported. The large size of the pump and the need for frequent refills has made families hesitant to have these pumps implanted. We know of no center using the pump for this indication, although theoretically it would be an ideal indication. The pump would allow controlling the spasticity and allow children to be as functional as possible. Part of the problem with dorsal rhizotomy is that too much tone is removed and children are left weak. With the pump, this could be modulated.

Clearly, the mainstay of surgical treatment of children with diplegia is direct correction of the deformities that are causing the functional impairment to gait. The goal should be to correct all the impairments that can be corrected with one surgery. The analysis starts distally and works proximally. If there is a varus foot deformity with equinus that seems to be causing toe walking, there is a temptation to suggest that this should be corrected. In early and middle childhood diplegia, unless the varus foot deformity is fixed, no surgery should be done on the tibialis anterior or tibialis posterior. Almost all these children will convert to planovalgus later, and any surgery on the foot at this age will only speed up that process. If children have a planovalgus deformity that is supple and are tolerating an orthotic, continuation of the orthotic is in order. If the deformity is severe, causing problems with orthotic wear, correction of the planovalgus is indicated, usually with a lateral column lengthening at this age. For severe fixed deformities, subtalar fusion is indicated.

Ankle dorsiflexion on physical examination will almost always demonstrate a discrepancy between gastrocnemius and soleus muscle contractures. Usually, the ankle is in plantar flexion at initial contact and comes to early dorsiflexion, but still lacks normal dorsiflexion. The ankle moment shows increased plantar flexion moment early in stance with a high power absorption in middle stance and low push-off power generation. These parameters indicate the need for gastrocnemius lengthening. The whole Achilles tendon should never be cut with a percutaneous tenotomy in children with diplegia. Although one study reportedly found no difference between open Z-lengthening of the Achilles tendon and doing a gastrocnemius-only lengthening,[68] there is no known or theoretical benefit to lengthening the soleus tendon if the muscle is not contracted.

Almost all children with diplegia have increased popliteal angles on physical examination and increased knee flexion at initial contact and during weight acceptance. Most will continue with increased knee flexion in midstance as well, which indicates hamstring lengthening is needed. If the knee goes into extension in midstance phase but has a very high popliteal angle of greater than 60° and knee flexion at initial contact of more than 40°, hamstring lengthening is still indicated, but usually only medial semitendinosus and semimembranosus lengthenings. However, if children have external tibial torsion, a biceps lengthening should also be added. If children's popliteal angles and knee flexion are intermediate between the two and they have full knee extension in midstance phase, only the semitendinosus should be lengthened. As the knee motion proceeds into swing phase, rectus dysfunction is diagnosed by prolonged swing phase rectus activity on EMG, low peak knee flexion, and late peak knee flexion in swing phase. If the walking velocity is greater than 80 cm/s and families complain of toe drag, a rectus transfer is indicated.

At the hip, a flexion contracture of more than 20° with anterior pelvic tilt of greater than 20° and decreased hip extension in early stance phase are indications for iliopsoas lengthening. If the indication is borderline, the procedure should be done if children are independent ambulators, but not if they are using walking aids or walk slower than 80 cm/s. Transverse plane deformities need to be assessed and should be addressed if the foot progression angle is more than 10° internal or 30° external. At this age, children almost never have an external progression foot angle; however, internal foot progression angle, which may be due to the internal tibial torsion or femoral anteversion or a combination of both, is common. On physical examination, significantly greater internal hip rotation compared with external rotation suggests increased femoral anteversion, and if this is combined with 20° or more of internal rotation of the hip on the kinematic evaluation, and especially if this occurs in early stance phase, it should be corrected with a proximal femoral derotation osteotomy. If the transmalleolar axis-to-thigh angle is internal, or the internal torsion measures more than 20° internal on the kinematic evaluation, a tibial derotation osteotomy is indicated. In some children, both will be present and both should be corrected. Do not overcorrect at one level to compensate for the other level. This compensatory overcorrection will lead to the knee joint axis being out of line with the forward line of progression and will likely deteriorate or increase as children grow, requiring later correction.

After a full gait assessment, children can have the specific surgical plan made. Each limb should be assessed separately, as many children with diplegia have some asymmetry and require different surgical procedures on each limb. In general, most children with diplegia need gastrocnemius lengthening with some hamstring lengthening. Very rarely is only a gastrocnemius lengthening indicated. The surgical procedure should be done so that children can be rapidly mobilized and returned to physical therapy for rehabilitation. Postoperatively, most children will continue to need some level of foot support, often with an AFO, to assist with dorsiflexion until the tibialis anterior develops muscle tone and correct length.

Middle Childhood, Early Crouch, and Recurvatum of the Knee

After the surgical correction and postoperative rehabilitation, which should be expected to last 1 year as an outpatient with gradually decreasing physical therapy, children with diplegia should be in a stable motor pattern for middle childhood. Often, these children will be more stable; however, they will also walk slower because they are now standing foot flat and do not have the falling gait that was present with the high prancing toe walking posture. Parents may see this slower gait as regression, but they have to be informed to expect this change, which will now allow the children to focus on developing a more stable gait. Children with diplegia in middle childhood tend to be drawn to several postural attractors. This is the age when prominent back-kneeing or crouched gait pattern will start to be seen consistently. This is the time when there may be sudden shifts in ankle position as the posture is being drawn to back-kneeing or crouch positions (Figure 6.46). With the correct soft-tissue balance, almost all children who are independent ambulators will tend to fall into a mild crouched position, which is the goal of treatment. This position is most functional when the crouch is mild, meaning midstance phase knee flexion is less than 20° to 25° and the children have an ankle dorsiflexion maximum of less than 20°. In middle childhood, this tends to be stable with children gaining confidence in walking ability with

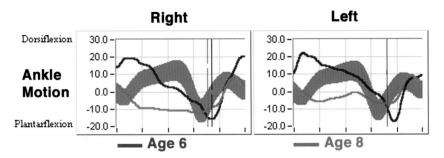

Figure 6.46. As growth occurs and muscle length changes along with changes in the muscle strength to body mass ratio changes, children often make sudden significant shifts in posture; this shows the concept of a shift from one strong attractor to another strong attractor. In this example, a child changed from a flat foot premature heel rise gait pattern to toe walking with ankle equinus. These relatively quick shifts are difficult to predict.

less falling and having longer community ambulator endurance. If the ankle dorsiflexion is increasing above 20°, a dorsiflexion resisting AFO or ground reaction AFO should be applied. If the midstance knee flexion goes above 30° and children develop increasing knee flexion contracture and progressive hamstring contracture, repeat muscle lengthening has to be considered. These contractures seldom become a problem until approximately 5 to 7 years after the initial surgery, when the children are in early adolescence. During middle childhood, there is little need for routine physical therapy for children who are independent ambulators. These children should be encouraged to get involved in sports activities, such as martial arts or swimming. For children who are dependent on walking aids, therapy directed at learning to use forearm crutches before the age of 10 years and weaning off the walker are recommended. Learning to use crutches may require a period of teaching by physical therapy during the summer, or during a time when it does not interfere with school work. Passive range of motion should not be routinely done by physical therapists, and children should be encouraged to do it themselves under the direction of the parents or caretakers.

Knee Recurvatum

Some children who fall into the back-knee attractor have a gastrocnemius that is a little too tight for the hamstrings, which can be easily controlled with an AFO that limits plantar flexion. These children need full calf-length articulated AFOs that block plantar flexion at 5° of dorsiflexion. Often, with full-time brace wear, the hamstrings will gain strength over time and the back-kneeing will slowly resolve as children grow. The second pattern of back-kneeing is children who go into the jump position, where the body is anterior to the hip and the knee joint axis. This pattern may be due to a missed iliopsoas contracture that was not lengthened or may result from a weak gastrocsoleus. The use of a solid AFO in 5° of dorsiflexion should provide a trial. Also, if there is decreased lordosis and more than 30° of hip flexion contracture, the hip flexor should be suspected as the primary cause. If the problem is a contracted hip flexor that was missed in the original operation, this may need to be lengthened to get children to stand upright. The third posture creating back-kneeing is taken by independent ambulators who back-knee in stance with hyperlordosis. In this posture, the HAT center of mass is behind the hip joint but in front of the knee joint. A trial with a solid AFO is the best treatment of this pattern. Most children who are independent ambulators in middle childhood respond well to AFO treatment for back-kneeing.

Back-kneeing in children who use walking aids, such as walkers or forearm crutches, is a major problem (Case 6.20). This back-kneeing may be due to a motor control problem in which individuals lean forward on the crutches, usually with hyperlordosis. With the center of mass of the HAT segment far forward of the hip and knee joint, there is a large knee external

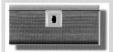

Case 6.20   Frederico

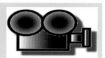

Frederico, a 7-year-old boy, presented with his mother who complained that he had severe back-kneeing when he walked with his walker or used his crutches. He had AFOs, which he complained did not help him and he did not want to wear them. On physical examination he had normal hip motion and knee popliteal angles of 40° bilaterally. Knee extended ankle dorsiflexion was −10° and knee flexed ankle dorsiflexion was +15°. Frederico had poor balance and could not stand without holding on. Kinematic evaluation showed increased knee flexion at foot contact, knee hyperextension with almost every step in midstance, early and decreased ankle dorsiflexion with significant early plantar flexion, and very little additional plantar flexion at toe-off. He had gastrocnemius lengthenings, which were the main cause of the back-kneeing; this was also the reason he could not tolerate the AFOs. He was then gradually weaned out of the AFOs, and gained knee control, although he still had a tendency to be either in crouch or convert into knee hyperextension in midstance.

extension moment on the knee. If individuals have any shortness of the gastrocsoleus, the knee will hyperextend and go into back-kneeing. Also, if individuals have weakness in the gastrocsoleus, they will back-knee. The primary treatment is to use AFOs that prevent plantar flexion; however, with the use of walking aids, AFOs often do not work well as individuals will simply allow the forefoot to rise from the floor. If the knee flexion moment is very high in midstance and individuals complain of knee pain or passive range of knee hyperextension demonstrates an increase of more than 10° to 15°, the only option is the use of a KAFO with an extension stop knee hinge. It is important to make sure that there is no contracture of the gastrocsoleus. Ankle dorsiflexion has to be 5° to 10° in knee extension or the gastrocnemius should be lengthened. Many individuals will continue to have back-kneeing but will remain stable and pain free over many years. Often, the back-kneeing will include a valgus extension thrust in midstance; however, the knee flexion moment is not too large, probably because weight bearing on the upper extremity through the walking aid helps to reduce the magnitude of the ground reaction force. Another way of understanding this is that as individuals move the center of mass of the HAT segment further forward, more weight is shifted to the arms. Although the extension moment at the knee is getting longer, there is a decreased amount of weight from the HAT segment carried by the feet, which decreases the magnitude of the extension moment.

There may be a role for dorsal rhizotomy in the middle childhood period; however, the rehabilitation of older children is even slower. Dorsal rhizotomy is even less indicated because more localized methods are available. Also, the use of intrathecal baclofen has had little or no exposure in this population age.

Adolescent, Young Adult Crouched Gait

During adolescence with the rapid onset of weight and height growth, the classic crouch gait develops, gets worse, and may prevent some children from functional ambulation if it is not treated appropriately. The crouch pattern may be seen in all levels of severity; however, it is primarily encountered in moderate and severe diplegia. The definition of a crouched gait is increased knee flexion in midstance with increased ankle dorsiflexion, and usually increased hip flexion. The toe walking knee flexion pattern is not seen in full adolescence or nearly adult-sized individuals. The muscles and joints are not strong enough to support the body weight for chronic ambulation with the typical early childhood toe walking pattern. If young children are left untreated, the natural history during late middle childhood, when knee flexion in stance increases and the foot starts to dorsiflex, causes collapsing through the midfoot and hindfoot as severe planovalgus foot deformities develop. During the time when children are growing rapidly and increasing weight quickly, midstance phase knee flexion will increase, and ankle dorsiflexion and hip flexion will also increase by a compensatory amount. Individuals who use walking aids tend to increase weight bearing on the walking aids during this time by increasing anterior lean (Case 6.21).

Many adolescents with mild crouch gait, defined as knee flexion in midstance between 10° and 25°, will not need any treatment or will need only single joint level treatment, such as correction of planovalgus feet. Almost all surgery should be done on individuals with moderate crouch, meaning midstance phase knee flexion of 25° to 45° Only rarely, and usually only in medically neglected patients, is surgery done in severe crouched gait with knee flexion in midstance greater than 45°. As with many other conditions, allowing the crouch to become severe means the treatment is less effective (see Case 6.7). The symptoms of increasing crouch include the complaint of knee pain as the stress rises on the knee extensor muscles to support weight bearing. Distal pole of the patella and tibial tubercle apophysitis may occur, especially during rapid growth. Walking endurance will decrease and the feet will start causing more pain with long-distance walking as the planovalgus develops larger pressure areas. The orthotics are no longer able to support the collapsing feet. All these progressive additive impairments combine to frustrate adolescents, and parents typically complain that the individual is losing motivation to walk.

Treatment

Appropriate treatment for crouched gait should focus on early detection and intervention before the problem becomes severe. Early detection means children should be followed closely, every 6 months during middle childhood. A full gait study should be available as a baseline and is usually obtained 1 year after the first surgery, which occurred between the ages of 5 and 7 years. Children's weight should be monitored on every clinic visit, and as they start gaining weight fast and complaining of high stress pain at the knees or the feet, another gait study is indicated. Also, the physical examination should be monitored, especially the passive knee extension and popliteal angle, to monitor progressive hamstring contractures or fixed knee flexion contractures. If there is a significant increase in either of these, a gait study should be made as well. Any significant change in community ambulatory endurance should prompt a full evaluation. Ambulatory children should not be allowed to become dependent on wheelchairs for community ambulation (Case 6.7). This level of deterioration makes the recovery and rehabilitation exceedingly more difficult.

The full evaluation of children with a significant increase in crouch or symptomatic loss of function from crouch should be carefully assessed to make sure all components of the crouched gait are found. All elements that are identified and are correctable should be corrected at the same time. The foot must be a stiff segment and be aligned within 20° of the forward line of movement and within 20° of right angle to the knee joint axis. This means if the foot has a significant planovalgus or a midfoot break, it must be corrected. A stable and correctly aligned foot is mandatory in the correction of

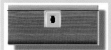

Case 6.21   Elizabeth

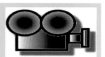

Elizabeth, a 14-year-old girl, presented with the concern that her walking had become so difficult that she could no longer walk around her junior high school. According to her parents, she did not even own a wheelchair when she was in grade school, as she was able to walk everywhere using a walker. They were concerned that she would completely lose her ability to walk. She had no previous surgeries and currently received no physical therapy. She had grown rapidly in the past 2 years, and in the past year, as she had spent more time in the wheelchair, she had gained a lot of weight. A physical examination demonstrated hip abduction to 20°, almost symmetric hip rotation with 40° internal and 30° external rotation; popliteal angles were 70°, the knees had 10° fixed knee flexion contractures, and the feet had severely fixed planovalgus deformities. The kinematics showed high knee flexion at foot contact and decreased knee flexion in swing phase, with a severely reduced knee range of motion (Figure C6.21.1). The pedobarograph showed severe planovalgus with external foot progression of 34° on the right and 19° on the left (Figure C6.21.2). Most weight bearing was in the medial midfoot (Figure C6.21.3). The main cause of the loss of ambulation appeared to be the crouch gait caused primarily by severe and progressive planovalgus foot de-

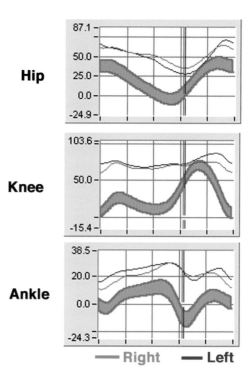

Figure C6.21.1

Left   Right

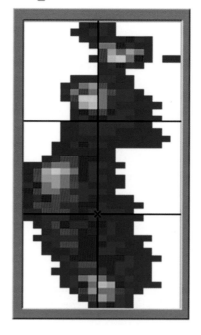

Figure C6.21.2

formities, which prevented the foot from functioning as a rigid moment arm, with the majority of the weight bearing on the medial midfoot (Figure C6.21.3). This lever arm disease needed to be corrected by stabilizing the foot so it was a stiff and stable structure, and it had to be aligned with the axis of the knee joint. Correction of the plano-

valgus with a triple arthrodesis both stabilized the foot and corrected the malalignment. Hamstrings were lengthened, and after a 1-year rehabilitation period, she was again doing most of her ambulation as a community ambulator using crutches. The foot pressure showed a dramatic improvement although there was still more weight

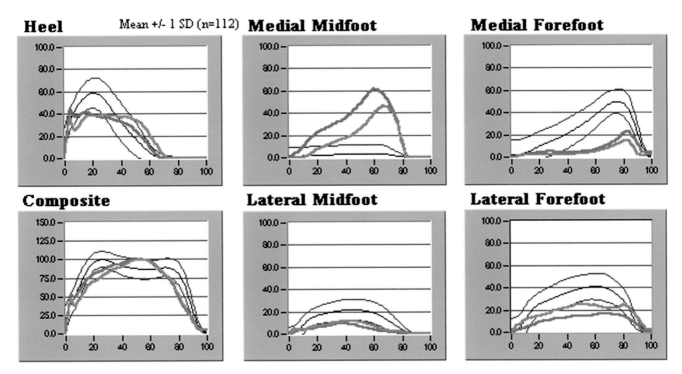

Figure C6.21.3

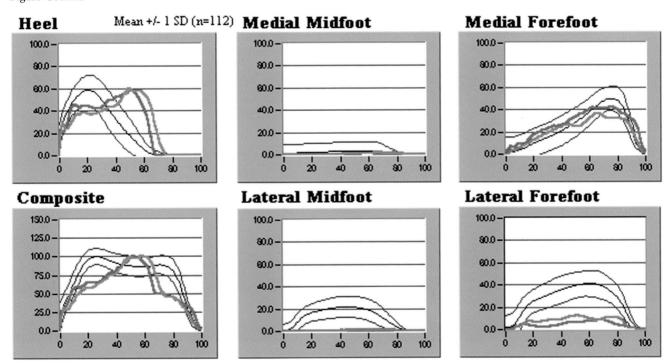

Figure C6.21.4

bearing on the medial forefoot than the lateral forefoot, indicating some mild residual valgus (Figure C6.21.4). There is also increased weight bearing on the heel, indicating continued weakness in the gastrocsoleus (Figures C6.21.4, C6.21.5). The kinematics demonstrate a good improvement in knee extension and ankle plantar flexion (Figure C6.21.6). Elizabeth would have become a permanent wheelchair user if her feet had not been corrected.

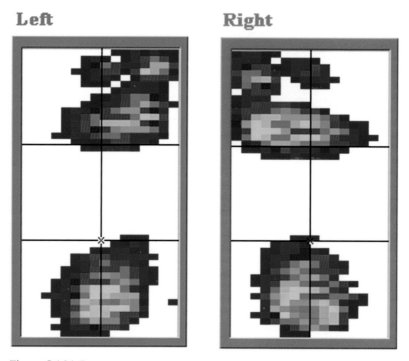

Figure C6.21.5

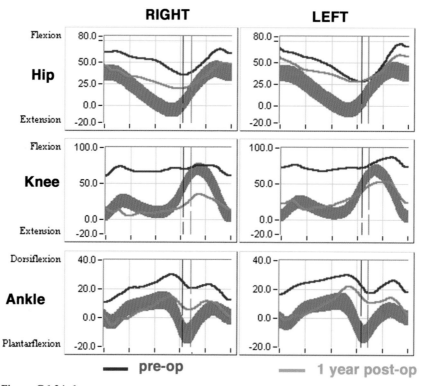

Figure C6.21.6

crouch because the ground reaction force has to be controlled through the foot as a functional moment arm.

Poor moment arm function of the foot causing the ground reaction force to be ineffective in producing knee extension is often one of the primary pathologies of a crouched gait pattern. The foot has to come to within neutral dorsiflexion in midstance so it can be placed in an orthosis, or the gastrocsoleus must provide the force needed to control the ground reaction force. If the gastrocnemius or soleus is contracted, it must be lengthened, but only to neutral dorsiflexion at the end range.

Never do uncontrolled, percutaneous tendon Achilles lengthenings in adolescent crouching individuals. These individuals will likely never be able to stand again without using a fixed AFO. Tibial torsion must be assessed next, and if it is contributing to the malalignment of the foot causing the foot to be out of line with the knee joint axis, a tibial derotation is required.

Physical examination of passive range of motion of the knee should allow extension to within 10° of full extension. If the fixed knee flexion contracture is between 10° and 30°, a posterior knee capsulotomy is required. If the fixed knee flexion contracture is greater than 30°, a distal femoral extension osteotomy is required. Distal hamstring lengthening is always indicated with crouched gait unless the procedure has been done in the preceding year. The indication to do a hamstring lengthening is a popliteal angle of more than 50° with an initial contact knee flexion of more than 25°, and knee flexion in midstance phase of more than 25°. If individuals have decreased knee flexion in swing phase or late knee flexion in swing phase with toe drag, a rectus transfer should be performed. Many clinicians are hesitant about doing rectus transfers in individuals with crouched posture; however, they must remember that the rectus is only 15% of the strength of the quadriceps and the muscle is not even active, except in pathologic cases in midstance phase. If children are very slow walkers in the quadriplegic category, rectus transfer has less benefit. This discussion presumes independent ambulators or ambulators who use walking aids but do not use wheelchairs for community ambulation. This type of ambulator will gain much more from the rectus transfer than the risk of weakness.[69] If children require a distal femoral osteotomy to correct fixed knee flexion contracture, a shortening of the patellar ligament is usually required as well (Case 6.22). Individuals with moderate crouch, defined as midstance phase knee flexion of 25° to 45°, will not need any shortening of the patellar ligament because the quadriceps will have enough excursion and will readjust when the pathomechanics are corrected. The next concern is the axis of the knee joint, which should be between 0° internal and 20° external at initial contact.

If there is significant internal rotation, meaning more than 5° to 10° of internal rotation at initial contact, and the physical examination shows significantly more internal than external rotation of the hip, the femoral internal rotation should be corrected. Usually, this correction is made by doing a femoral derotational osteotomy, but if there is a question of the source of the internal rotation, a CT scan of the femur should be obtained to evaluate the source of the internal rotation. Last, the hip flexor will need lengthening if the hip flexion contracture is more than 20° and midstance phase hip extension is less than −30°. If there is more than 30° of anterior pelvic tilt but less hip flexion, hip flexor lengthening is also indicated, usually doing an intramuscular lengthening of the iliopsoas. While assessing the crouched pattern, it is important to assess each lower extremity independently, as the surgery will often need to be asymmetric. Correction of the torsional malalignments is extremely important for the correct mechanical function of the lower extremity, especially when there is decreased motor control.

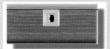 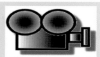

Case 6.22 Brandon

Brandon, a 3-year-old boy, started to walk using a walker while in physical therapy. He did well walking in his school environment; however, his mother reported that he refused to use the walker at home. During the next several years his grandmother cared for him; then, at age 7 years, he again returned to his mother and his initial school. He had developed significant knee flexion deformities that made walking difficult; however, he moved freely on the floor in reciprocating quadruped crawl. A popliteal angle of 90° and 30° knee flexion contractures were found on physical examination. He had knee capsulotomies and hamstring lengthening bilaterally; however, the stress of the surgery and a breakdown in the social service system led to very little physical therapy. By the time he returned to school 4 months later, and the school got him back to the clinic, his knee flexion contractures were slightly worse than preoperatively. Over the next several years, he was in school but received only sporadic therapy. At age 10 years, his mother was very concerned because he crawled everywhere, but he was getting bigger and he refused to stand on his feet. In the classroom and at home he did a lot of knee walking and had several episodes of severe knee bursitis, which required his mother to try to keep him off his knees. His mother's main concern was that soon she could not care for him if she had to carry him everywhere. At this time, he was in a self-contained special needs classroom with a teacher's aide. He had moderate mental retardation, functioning at the 3-year-old level. On physical examination he had a popliteal angle of 100° and fixed knee flexion contractures of 60° bilaterally (Figure C6.22.1) but excellent knee flexion (Figure C6.22.2). He had a large callus on the anterior knee, demonstrating that he did a lot of knee walking (Figure C6.22.3). His hip motion and hip radiographs were normal, and his feet were in planti-

grade and without deformity. Knee radiographs showed no abnormalities (Figure C6.22.4). Observation of his movement on the floor showed that he was very proficient as a reciprocal quadruped crawler and a very functional independent knee walker. Based on the assessment that he had excellent balance with good motor control and motor planning skills, he had hamstring lengthening, distal femoral extension osteotomy, patellar tendon plication, and transfer of the rectus to the sartorius (Figures C6.22.5, C6.22.6). After the osteotomy healed (Figure C6.22.7) and after a 1-year rehabilitation period, he was able to walk in the school and home using a posterior walker with full knee extension. Limited knee flexion prevented proficient crawling or knee walking, which drove him toward walking with the walker. In the second year after this procedure, Brandon developed scoliosis, which required a spinal fusion, and that required another year of rehabilitation. It is expected that he will continue to make more gains in his walking ability over the next several years as his motivation to walk improves. The mental retardation is a significant factor in the speed of the rehabilitation but probably not in the final outcome.

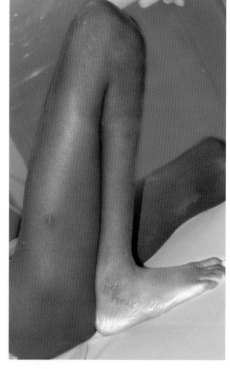

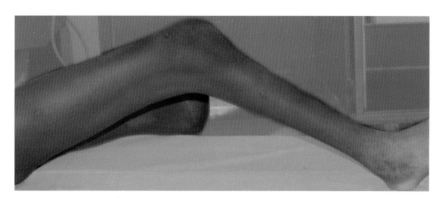

Figure C6.22.1   Figure C6.22.2

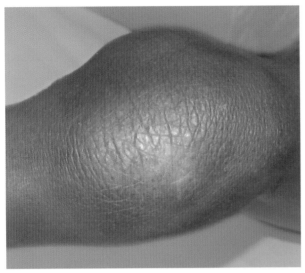

Figure C6.22.3

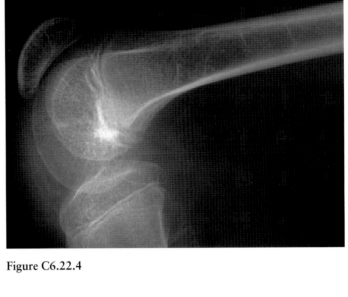

Figure C6.22.4

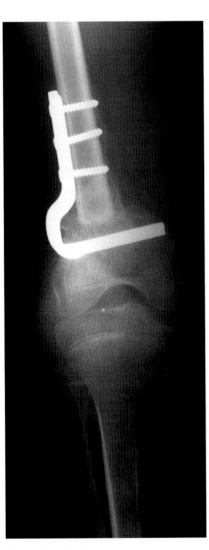

Figure C6.22.5

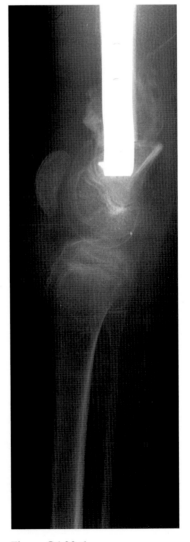

Figure C6.22.6

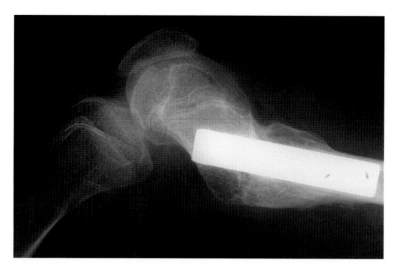

Figure C6.22.7

Performing the Crouched Gait Surgery

The surgery for crouched gait often involves many procedures at different joints. The preferred order is to start at the hip and correct the hip rotation, with iliopsoas lengthening if needed. Then the knee is addressed by hamstring lengthening followed by knee capsulotomy or femoral extension if indicated. The foot deformity is corrected next, then an intraoperative assessment of the torsional alignment is used to make the final determination of the need for a tibial osteotomy. After the tibial osteotomy, another intraoperative assessment should be made to show that the hip fully extends and the knee can be fully extended and lies in approximately 10° of external rotation. The foot-to-thigh alignment should be 20° external to neutral with neutral dorsiflexion. Postoperative rehabilitation should start in the hospital with the goal of having children at least standing before discharge and plan for immediate home rehabilitation. Parents need to expect that the acute rehabilitation will take 3 months until these individuals are close to their preoperative function, and then it will take at least 1 year of rehabilitation to reach maximum function. If there is weakness or a tendency for the gastrocsoleus not to have good strength, a ground reaction AFO has to be used postoperatively. This is the ideal time to use the articulated ground reaction AFO, which will allow the gastrocsoleus to gain strength, and over 1 to 2 years, the orthotic can be weaned away and the correction will be maintained.

The outcome of surgery for crouched gait is excellent if there is a complete diagnosis, correction of all deformities, and follow-through with good rehabilitation. If the surgery is done at adolescence near the end of growth or when individuals are well into adolescence, the correction will be permanent and no additional procedures will be needed.

Back-Kneeing as Adolescents or Young Adults

Back kneeing continues to be a problem in adult-sized individuals, primarily in those using walking aids. The same treatment is used as noted in the section on middle childhood. A few individuals who walk independently will back-knee, and they are usually the individuals with severe weakness of the gastrocsoleus, and have often had tendon Achilles transections.

Spasticity Reduction in Adolescents and Young Adults

Some adolescents have very limited motion because of severe spasticity but are nevertheless good ambulators. The use of intrathecal baclofen is a reasonable option; however, it often unmasks weakness when the spasticity is reduced. There have been no objective reports on the effects of intrathecal baclofen on gait in this age. In our personal limited experience, individuals will have a mild increased crouch and may slow their gait slightly. The patients, however, report feeling more comfortable and find dressing and other activities of daily living easier. Dorsal rhizotomy is not indicated in this group, as the risks far outweigh any benefits that could be expected.

Quadriplegic Gait

By definition, most children with quadriplegia do not ambulate. However, there are many children who have some ambulatory ability. These children are often called severe diplegia or mild quadriplegia, and for the purpose of this discussion, we will consider these individuals to have quadriplegic pattern involvement. By definition, these are individuals who use walking aids and are usually limited to household ambulation. Other ways to define this population are patients with a standing (dimension D) on the GMFM of less than 25%, a walking speed less than 50 cm/s, or an oxygen cost that is greater than 0.8 ml of oxygen per kilogram per meter walked. Many of these are children or adolescents who used a gait trainer in early childhood and are transitioned to a walker adapted with forearm supports in middle childhood. At adolescence, these individuals are usually transfer ambulators, able to move in their home environment and do weightbearing transfers. Many of these individuals have high tone from spasticity and many in the late 1980s and early 1990s had dorsal rhizotomies. The typical experience of this group with rhizotomy, in which spasticity was removed, is that these children can no longer stand or walk, except with the assistance of a gait trainer. If the rhizotomy is less aggressive, leaving some spasticity, most of the spasticity will return over a few years and these children will be back where they started. Rhizotomy is not indicated for this population. The use of the intrathecal baclofen pump, especially for middle childhood and adolescence, is an excellent option. Correctly adjusting the pump so there is enough spasticity to stand but not cause problems requires trial and error.

Early Childhood

In early childhood the children should be placed in standers, and as they develop coordination, start in gait trainers. Many of these children are at high risk for developing spastic hip disease and need to be monitored for the prevention of spastic hip disease. Encouraging ambulation in a gait trainer may not allow individuals to move to walking with an unsupported walker; however, it still gives them a sense of movement and weight bearing. Usually, these children are provided distal support with a solid ankle AFO so they can focus on proximal motor control at the hip and knee. There is really nothing to be gained by using articulated AFOs for these children. Often, these children will have significant scissoring with adduction in initial swing phase. If the adductors are very spastic and contracted, these children may benefit from adductor lengthening; however, this is often not due to spasticity but is a motor control problem. The best way to address this motor control problem is to use lateral ankle restraints, which are available on many commercial gait trainers. If severe equinus limits orthotic tolerance, the use of Botox may help, or surgical lengthening is required. Aggressive attempts to lengthen muscles, correct foot deformities, and correct torsional malalignments in young children less than 6 or 7 years of age often leads to disappointment unless an evaluation has clearly demonstrated that the musculoskeletal impairment is the direct cause of the limited function. Often, parents will identify some problem, such as scissoring, and focus on the assumption that if this problem were removed, the children could walk. If adductor lengthening is performed in these children but they still can adduct, the scissoring is seldom improved. These children's central motor control generators are using a flexor posture that causes the legs to scissor but is not directly responsible for simple, single-muscle overactivity. The scissoring is part of the primitive stepping mass reflex that children are using to advance the limbs. Often, as these children mature, they learn to overcome scissoring and subsequently will slowly do less scissoring. If the musculoskeletal impairment is blocking progress, it is reasonable to correct the deformity, usually around 5 to 7 years of age at the youngest. If there is a question of the significance of the musculoskeletal impairment, it may be beneficial to wait until 8 to 10 years of age when a better assessment can be made, with more time to evaluate how these children are changing.

Middle Childhood Quadriplegic Ambulators

In middle childhood, most children will reach a plateau with motor function. An evaluation of the benefits of correction of musculoskeletal deformities should be performed. If there are limitations that are significantly impairing the children, correction should be made. Correcting the contractures that are causing impairments is often beneficial, and these contractures may include equinus contractures, hamstring contractures, knee flexion contractures, hip flexion contractures, and adductor contractures. Sometimes the parents report that these releases help the caretakers provide personal hygiene more easily, such as easier bathing or dressing. Severe planovalgus foot deformities merit correction when they limit orthotic wear. During this time, if children have good cognitive function, a decision should be made to focus less on walking and more on cognitive learning and fine motor skills. If children have moderate or severe mental retardation, continuing to focus on ambulation is a reasonable option. Some of the children with severe mental retardation will make significant progress in ambulatory skills in middle childhood, even up to age 12 or 13 years. As children approach adolescence, the gait trainer is less useful because the device has to be so large that it does not fit through doors and cannot be functionally used in most homes. Caretakers and parents are encouraged to continue to walk holding the hands of the patients, so as not to lose the ability to do weightbearing transfers. Correction of foot deformities and knee contractures should also be directed at the goal of maintaining these individuals' ability to do standing weightbearing transfers.

Adolescent Quadriplegic Ambulation

Adolescence is when individuals will continue to do household ambulation if they can walk with a standard walker, but usually stop walking if it requires the use of a gait trainer. Most individuals will be able to maintain weight bearing as a transfer ability. If the limitation is due to a musculoskeletal deformity, correction should be considered. Typical problems that occur at this age are severe planovalgus feet, which limit the ability of individuals to stand or wear AFOs. This correction is easy to maintain and will not be lost at this age. The second most common major problem is hamstring contractures and fixed knee flexion contractures. If children are growing rap-

idly, the hamstrings will often rapidly recontract after lengthening. If there is
a severe knee flexion contracture of more than 30°, this too gets worse. As
the knee flexion contracture goes over 30° to 40°, standing rapidly becomes
more difficult. Correcting the knee flexion contracture is a difficult decision
because the contracture may make standing more difficult, but if individuals can only stand and spend most of their time sitting in their wheelchairs,
correction of knee flexion contracture is not likely to be successful, as the
knee will just recontract. Therefore, correction of significant knee flexion
contractures should be reserved for individuals who do some community
ambulation, or who surgeons believe have the ability to do some community
ambulation. Correction of torsional malalignment, such as tibial torsion or
femoral anteversion, is indicated if the correction will improve an individual's ability to sit. Often, the benefit from treatment for sitting takes precedence over problems of ambulation unless it is a very severe torsional malalignment. The problems of stiff leg gait with rectus spasticity are often much
less of a problem in this group of individuals than individuals who are full
community ambulators with faster walking speed. Also, the quadriplegic
pattern involved individuals have a high tendency for recurrence of knee
stiffness in swing phase, sometimes even recruiting the vastus muscles to keep
the knees stiff during swing phase if the rectus is removed. It seems these individuals with limited ambulatory ability need the knee stiffness to be able
to provide stability and control of their standing.

One of the problems that occurs with these quadriplegic patterns is caretakers who insist the children used to walk everywhere but now they can no
longer walk, except in the house. Parents and caretakers tend to forget how
these children walked 3 years prior, and most often, the video record will
show that there is little difference. If there is a real difference and it is due to
progressive musculoskeletal problems, these deformities must be corrected.
If the deterioration cannot be explained by musculoskeletal changes, a full
neurologic workup is indicated to determine if there is any pathology not
previously diagnosed. Forgetting how these children walked is a very important reason for having video records of ambulation, even in children with
limited walking ability. Video records are an important and relatively cheap
tool to assess change in ambulatory ability for children with some ambulatory ability during development.

The outcome of treating gait problems in children with limited ambulatory ability is the same as it is for children with more function. These children should not lose substantial ambulatory ability that they gained. If they
do lose ambulatory ability, the cause should be found.

Movement Disordered Gait

Athetosis

Gait problems in individuals with movement disorders can be especially difficult to address. Individuals with athetosis often have spasticity associated
with the athetosis, which works as a shock absorber on the pathologic movement. Individuals with athetosis may develop significant deformities that
make ambulation more difficult, and there is merit in addressing these problems. Therapy to improve athetoid gait is limited but sometimes adding resistance through the use of ankle weights or a weighted vest can be helpful.
Procedures that will provide stability have the most reliable outcome. For
example, correction of planovalgus feet with a fusion is a reliable procedure.
There is no benefit of trying muscle balancing or joint preservation treatment
in the face of athetosis.

Knee flexion contracture is the most common problem at the knee level, and may lead to significant fixed knee flexion contracture. Although the postoperative course may be difficult, the outcome of the surgical treatment of fixed knee flexion contractures is usually good. Often, these patients have very high cognitive function and are very hesitant to undertake the correction, even if severe deforming musculoskeletal problems are clearly limiting their activities. Both a full analysis and an experienced surgeon will usually be able to convince them of the benefit if the problem is clear and straightforward. These patients also need an explanation of the corrections planned, which are limited to bony correction, joint fusion, or muscle lengthening. There is no role for tendon transfer in individuals with significant athetosis. Most of the surgery should be planned in late middle childhood or adolescence, as these individuals seldom have fixed deformities that cause problems earlier.

Dystonia

The first and most important thing to address in individuals with dystonia is to diagnose the dystonia and make sure it is not misinterpreted as spasticity. Diagnosing dystonia was addressed fully in the motor control chapter. Often, a foot will look like it has severe varus deformity, then on another day, the foot will be in valgus. If surgeons do not have a video record and are not very attentive, a presumption of a spastic equinovarus foot deformity may easily be made. These feet may look like ideal feet for tendon transfers because they are supple; however, tendon transfers tend to cause severe overreaction in the opposite direction. There is no role for tendon transfer in dystonia. We had one patient in whom we did a rectus transfer, not recognizing that it was dystonia and not spasticity. This individual spent 9 months with a flexed knee every time she tried to walk. With persistent therapy and bracing, and under the threat of reversing the transfer, the muscle suddenly went silent and knee flexion in stance stopped. Botulinum toxin is an extremely effective agent to block the muscle effects of dystonia, with its major side effect being that it only works for three to four injection cycles, then the body becomes immune. If the individual has a foot deformity that is symptomatic, the correct treatment is fusion, usually a triple arthrodesis with transection of the offending muscles. Very little other surgery except for fusion is of benefit in ambulatory individuals with dystonia.

Ambulatory problems related to chorea and ballismus are rare, and we have never had occasion in which surgery was required. Again, if there is foot instability, a fusion would be a reasonable option.

Complications of Gait Treatment

There are many real and potential complications in the treatment of gait problems in children with CP. Often, there is the presumption that nonoperative treatment has no complications; however, this is false. The most severe complication of nonoperative treatment is to continue to treat a deformity that is clearly getting worse but the progression is ignored (Case 6.7). A typical example is a child who is increasing in crouch with increasing knee flexion contracture, but there is no decision to address the problem. When the knee flexion contracture finally gets to the point that the child can no longer walk, a decision has to be made to put him in a wheelchair or try surgery. This poor judgment will be the direct cause of the child being in a wheelchair for the remainder of his life, or it may be the direct cause of the complications, which are incurred much more commonly in correcting severe knee flexion contractures than in correcting milder deformities. Individuals who are good community ambulators at age 7 or 8 years of age do not go into wheelchairs at age 15 years unless there is some complication or supervening medical problem unrelated to CP. Also, the use of inappropriate orthotics can lead to severe skin breakdown or permanent scars on the calf from breakdown of the subcutaneous fat layer. Another complication of nonoperative management is to have children in walking aids that are inappropriate. This means that children should have the correct training before being allowed to use crutches or walkers. Parents have to be informed of the risks of walking aids, such as being aware of wet floors with the use of crutches or open stair doors for individuals with poor judgment.

Complications of Gait Analysis

Complications that arise in the analysis of gait for preoperative planning are usually recognized by the analysis team. Parents or caretakers should be asked if the current gait is representative of the child's home and community ambulation. Children spend enough time during the analysis that experienced therapists will also see how constant and representative their gait is during the whole evaluation. Children may be able to walk for doctors or therapists in a 10-minute clinic examination, but this walk can almost be impossible for them to maintain for a 2-hour laboratory evaluation. Also, the current standard is to evaluate multiple gait cycles, with 10 to 15 cycles usually being evaluated. Evaluating multiple gait cycles also removes the concern about a representative specific cycle. Some children, especially those with behavior problems, have trouble with the level of cooperation that is required to get a full gait analysis. Also, it is difficult to get a full evaluation in children before age 3 years because of the cooperation required. Another complication to watch out for in evaluating gait data is to recognize the sensitivity of the rotational measures to proper marker placement on the extremities. Therefore, hip rotation and tibial torsion have to always be compared with the physical examination and with the knee varus-valgus measures on the kinematics as an assurance of accuracy. If the knee joint axis is incorrect, the knee will demonstrate increased varus-valgus movement as the knee flexes. There also needs to always be a careful evaluation of EMG patterns with the thought that leads may have gotten switched. If the pattern is really confusing, consider lead mix-up as a possibility and have the EMG repeated.

Complications of Surgery Planning

Complications of surgery planning are mostly related to not identifying all the problems or misinterpreting a compensatory problem for a primary problem. A common example of missing problems is not identifying the spastic rectus in the crouched gait pattern, missing internally rotated hips in children with an ipsilateral posterior rotation of the pelvis, and missing internal tibial torsion when there is severe planovalgus deformity that needs to be corrected (Case 6.23). Some common misinterpreted secondary problems are the midstance phase equinus on the normal side of a child with hemiplegia, hip flexor weakness in children with increased hip flexion and anterior pelvic tilt but high lordosis as they rest on the anterior hip capsule, weakness of the quadriceps as a cause of crouch, and intraarticular knee pathology as a cause of knee pain in adolescents with crouched gait. Many decisions on specific data are somewhat arbitrary, but having the data is an excellent way to develop an understanding of what the data mean. As a clinical decision is made, the result is then evaluated after the rehabilitation period, and understanding of the significance of the data is developed. Also, some of the errors in interpretation are related to not taking natural history into account. An example is the response of the common equinovarus foot position seen in early childhood. If these children are diplegic, the natural history is for this deformity

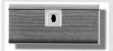

Case 6.23   Nikkole

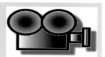

Nikkole, a 4-year-old girl, was evaluated with the concern that she was having trouble controlling her feet. According to her mother she had made good progress in her walking ability in the past 3 months. Her hip radiographs were normal. She was continued in her physical therapy program to work on balance and motor control issues. Her mother was taught how to use walking sticks to help Nikkole with motor control and balance development. She continued to make good progress until age 6 years, when she plateaued in her motor skills development. At that time she had a full evaluation. On physical examination she was noted to have hip abduction of 25°, and hip internal rotation of 70° on the right and 78° on the left. Hip external rotation was 5° on the right and 12° on the left. Popliteal angles were 65° on the right and 73° on the left. An Ely test was positive at 60°. Extended knee ankle dorsiflexion was −8° on the right and −10° on the left. Flexed knee ankle dorsiflexion was 5° on the right and 3° on the left. Observation of her gait demonstrated that she was efficient in ambulating with a posterior walker. However, she had severe internal rotation of the hips, with knee flexion at foot contact and in midstance, and a toe strike without getting flat foot at any time. The kinematics confirmed the same and the EMG showed significant activity in swing phase of the rectus muscles. There was minimal motion at the knee with ankle equinus and lack of hip extension and internal rotation of the hip (Figure C6.23.1). She had femoral derotation osteotomies, distal hamstring lengthenings, and gastrocnemius lengthenings. A rectus transfer was also recommended, but because of the fear of causing further crouch, she did

not receive this procedure. Following the rehabilitation, she was taught to use Lofstrand crutches, with which she became proficient. Her main problem after the rehabilitation was a severe stiff knee gait, but because of the trauma of the surgery, neither she nor her mother was willing to have another operative procedure unless it was absolutely needed; they felt she was doing much better and they were happy. This case is also a good example of a family that is happy because of the excellent gains, even though the surgeon would grade this outcome as disappointing because of the severe stiff knee gait, which should have been treated at the initial procedure.

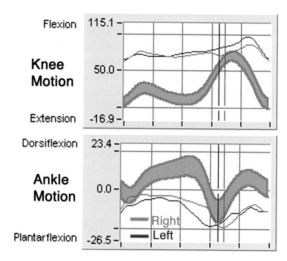

Figure C6.23.1

to completely reverse and become a planovalgus foot, so aggressive treatment should seldom be considered for the early childhood equinovarus posture. Another error is in not considering the energy cost of walking. Children who use 2 ml oxygen per kilogram per meter walking are not going to be community ambulators, and judgment has to be directed as to their real function, which will primarily be sitting in a wheelchair. Also, children's general condition should be considered as the complaints related to walking may be in part result from very poor conditioning and not specific deformities.

Interrelated Effect of Multiple Procedures

When interpreting gait data, there should be an awareness of the impact of adding procedures together. Most procedures are relatively independent of each other; however, there are some interactions. Understanding the impact of multiple concurrent procedures is somewhat like understanding drug interactions. Some specific combinations to watch out for include tibial derotation for internal tibial torsion in the ipsilateral side of a foot that is having posterior tibial tendon surgery for equinovarus. In a small series of 10 limbs, 8 failed and required repeat surgery, all with overcorrection.[70] Based on this, we recommend choosing the deformity that seems to be the worst, or primary, deformity. Another procedure interaction is planovalgus foot correction so that the heel is in neutral through the use of a subtalar fusion, then doing a supramalleolar osteotomy to correct ankle valgus. This combination of procedures will leave the heel with a residual varus deformity, which is highly undesirable. Another interaction of procedures is that patients who have external tibial torsion that is not being corrected should not have only medial hamstring lengthening, as this will further imbalance the external rotation torque by allowing the biceps femoris muscle to create additional external torque through the knee joint.

Complications of Surgical Execution

The most common complication of surgical execution is overcorrection of a deformity, especially in correction of femoral anteversion. Undercorrection may also occur in femoral rotation. The reason undercorrection occurs is that the femur is somewhat square, and often the plate used for fixation wants to set on the corner, but as the screws are tightened, it may rotate 10° or 15° in one direction or the other. Careful intraoperative evaluation after the fixation is important, and if the rotation is not corrected, it can be corrected immediately. Other intraoperative problems are specific to the procedure, such as recognizing that the foot will never look better than it does immediately after the surgery has been performed in the operating room; therefore, if the foot is still in valgus, it will be so when the cast is removed. Three months and 12 months after surgery, this valgus will only get worse, not better. Correcting residual problems in the operating room is much easier than deciding to come back and correct them with a separate surgical procedure or a revision procedure.

Complications of Rehabilitation

The major problem with rehabilitation is the lack of follow-through by families, or failure of families to be able to pay or get their insurance companies to pay for the therapy that is required. Most children can be rehabilitated as outpatients; however, there are a few especially complicated cases that really benefit from inpatient rehabilitation. The need for postoperative rehabilitation should be discussed with families, and an understanding of how and who will provide this is important even before undertaking the surgery. It is important to have therapists who clearly understand the goals for these children's function, as it is of little benefit to have therapists spend a great deal of time working on sitting transfers when the goal of the surgery was to get the children walking. Postoperatively, the physical therapy has to be directed at the goal that was preoperatively defined through communication with the surgeon, who should be able to clearly articulate what the goals of the surgery were. Other issues in the postoperative period that may cause problems are postoperative pain and subsequent depression. Postoperative pain and depression need to be treated aggressively if they are interfering with the ability of patients to cooperate with the rehabilitation program. Often, using the correct pain medication and adding an antidepressant can be very helpful.

Monitoring the Outcome of Gait Development and Treatment

Monitoring the outcome of gait treatment is an area where a clear consensus of a goal has not developed. In general, the goal is to make the different patterns of gait impairments move toward the normal means. Therefore, children who walk at 60 cm/s are considered improved if, following the treatment, they walk 90 cm/s. Likewise, children who go from 90 cm/s to 60 cm/s would be considered worse. This goal can be applied to joint motions, such as midstance phase knee flexion, maximum knee flexion in swing, or terminal stance power generation at the ankle. However, there are situations where this might not be exactly true, as in the example of a 5-year-old with a high toe walking prancing gait pattern who can only move fast or fall over. He may have a walking speed of 90 cm/s; however, after soft-tissue lengthening, the foot is flat and he can stand in one place and start and stop without falling, although the velocity has dropped to 60 cm/s. This child has clearly improved in the sense of stability, and even though the change in speed seems to be demonstrating the opposite, it is not a reflection of the goal of the initial treatment. The change in perspective of a specific child, the child's age, the functional ability, and the goal of the surgery have to be considered. It is not very effective to measure the volume of a fluid with a thermometer, and in this same way, the measurement tool must reflect the treatment goal. Often, parents complain that the children do not walk better after an adductor lengthening performed as part of the preventive treatment of spastic hip disease. The parents need to be initially told that the goal was to prevent hip subluxation and not make their child walk better. At the same time, children are not expected to walk worse after the adductor lengthening, but the surgery was not directed at improving gait and therefore gait improvement should not be expected.

Energy Use Measurement

Another measure that has been advocated for assessing outcome of gait treatment is the energy efficiency measured by oxygen consumption. There have been suggestions of using physiologic cost index to measure energy efficiency in children with CP[71, 72]; however, this has so much variability that it is of no use in these children.[36, 73] If children have a high oxygen cost of walking, then an improvement is desired; however, this is also a relative measure because a very energy efficient gait can at the same time be completely nonfunctional. This nonfunctional but energy-efficient gait is commonly seen in children with primary muscle disease.[37] There have been oral reports that rhizotomy is effective in decreasing the energy cost; however, it makes children act like muscle disease patients rather than spastic patients. The improvement in oxygen cost of walking has to be confirmed with an increased physical functionality, meaning children can do more in their environment. There has been increased interest in developing tools to assess children's function as related to their environment. The pediatric MODEMS questionnaire has been developed for use with children with physical disabilities. There has not been much reported use of this instrument in children with CP. Another scale, developed at the Gillette Hospital, the Gillette Functional Assessment Questionnaire, asks parents to grade children's ambulatory ability on a 10 functional level scale.[74] This same group has developed a scale or normality in the gait motion data, using principal component analysis of 16 gait variables.[75] The GMFM and the Pediatric Evaluation of Disability Inventory (PEDI) are two other measures that can be used to give some measure of functional ability.

At this time, a parent-reporting questionnaire with technical data from the gait analysis has to be combined as a measure of outcome. The outcome should also be considered over the child's whole growth and development, not only for a 1-year follow-up period. This measure of outcome has to include obtaining as much information as possible about the natural history of the condition. Measuring outcome is an area that will require much work in the future but it is crucial if the treatment algorithm for the gait impairment secondary to CP is to improve in a way that is documented.

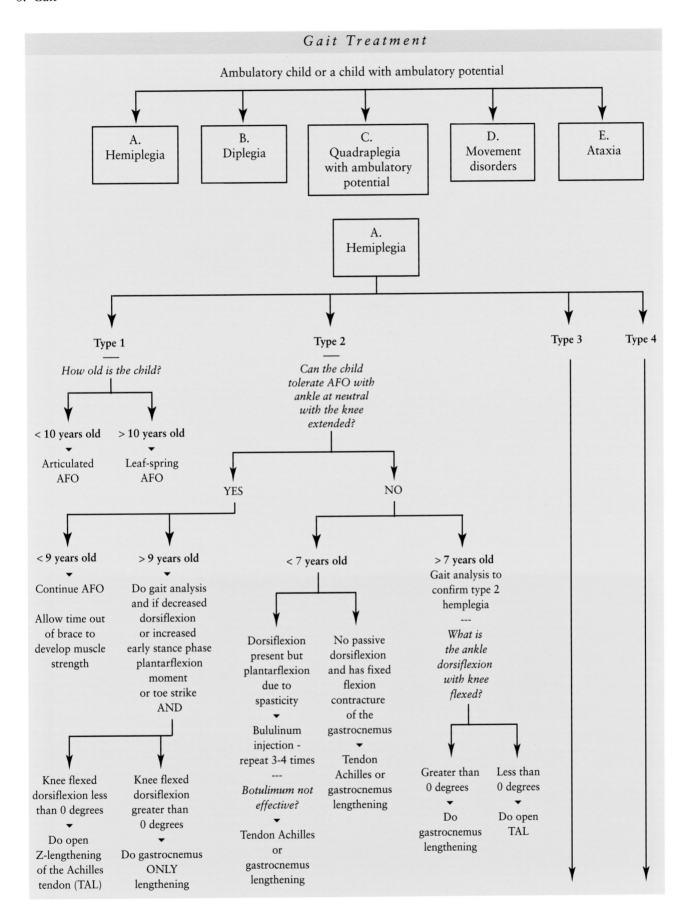

Gait Treatment

Ambulatory child or a child with ambulatory potential

A. Hemiplegia
B. Diplegia
C. Quadraplegia with ambulatory potential
D. Movement disorders
E. Ataxia

A. Hemiplegia

Type 1 — *How old is the child?*

< 10 years old → Articulated AFO

> 10 years old → Leaf-spring AFO

< 9 years old → Continue AFO

Allow time out of brace to develop muscle strength

Knee flexed dorsiflexion less than 0 degrees → Do open Z-lengthening of the Achilles tendon (TAL)

> 9 years old → Do gait analysis and if decreased dorsiflexion or increased early stance phase plantarflexion moment or toe strike AND

Knee flexed dorsiflexion greater than 0 degrees → Do gastrocnemus ONLY lengthening

Type 2 — *Can the child tolerate AFO with ankle at neutral with the knee extended?*

YES

NO

< 7 years old

Dorsiflexion present but plantarflexion due to spasticity → Bululinum injection - repeat 3-4 times --- *Botulimum not effective?* → Tendon Achilles or gastrocnemus lengthening

No passive dorsiflexion and has fixed flexion contracture of the gastrocnemus → Tendon Achilles or gastrocnemus lengthening

> 7 years old
Gait analysis to confirm type 2 hemplegia

What is the ankle dorsiflexion with knee flexed?

Greater than 0 degrees → Do gastrocnemus lengthening

Less than 0 degrees → Do open TAL

Type 3

Type 4

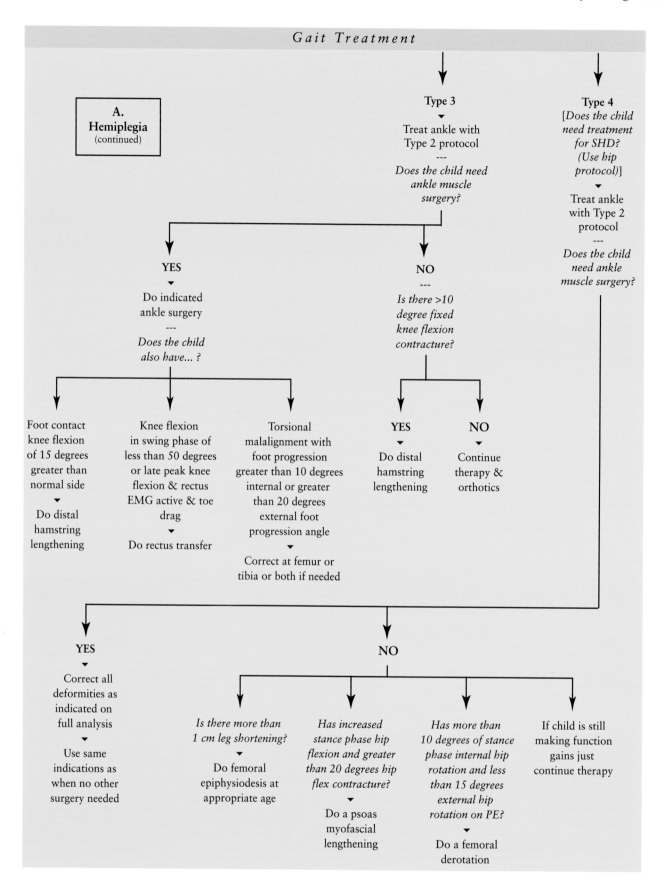

Gait Treatment

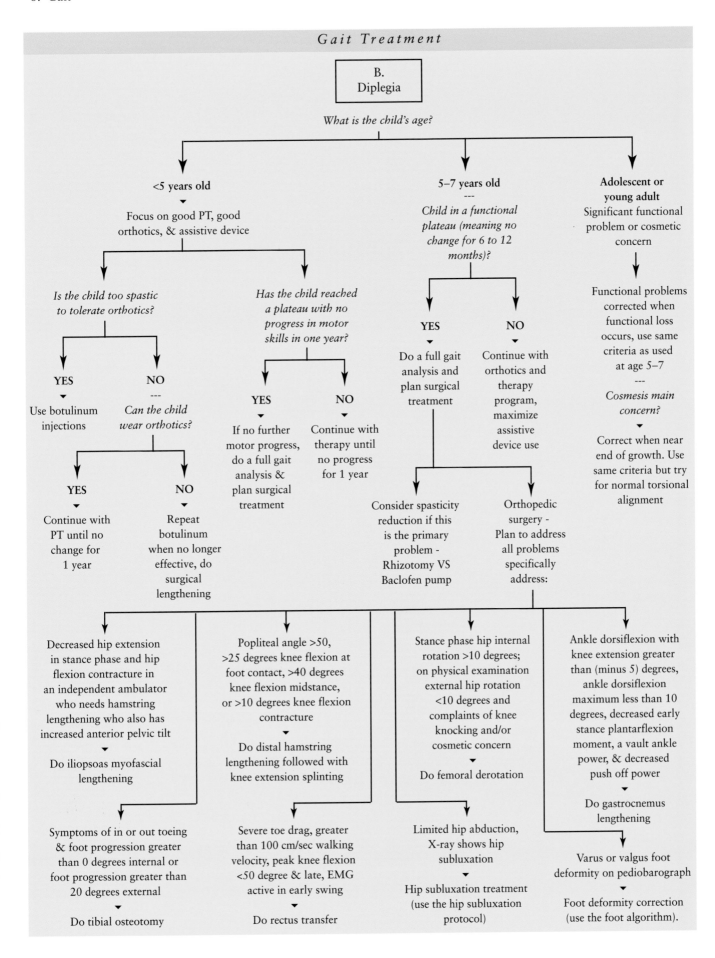

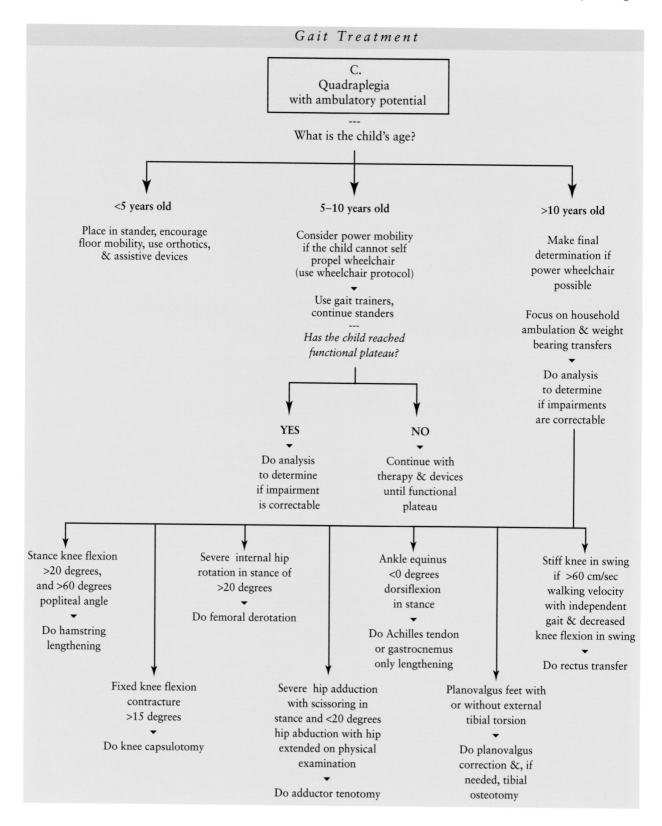

Gait Treatment

C.
Quadraplegia
with ambulatory potential

What is the child's age?

<5 years old

Place in stander, encourage
floor mobility, use orthotics,
& assistive devices

5–10 years old

Consider power mobility
if the child cannot self
propel wheelchair
(use wheelchair protocol)

Use gait trainers,
continue standers
---
*Has the child reached
functional plateau?*

>10 years old

Make final
determination if
power wheelchair
possible

Focus on household
ambulation & weight
bearing transfers

Do analysis
to determine
if impairments
are correctable

YES

Do analysis
to determine
if impairment
is correctable

NO

Continue with
therapy & devices
until functional
plateau

Stance knee flexion
>20 degrees,
and >60 degrees
popliteal angle

Do hamstring
lengthening

Severe internal hip
rotation in stance of
>20 degrees

Do femoral derotation

Ankle equinus
<0 degrees
dorsiflexion
in stance

Do Achilles tendon
or gastrocnemius
only lengthening

Stiff knee in swing
if >60 cm/sec
walking velocity
with independent
gait & decreased
knee flexion in swing

Do rectus transfer

Fixed knee flexion
contracture
>15 degrees

Do knee capsulotomy

Severe hip adduction
with scissoring in
stance and <20 degrees
hip abduction with hip
extended on physical
examination

Do adductor tenotomy

Planovalgus feet with
or without external
tibial torsion

Do planovalgus
correction &, if
needed, tibial
osteotomy

References

1. Perry J. Gait Analysis: Normal and Pathologic Function. Thorofare, NJ: Slack, 1992.
2. Harris G, Smith PA. Human Motion Analysis; Current Applications and Future Directions. New York: The Institute of Electrical and Electronic Engineers, 1996.
3. Gage J. Gait analysis in Cerebral Palsy. London: Mac Keith Press, 1991.
4. Burke RE, Levine DN, Tsairis P, Zajac FE III. Physiological types and histochemical profiles in motor units of the cat gastrocnemius. J Physiol (Lond) 1973;234:723–48.
5. Gordon DA, Enoka RM, Stuart DG. Motor-unit force potentiation in adult cats during a standard fatigue test. J Physiol (Lond) 1990;421:569–82.
6. Chamberlain S, Lewis DM. Contractile characteristics and innervation ratio of rat soleus motor units. J Physiol (Lond) 1989;412:1–21.
7. Cavagna GA, Dusman B, Margaria R. Positive work done by a previously stretched muscle. J Appl Physiol 1968;24:21–32.
8. Miller F, Moseley CF, Koreska J. Spinal fusion in Duchenne muscular dystrophy. Dev Med Child Neurol 1992;34:775–86.
9. Jozsa L, Kannus P, Jarvinen TA, Balint J, Jarvinen M. Number and morphology of mechanoreceptors in the myotendinous junction of paralysed human muscle. J Pathol 1996;178:195–200.
10. Castle ME, Reyman TA, Schneider M. Pathology of spastic muscle in cerebral palsy. Clin Orthop 1979:223–32.
11. Ito J, Araki A, Tanaka H, Tasaki T, Cho K, Yamazaki R. Muscle histopathology in spastic cerebral palsy. Brain Dev 1996;18:299–303.
12. Wiley ME, Damiano DL. Lower-extremity strength profiles in spastic cerebral palsy. Dev Med Child Neurol 1998;40:100–7.
13. Damiano DL, Abel MF. Functional outcomes of strength training in spastic cerebral palsy. Arch Phys Med Rehabil 1998;79:119–25.
14. Damiano DL, Kelly LE, Vaughn CL. Effects of quadriceps femoris muscle strengthening on crouch gait in children with spastic diplegia. Phys Ther 1995; 75:658–67; discussion 668–71.
15. Pearson AM. Muscle growth and exercise. Crit Rev Food Sci Nutr 1990;29: 167–96.
16. Ziv I, Blackburn N, Rang M, Koreska J. Muscle growth in normal and spastic mice. Dev Med Child Neurol 1984;26:94–9.
17. Thompson NS, Baker RJ, Cosgrove AP, Corry IS, Graham HK. Musculoskeletal modelling in determining the effect of botulinum toxin on the hamstrings of patients with crouch gait. Dev Med Child Neurol 1998;40:622–5.
18. Gros C, Frerebeau P, Perez-Dominguez E, Bazin M, Privat JM. Long term results of stereotaxic surgery for infantile dystonia and dyskinesia. Neurochirurgia (Stuttg) 1976;19:171–8.
19. Koman LA, Mooney JF III, Smith BP. Neuromuscular blockade in the management of cerebral palsy. J Child Neurol 1996;11(Suppl 1):S23–8.
20. Videman T. An experimental study of the effects of growth on the relationship of tendons and ligaments to bone at the site of diaphyseal insertion. Acta Orthop Scand Suppl 1970:1–22.
21. Roll JP, Vedel JP, Ribot E. Alteration of proprioceptive messages induced by tendon vibration in man: a microneurographic study. Exp Brain Res 1989;76: 213–22.
22. Booth CM, Cortina-Borja MJ, Theologis TN. Collagen accumulation in muscles of children with cerebral palsy and correlation with severity of spasticity. Dev Med Child Neurol 2001;43:314–20.
23. Fettweis E. Spasm of the adductor muscles, pre-dislocations and dislocations of the hip joints in children and adolescents with cerebral palsy. Clinical observations on aetiology, pathogenesis, therapy and rehabilitation. Part II. The importance of the iliopsoas tendon, its tenotomy, of the coxa valga antetorta, and correction through osteotomy turning the hip into varus (author's transl). Z Orthop Ihre Grenzgeb 1979;117:50–9.

24. Kolban M. Variability of the femoral head and neck antetorsion angle in ultra-sonographic measurements of healthy children and in selected diseases with hip disorders treated surgically. Ann Acad Med Stetin 1999;Suppl:1–99.

25. Catanese AA, Coleman GJ, King JA, Reddihough DS. Evaluation of an early childhood programme based on principles of conductive education: the Yooralla project. J Paediatr Child Health 1995;31:418–22.

26. Burtner PA, Woollacott MH, Qualls C. Stance balance control with orthoses in a group of children with spastic cerebral palsy. Dev Med Child Neurol 1999; 41:748–57.

27. Brogren E, Hadders-Algra M, Forssberg H. Postural control in children with spastic diplegia: muscle activity during perturbations in sitting. Dev Med Child Neurol 1996;38:379–88.

28. Chao EY. Justification of triaxial goniometer for the measurement of joint rotation. J Biomech 1980;13:989–1006.

29. Grood ES, Suntay WJ. A joint coordinate system for the clinical description of three-dimensional motions: application to the knee. J Biomech Eng 1983;105: 136–44.

30. Spoor CW, Veldpaus FE. Rigid body motion calculated from spatial co-ordinates of markers. J Biomech 1980;13:391–3.

31. Delp SL, Hess WE, Hungerford DS, Jones LC. Variation of rotation moment arms with hip flexion. J Biomech 1999;32:493–501.

32. Delp SL, Arnold AS, Speers RA, Moore CA. Hamstrings and psoas lengths during normal and crouch gait: implications for muscle-tendon surgery. J Orthop Res 1996;14:144–51.

33. Hoffinger SA, Rab GT, Abou-Ghaida H. Hamstrings in cerebral palsy crouch gait. J Pediatr Orthop 1993;13:722–6.

34. Enoka RM, Rankin LL, Stuart DG, Volz KA. Fatigability of rat hindlimb muscle: associations between electromyogram and force during a fatigue test. J Physiol (Lond) 1989;408:251–70.

35. Bowen TR, Cooley SR, Castagno PW, Miller F, Richards J. A method for normalization of oxygen cost and consumption in normal children while walking. J Pediatr Orthop 1998;18:589–93.

36. Bowen TR, Lennon N, Castagno P, Miller F, Richards J. Variability of energy-consumption measures in children with cerebral palsy. J Pediatr Orthop 1998; 18:738–42.

37. Bowen TR, Miller F, Mackenzie W. Comparison of oxygen consumption measurements in children with cerebral palsy to children with muscular dystrophy. J Pediatr Orthop 1999;19:133–6.

38. Rose J, Medeiros JM, Parker R. Energy cost index as an estimate of energy expenditure of cerebral-palsied children during assisted ambulation. Dev Med Child Neurol 1985;27:485–90.

39. Rose SA, DeLuca PA, Davis RB III, Ounpuu S, Gage JR. Kinematic and kinetic evaluation of the ankle after lengthening of the gastrocnemius fascia in children with cerebral palsy. J Pediatr Orthop 1993;13:727–32.

40. Saraph V, Zwick EB, Uitz C, Linhart W, Steinwender G. The Baumann procedure for fixed contracture of the gastrocsoleus in cerebral palsy. Evaluation of function of the ankle after multilevel surgery. J Bone Joint Surg Br 2000;82: 535–40.

41. Simon SR, Deutsch SD, Nuzzo RM, et al. Genu recurvatum in spastic cerebral palsy. Report on findings by gait analysis. J Bone Joint Surg [Am] 1978;60: 882–94.

42. Ounpuu S, Muik E, Davis RB III, Gage JR, DeLuca PA. Rectus femoris surgery in children with cerebral palsy. Part I: The effect of rectus femoris transfer location on knee motion. J Pediatr Orthop 1993;13:325–30.

43. Chambers H, Lauer A, Kaufman K, Cardelia JM, Sutherland D. Prediction of outcome after rectus femoris surgery in cerebral palsy: the role of cocontraction of the rectus femoris and vastus lateralis. J Pediatr Orthop 1998;18:703–11.

44. Ounpuu S, Muik E, Davis RB III, Gage JR, DeLuca PA. Rectus femoris surgery in children with cerebral palsy. Part II: A comparison between the effect of trans-

fer and release of the distal rectus femoris on knee motion. J Pediatr Orthop 1993;13:331–5.

45. McCarthy RE, Simon S, Douglas B, Zawacki R, Reese N. Proximal femoral resection to allow adults who have severe cerebral palsy to sit. J Bone Joint Surg [Am] 1988;70:1011–6.

46. Miller F, Cardoso Dias R, Lipton GE, Albarracin JP, Dabney KW, Castagno P. The effect of rectus EMG patterns on the outcome of rectus femoris transfers. J Pediatr Orthop 1997;17:603–7.

47. Thometz J, Simon S, Rosenthal R. The effect on gait of lengthening of the medial hamstrings in cerebral palsy. J Bone Joint Surg [Am] 1989;71:345–53.

48. Atar D, Zilberberg L, Votemberg M, Norsy M, Galil A. Effect of distal hamstring release on cerebral palsy patients. Bull Hosp Jt Dis 1993;53:34–6.

49. Damron T, Breed AL, Roecker E. Hamstring tenotomies in cerebral palsy: long-term retrospective analysis. J Pediatr Orthop 1991;11:514–9.

50. Hsu LC, Li HS. Distal hamstring elongation in the management of spastic cerebral palsy. J Pediatr Orthop 1990;10:378–81.

51. McHale KA, Bagg M, Nason SS. Treatment of the chronically dislocated hip in adolescents with cerebral palsy with femoral head resection and subtrochanteric valgus osteotomy. J Pediatr Orthop 1990;10:504–9.

52. DeLuca PA, Ounpuu S, Davis RB, Walsh JH. Effect of hamstring and psoas lengthening on pelvic tilt in patients with spastic diplegic cerebral palsy. J Pediatr Orthop 1998;18:712–8.

53. Sutherland DH, Zilberfarb JL, Kaufman KR, Wyatt MP, Chambers HG. Psoas release at the pelvic brim in ambulatory patients with cerebral palsy: operative technique and functional outcome [see comments]. J Pediatr Orthop 1997;17:563–70.

54. Tylkowski CM, Rosenthal RK, Simon SR. Proximal femoral osteotomy in cerebral palsy. Clin Orthop 1980:183–92.

55. Joseph B. Treatment of internal rotation gait due to gluteus medius and minimus overactivity in cerebral palsy: anatomical rationale of a new surgical procedure and preliminary results in twelve hips. Clin Anat 1998;11:22–8.

56. Metaxiotis D, Accles W, Siebel A, Doederlein L. Hip deformities in walking patients with cerebral palsy. Gait Posture 2000;11:86–91.

57. Hullin MG, Robb JE, Loudon IR. Gait patterns in children with hemiplegic spastic cerebral palsy [see comments]. J Pediatr Orthop B 1996;5:247–51.

58. Winters TF Jr, Gage JR, Hicks R. Gait patterns in spastic hemiplegia in children and young adults. J Bone Joint Surg [Am] 1987;69:437–41.

59. Renders A, Detrembleur C, Rossillon R, Lejeune T, Rombouts JJ. Contribution of electromyographic analysis of the walking habits of children with spastic foot in cerebral palsy: a preliminary study. Rev Chir Orthop Reparatrice Appar Mot 1997;83:259–64.

60. O'Malley MJ, Abel MF, Damiano DL, Vaughan CL. Fuzzy clustering of children with cerebral palsy based on temporal-distance gait parameters. IEEE Trans Rehabil Eng 1997;5:300–9.

61. Lin CJ, Guo LY, Su FC, Chou YL, Cherng RJ. Common abnormal kinetic patterns of the knee in gait in spastic diplegia of cerebral palsy. Gait Posture 2000;11:224–32.

62. McLaughlin JF, Bjornson KF, Astley SJ, et al. Selective dorsal rhizotomy: efficacy and safety in an investigator-masked randomized clinical trial [see comments]. Dev Med Child Neurol 1998;40:220–32.

63. Boscarino LF, Ounpuu S, Davis RB III, Gage JR, DeLuca PA. Effects of selective dorsal rhizotomy on gait in children with cerebral palsy. J Pediatr Orthop 1993;13:174–9.

64. Peacock WJ, Staudt LA. Functional outcomes following selective posterior rhizotomy in children with cerebral palsy. J Neurosurg 1991;74:380–5.

65. Vaughan CL, Berman B, Peacock WJ. Cerebral palsy and rhizotomy. A 3-year follow-up evaluation with gait analysis. J Neurosurg 1991;74:178–84.

66. Thomas SS, Aiona MD, Buckon CE, Piatt JH Jr. Does gait continue to improve 2 years after selective dorsal rhizotomy? J Pediatr Orthop 1997;17:387–91.

67. Marty GR, Dias LS, Gaebler-Spira D. Selective posterior rhizotomy and soft-tissue procedures for the treatment of cerebral diplegia. J Bone Joint Surg Am 1995;77:713–8.

68. Yngve DA, Chambers C. Vulpius and Z-lengthening. J Pediatr Orthop 1996; 16:759–64.

69. Gage JR. Surgical treatment of knee dysfunction in cerebral palsy. Clin Orthop 1990:45–54.

70. Liggio F, Kruse R. Split tibialis posterior tendon transfer with concomitant distal tibial derotation osteotomy in children with cerebral palsy. J Pedaitr Orthop 2001;21:95–101.

71. Carmick J. Clinical use of neuromuscular electrical stimulation for children with cerebral palsy. Part 1: Lower extremity [see comments] [published erratum appears in Phys Ther 1993;73(11):809]. Phys Ther 1993;73:505–13; discussion 523–7.

72. Nene AV, Evans GA, Patrick JH. Simultaneous multiple operations for spastic diplegia. Outcome and functional assessment of walking in 18 patients. J Bone Joint Surg [Br] 1993;75:488–94.

73. Boyd R, Fatone S, Rodda J, et al. High- or low-technology measurements of energy expenditure in clinical gait analysis? Dev Med Child Neurol 1999;41:676–82.

74. Novacheck TF, Stout JL, Tervo R. Reliability and validity of the Gillette Functional Assessment Questionnaire as an outcome measure in children with walking disabilities. J Pediatr Orthop 2000;20:75–81.

75. Schutte LM, Narayanan U, Stout JL, Selber P, Gage JR, Schwartz MH. An index for quantifying deviations from normal gait. Gait Posture 2000;11:25–31.

SECTION II

Rehabilitation Techniques

Many interventions have been applied to treat cerebral palsy, but when all is said and done we are still dealing with a nervous system that is impaired in many different ways. Some of the interventions that we are applying to children with cerebral palsy (CP) are really attempts at remediation of the consequences of weakness or abnormal tone. The interventions we apply have their own side effects and limitations. As a consequence, we can fall into a trap and apply these interventions with an intensity that sends an unfair signal to the child and family. That signal is that we can make the child normal. We do not make damaged nervous systems normal. In many cases, we simply teach and/or trick the child's nervous system to cope and provide strategies that alter some of the side effects and, in some cases, simply delude ourselves.

1. Neurodevelopmental Therapy
Elizabeth Jeanson, PT

In the 1960s and early 1970s, pediatric therapists for CP appeared distinct from therapists who trained on poliomyelitis cases and from there quickly developed a cadre of therapists who practiced neurodevelopmental therapy (NDT). Neurodevelopmental treatment has gone through a long evolution over the years. Time has forced it to become more eclectic and become one of the most commonly used intervention strategies for children from infancy through adulthood with CP.[1] Since the conception of NDT by Dr. Karl and Mrs. Berta Bobath in the 1940s, the scientific community's understanding of the brain and the conceptual framework of NDT has evolved. As our understanding of how the brain inspires and controls movement evolves, so does the theory of NDT into what is currently accepted as the Dynamic Systems Theory. In this way NDT is a "living concept."[2] It adapts and grows as knowledge of the brain's function is revealed.

Using the Dynamic Systems Theory, NDT-trained therapists are able to use a variety of handling techniques. These specialized techniques encourage active use of appropriate muscles and diminish involvement of muscles not necessary for the completion of a task. Child-directed and -initiated movement tasks are critical to the success of neurodevelopmental treatment.[2] Therapists practicing NDT set functional individual session goals, which build upon each other to facilitate new motor skills or improve the efficiency of learned motor tasks. Improvements in efficiency can include decreased energy used during a task, decreased work required of the muscles during a task, and habituation of new patterns of movement. These tasks are specific to and driven by the functional needs of the child. In NDT the child takes an active role in treatment design. The therapist must be constantly evaluating their input into the child's movement with the goal of active, habituated, independent movement.

NDT is a problem-solving approach focusing on the individual's current needs while aiming for the long-term goal of function across the lifespan.[2] Occupational, speech, and physical therapists as well as educators can use NDT. The benefits of utilizing NDT include improved ability to perform functional activities appropriate to the needs of the individual, active participation of the child, improved strength, flexibility, and alignment, and improved function over a lifespan. NDT is not an exclusive treatment for individuals with CP.

NDT-trained therapists have completed an 8-week pediatric or a 3-week adult course, and some, an additional 3-week infant postgraduate course.

Practicing therapists can be found in every community. Therapists can learn about the theory and techniques at a variety of continuing education courses offered throughout the year and over the course of many years.

2. Strengthening Exercises
Diane Damiano, PhD

In past years, several clinical myths existed about what one should never provide to patients with CP, such as "no plastic for spastics" when prescribing orthoses or "never strengthen spasticity." Recent research has provided evidence to dispel these myths and bring a new level of awareness of how children with CP can be helped. It has always been known that increased tone is not the only or even the most significant impairment of CP, but that there is poor recruitment of muscle unit activity and inconsistent maintenance of maximum efforts. Research that investigates muscle strengthening has contributed to this understanding.

More than 50 years ago, Phelps proposed that resisted exercise "to develop strength or skill in a weakened muscle or an impaired muscle group" was an integral part of treatment in CP.[3] Shortly thereafter, physical therapists denounced strengthening for their patients with upper motor neuron syndromes based primarily on the clinical concern that such strong physical effort would exacerbate spasticity. However, scientific evidence has been accumulating in recent years that dispels this contention and supports the effectiveness of strength training for improving motor function in CP as well as in other neuromotor disorders. Muscle strength is related to motor performance and should be an integral part of a rehabilitation program that addresses other impairments which inhibit motor performance in this population, such as muscle–tendon shortening, spasticity, and coordination deficits.

It has been shown that even highly functional children with spastic CP are likely to have considerable weakness in their involved extremities compared to age-related peers, with the degree of weakness increasing with the level of neurologic involvement.[4,5] If a child has at least some voluntary control in a muscle group, the capacity for strengthening exists. In the absence of voluntary control, strength training is more problematic, but may be facilitated by the use of electrical stimulation or by strengthening within synergistic movement patterns. However, strengthening is only justifiable if the ultimate goal is to improve a specific motor skill or function. Therefore, a child with little or no capacity for voluntary muscle control is unlikely to experience substantial functional benefits from a strength-training program. Most ambulatory children with CP have the capacity to strengthen their muscles, although poor isolated control or inadequate length in the ankle dorsiflexor or the hamstring muscles may limit progress in some patients. Nonambulatory children may also experience improvements in their ability to use their upper extremities, transfer more effectively, or engage more actively in recreational and fitness activities. Invasive procedures such as muscle–tendon lengthening, selective dorsal rhizotomy, intrathecal baclofen pump implantation, or botulinum toxin injections may improve muscle length and/or control so that muscles can then be strengthened more effectively. In turn, strength training may serve to augment or prolong the outcomes of these procedures.

To participate in a strength-training program, the child must be able to comprehend and to consistently produce a maximal or near-maximal effort. Children as young as 3 years of age may be capable of this, but waiting to augment the program until the child is age 4 or 5 years is more realistic.

Motivational and attentional factors can also affect a program's success. Family compliance with the treatment schedule and protocol is also critical.

The same physiologic principles that underlie the development of muscle strength apply whether or not a person has CP. Load is the stimulus for increasing strength and it should be close to an individual's maximum to achieve measurable gains. In practical terms, this would mean that a person should be able to lift a specified load two to three times before experiencing fatigue or a decrement in performance. Data on the specific treatment regimens to differentially train for strength, endurance, or power in this population, or which muscles can and should be strengthened to impart the greatest functional benefits, are not yet available specifically for CP, although useful guidelines may be found in the literature.[6,7] The number of repetitions and how these are grouped in a session will vary depending on the desired functional goals. For example, if the focus were on strengthening, an optimal program would be to use high loads with a low number of repetitions (3 to 8) arranged in multiple sets with a rest between each set. In contrast, if the therapist is more interested in improving muscle endurance, the load does not need to be quite so high, but repetitions should be greater (8 to 20) before resting. As the patient improves, the load and/or the number of repetitions can be increased depending again on the therapist's goal. If the goal is to try to increase strength, the recommended frequency of sessions is three times a week.

It seems logical that muscles across the joint from those that tend to be spastic are good candidates for strengthening. In spastic CP, for example, one might consider strengthening any or all of the following: elbow extensors, forearm pronators, wrist extensors, hip extensors and abductors, knee extensors, and ankle dorsiflexors. However, weakness can be present in other muscles that may also disrupt performance, such as the ankle plantar flexors or hip flexors, which are important power producers in gait. Both absolute and relative strength across a joint should be considered when designing protocols to avoid exacerbating muscle imbalance and contractures. Sample isotonic and isokinetic training programs are shown in Tables R1 and R2. Strengthening does not necessarily require weights, or devices, but can be achieved through multiple activities so long as the intensity of the load is sufficiently high to stress the muscle. Some other options for strength training include treadmill training, aquatic resistive exercise, and many different sports and recreational activities.

Weight training is deemed to be safe for children of all ages when performed properly.[8] Before the completion of physical growth, training loads should not exceed maximum to avoid damaging developing musculoskeletal structures. Other safety considerations include a more gradual buildup in the amount of resistance for children who are particularly weak or inactive, not allowing a child to lift weights without adult supervision, and not letting

Table R1. Sample isotonic program.

GOAL: Increase hip flexor and knee extensor strength for faster, more upright gait pattern

LOAD: Use free ankle weights at 80% maximum

FREQUENCY/DURATION: 3 times per week for 8 weeks

SESSION: 4 sets of 5 repetitions each (total = 20) for both muscle groups on right and left legs

POSITION: Hip: Supported standing while lifting leg as in high "marching"; knee: sitting on chair with feet off the ground while extending knee slowly

PROGRESS: Strength measured and load increased every 2 weeks throughout program

Table R2. Sample isokinetic program.

GOAL: Increase torque and rate of torque production in knee extensor and ankle dorsiflexor muscles on a hemiplegic extremity to improve gait

LOAD: Accommodating resistance with "window" set at 80%–90% of maximum effort

FREQUENCY/DURATION: Three times per week for 8 weeks

SESSION: Ten repetitions (concentric) at 2 speeds (30, 60/sec) with rests as needed; 10 repetitions (eccentric) at 30°/sec for each muscle group

POSITION: Semireclining sitting position on device using standard knee and ankle attachments and protocols

PROGRESS: Increased to higher speed by 30 as soon as person can exert force to match speed of machine throughout the range (concentric only)

a weight dangle on a limb in the absence of muscle effort or external support. Children should not exercise the same muscle group on consecutive days. If excessive soreness is present or persists, or if muscle tightness worsens as a result of the strengthening program, the protocol should be modified. The presence of a seizure disorder may also preclude participation for some patients if these are poorly controlled by medication and are exacerbated by increased physical effort. Physician approval should be obtained before initiating a weight-training program with any child.

Both isotonic and isokinetic training programs have been shown to increase strength and motor function in CP, as quantified by the Gross Motor Function Measure.[9–14] Gait improvements that have been reported include increased velocity at free and fastest speed, primarily through increased cadence, increased active motion in the muscles trained, and greater stability in stance.[9,11,14–16] Improved self-perception has also been noted,[10] but more research is needed to examine these and other effects from specific programs and activities.

Weakness limits functional performance in CP, but can be improved through training. Therapists should also be more proactively involved in prevention of secondary impairments and promotion of wellness and fitness in their patients. Strength and endurance training are important components of fitness, and may promote more optimal health across the lifespan and increase participation in recreational, social, and occupational activities in children and adults with CP.

3. Balance Interventions
Betsy Mullan, PT, PCS

The impairments of motor control and tone in and of themselves can present a balance problem to patients, or there can even be further impairments of the vestibular and sensory system, which affect balance and equilibrium, thus creating an even more complicated picture.

Balance cannot be separated from the action of which it is an integral component or from the environment in which it is performed.[17] Normal balance development involves three systems: the vestibular, visual, and somatosensory. Initially, vision is critical to postural control development, peaking during times when major gross motor development skill transitions occur in sitting to crawling, crawling to standing, and standing to walking.[18] Postural responses, such as those of children on a moving platform, vary with the age of the child. The apparent integration of the visual, vestibular, and somatosensory inputs appears to occur by 4 to 6 years of age, with the responses of the 7- to 10-year-old group being similar to adults.[19]

Cerebral palsy is a disorder with multisystem impairments, which may affect the visual, vestibular, and/or somatosensory systems. Nasher et al. found inappropriate sequencing of muscle activity, poor anticipatory regulation of muscle sequencing during postural control, and postural stability that was frequently interrupted by destabilizing synergistic or antagonistic muscle activity in individuals with CP.[20] It is evident that physical therapists working with individuals with CP need to assess as well as address these balance issues, keeping in mind the action that is required and the environment in which it is being performed.

Balance is a component of most, if not all, developmental assessments including the Gross Motor Function Measure, the Bruininks–Osterestky Test of Motor Proficiency, the Peabody Developmental Motor Scales, and the WeeFIM. These tests can be useful in helping the therapist ascertain whether the balance issue is visual (eyes open or closed), vestibular, or somatosensory (is the surface moving or not). It is also important to evaluate the child's balance needs and deficits relative to their task demands (sitting independently for dressing versus going to school and navigating the busy hallways), as well as the child's and parents' concerns and goals. This information can then be utilized to customize a treatment program.

Interventions should include various handling and treatment techniques mentioned elsewhere in this volume to help the child achieve success. Environments must be structured and tasks created in both open and closed situations to allow the greatest carryover to functional life skills. Closed tasks[21] are those whose characteristics do not change from one trial to the next; these require less information processing with practice. Open tasks[21] require more information processing. In closed environments[21] in which surroundings are fixed, children do not need to fit their balance into external timing, but can manage the situation at their own speed. Open environments require more attention and information processing.

Clinicians should keep in mind the action requiring balance, as well as the environment in which the child needs to function,[17] to appropriately assess and plan interactions to maximize a child's function in their environment.

4. Electrical Stimulation Techniques
Adam J. Rush, MD

An area that has received a great deal of press and a great deal of anecdotal experience is the role of electrical stimulation in CP. A review of the literature is very confusing, and there is great inconsistency from one medical center to the next as to what they are referring. Dr. L.J. Michaud probably has the most lucid discussion of electrical stimulation in CP.[22]

Making recommendations regarding which children should receive neuromuscular electrical stimulation (NMES) or transcutaneous electrical stimulation (TES) is a problem. Although there is no literature indicating that any particular group of children were likely to be harmed by it, or less likely to benefit, most children studied were mild to moderately affected by CP and seemed to have fairly good cognition. Furthermore, the worst side effect reported was a local skin reaction from the stimulating pads. Therefore, one could say that this is a harmless intervention that might be attempted in any child with CP. However, studies have not been performed comparing various regimens with each other.

We appear to have a recurring theme of therapists applying NMES and choosing their stimulation parameters based on personal experience, rather than based on good science. Dr. Michaud's article suggests the following, which strikes one as a reasonable place to begin: stimulus frequency, 45 to 50 Hz; stimulus intensity, maximum tolerated; on/off times, 10/50 seconds, or triggered; ramps, 1 to 5 seconds, or to comfort; treatment duration, 10 to 15 repetitions; frequency, 3 to 5 days per week.[22]

There are a number of studies regarding the relative utility of resistance exercise, NMES, or both.[23] Results vary, but they could be summarized to say that NMES is better than nothing, and not quite as good as resistance exercise alone, but that doing both is redundant.

5. Hippotherapy
Stacey Travis, MPT

Children benefit from movement and novelty. There have been some improvements in limb placement and balance and equilibrium seen in children who worked on the Bobath balls during neurodevelopment therapy. Hippotherapy gives them, if you will, a hairy, olfactory-stimulating, warm, four-legged Bobath ball platform on which a trained therapist can capitalize on motor control, stretching, and equilibrium as the therapist works with the child.[24-33] The North American Riding for the Handicapped Association (NARHA) has defined hippotherapy as "The use of the movement of a horse as a tool by physical therapists, occupational therapists, and speech-language pathologists to address impairments, functional limitations and disabilities in patients with neuromusculoskeletal dysfunction. This tool is used as part of an integrated treatment program to achieve functional outcomes."[33]

Years of traditional, clinic-based therapy can become tedious and ineffective for both the therapist and the child. Hippotherapy provides therapists and their patients with a novel and effective treatment modality that can spark new interest and enthusiasm. Hippotherapy is used for rehabilitation and is not to be confused with therapeutic riding. Therapeutic riding is not a formal treatment and focuses on recreation or riding skills for disabled riders.[27] Hippotherapy subjects must have an initial evaluation, progress notes, and a discharge note, just as any therapy patients.[25] It is important to note that this treatment may not be suitable or safe for children with spinal instability, severe osteoporosis, hip dislocation, uncontrolled seizures, spinal fusion, poor static sitting balance (in children >70 pounds), or increased tone after riding.[33] Individuals with CP have little experience with rhythmic movements because of impairments that limit their ability to reverse the direction of movement.[26] Researchers postulate that a walking horse simulates the triplanar movement of the human pelvis during gait, while the warmth and rhythm of the horse decrease tone and promote relaxation.[24,29] Theoretically, hippotherapy enables a child with CP to experience rhythmic movement by decreasing impairments and allowing for the self-organization of the movement patterns into functional movement strategies.[29] Researchers have supported this theory by reporting a number of observable benefits of hippotherapy[24-31,33] (Table R3).

The majority of the existing research on hippotherapy consists of subjective studies.[24,27,28] Results of hippotherapy are difficult to measure objectively due to a lack of valid and reliable instruments. Poor methodology and small sample sizes in the current research cause the results to be insignificant or inconclusive. Fortunately, despite this lack of objectivity, third-party reimbursement has been commonly received for hippotherapy sessions from a wide variety of insurance companies since 1982.[30]

A typical hippotherapy session lasts from 45 minutes to an hour. Current research is lacking a consensus on a definitive frequency or duration for this

Table R3. Benefits of hippotherapy.

Improves joint co-contraction	Increases attention span
Decreases tone	Mobilizes pelvis, hips, and spine
Decreases energy expenditure with movement	Increases muscle ROM, flexibility, and strength
Improves stability	Increases body awareness
Facilitates weight–shifting	Improves balance
Facilitates postural and equilibrium responses	Improves posture/alignment
	Increases listening and vestibular skills
Increases visual perception	Improves gait
Increases self-confidence	Improves speech and language
Improves respiration	Improves relationships
Increases coordination	

treatment, but preliminary studies recommend at least 30-minute sessions, two times per week, for at least 10 weeks.[33] Depending on the child, preparation activities may be necessary before mounting the horse.[33] These activities may include stretching or relaxation techniques to prepare the child's body to be ready for the horse. Hippotherapy does not typically use a saddle, but rather a sheepskin or soft pad.[24,30] This pad allows the child to be treated in almost any position on the horse's back (e.g., supine, prone, quadruped, sitting, side sitting, kneeling) (Figure R1). On the horse, the child wears a helmet and is accompanied by three adults: a therapist, a side walker, and a lead.[32,33] The therapist may ride along with the child or handle the child from beside the horse. The lead's main responsibility is guiding the horse. He/she walks alongside the horse, even with its eye. The side walker helps the therapist position and focus the child. He/she walks beside the rider's knee using an arm-over-thigh hold. The therapist can use toys or games (rings, balls, slinky) to work on various activities in different positions, or vary the terrain the horse is walking on to further challenge the child. Following the treatment on the horse, the session should end with similar activities on land to promote functional carryover.[30]

The American Hippotherapy Association has set specific guidelines, qualifications and responsibilities for the therapist using this modality.[25,33] It is recommended that only a properly trained therapist perform this type of treatment.

6. Aquatic Therapy
Jesse Hanlon, BS, COTA, and Mozghan Hines, LPTA

The therapeutic use of water lies in the art of careful selection to use the many physical properties of water in the most appropriate way to produce a sensible result. Misuse or careless application can mean that well-intended therapy fades into merely tender loving care. Aquatic therapy provides countless opportunities to experience, learn, and enjoy new movement skills, which leads to increase functional skills, mobility and builds self-confidence.

The relief of hypertonus in the spastic type of CP is one of the major advantages of aquatic therapy. When a body is immersed in warm water (92° to 96°F), its core temperature increases, causing reduction in gamma fiber activity, which in turn reduces muscle spindle activity, facilitating muscle

Figure R1. Hippotherapy is preformed on horseback with a thin soft saddle. Work on balance and motor coordination is often preformed with the child seated backward on the horse (A). Upright sitting stresses balance reactions. Performing hippotherapy requires three staff people. One individual leads the horse while the therapist works with the child, standing alongside the horse. A third assistant is required on the side opposite the therapist to prevent the child from falling and to assist the child in changing positions (B).

A

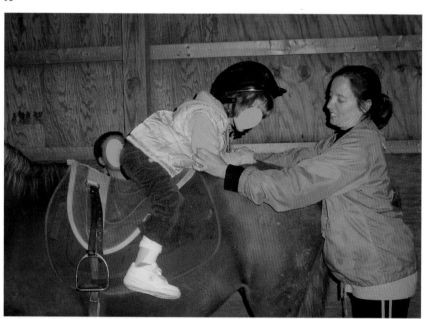

B

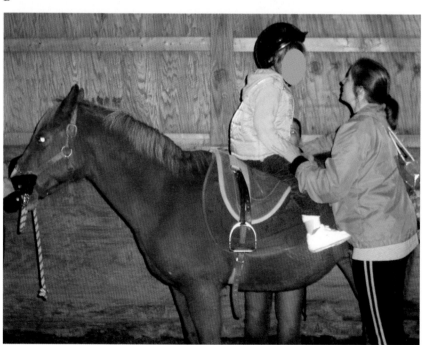

relaxation and reducing spasticity, thus resulting in increased joint range of motion and consequently creating better postural alignment.

Buoyancy, viscosity, turbulence, and hydrostatic pressure are properties of water that can provide assistance or resistance to a body. The property of buoyancy can be utilized in many different ways. Buoyancy can simply be defined as an upward force that counteracts the effect of gravity, providing weight relief. When a body is submerged up to the seventh cervical vertebra, or just below the chin, a person weighs 10% of their body weight on land; at chest level, 30% of body weight on land; and at just below waist, 50% of

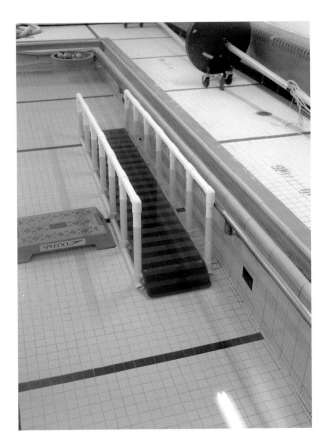

Figure R2. A great way to start gait training, especially after surgical procedures, is pool walking. This means the pool needs to have handles available in the water at the correct height.

body weight on land. For a gradual increase in weightbearing activities, the individual can be progressively moved to shallower water, starting in deep water using flotation devices. In addition to providing weight relief from gravitational forces, buoyancy can support movements, which facilitates learning functional skills such as sitting, standing, rolling, or walking before their achievement on land (Figure R2). The buoyant affect of immersion in water is a useful tool after orthopaedic surgery to treat weakness, painful joints, or decreased weight bearing through the lower extremities.

Due to its hydrostatic pressure, water is a natural brace to the trunk and a compression garment for lower extremities. This makes it possible for patients with postoperative edema to exercise in the water without wearing a pressure garment, and assists the therapist when working toward the goal of weaning an individual from a trunk brace, such as a thoracic lumbar spine orthosis (TLSO), after spinal surgery. Hydrostatic pressure also challenges breath control and voice projection while strengthening the respiratory muscles.

The viscosity of water acts as resistance to movement, meaning the faster the motion, the greater the resistance. This isokinetic trait of water is helpful in smoothing out ataxic movements and improving balance reactions by allowing increased response time. Hand paddles, walking boots, fins, and flotation devices can be added to maximize water's resistance in a progressive resistive strengthening program. Sensory and vestibular issues can also be addressed in an aquatics environment. Underwater swimming, splashing, water play, and pouring are examples of sensory exercises. The vestibular system can be challenged through activities such as spinning in an innertube, flips underwater, the game of Marco Polo, and diving for rings (see Table R3).

Research findings were presented by D.E. Thorpe et al. of the University of North Carolina at Chapel Hill on the effects of aquatic resistive exercises on a variety of factors in persons with CP at the American Physical Therapy Association's annual conference held in Texas in 2001.[34] Strength, balance, energy expenditure, functional mobility, and perceived competence of individuals were measured using standardized testing performed before, after, and 1 week after an aquatic progressive resistive exercise program. The nine subjects between 7 and 31 years of age with spastic diplegic CP performed stretching, resistive exercises with equipment, swimming skills, and lower extremity strengthening three times per week for 10 weeks. The study results demonstrated that the subjects had a significant increase in strength of their knee and hip extensors with retained hip extension, but not knee extension, at 1 week posttherapy. Gait velocity significantly improved immediately and at 1 week posttherapy CP. An example of a typical patient who can benefit from aquatic therapy is Heather who is status postmultiple orthopaedic procedures performed to correct severe progression of her bilateral foot deformities. The surgical procedures included bilateral tibial osteotomies, lateral column lengthenings, first metatarsal osteotomies and gastrocnemius recessions. Heather wore bilateral short-leg casts for 8 weeks. Her primary mode of locomotion was a power wheelchair. Physical therapy three times per week was initiated 5 days after surgery with focus on transfer training, increasing range of motion, strengthening, and ambulation training.

Clinical findings after land therapy and before pool therapy included that Heather was nonambulatory, transferred from a wheelchair to a mat with the maximum assistance of one, and her standing tolerance with a walker and contact guard was for 30 seconds. Her short-leg casts were removed 8 weeks after surgery. Aquatic therapy was initiated 2 days later with focus on walking in chest-deep water with the assistance of one for 30 feet. Strengthening exercises included wall squats, marching, biking, supine recover, and abdominal exercises. During land therapy 5 days after the start of aquatic therapy, Heather reported improved ease in weight bearing with two-person assistance. She was able to ambulate in parallel bars while wearing bilateral knee immobilizers for 6 feet times two with the moderate assistance of two. Heather continued land therapy one time per week and aquatic therapy two times per week for an additional 20 weeks. Presently she is able to ambulate 80 feet with a Kaye walker with minimal assistance. She is also able to take three to four backward steps. This is a skill she was never able to perform. In the pool she is able to walk backward 30 feet with minimal assistance. She currently transfers independently using a sliding transfer technique.

Table R4. Aquatic therapy: contraindications and precautions.

Contraindications	Precautions
Open wounds	Seizure disorder: controlled with medication
Communicable rashes (pseudomonas, streptococcus)	Respiratory compromise: vital capacity of 1.5 liters or less
Infections (respiratory, urinary, ear, blood)	Osteotomies, ileostomies, urostomies, "G" and "J" tubes, suprapubic appliances
Fever	
Uncontrolled seizure activity	External fixator
Tracheotomies	Behavior problems (children, head injuries, uncontrolled fear)
Cardiac failure	
Active joint disease (rheumatoid arthritis, hemophilia)	Hypersensitivity
Menstruation without internal protection	Autonomic dysreflexia
	Uncontrolled high or low blood pressure

Table R5. Recommended swimming strokes based on neurodevelopmental approach.

Severe Quadriplegia (spastic, athetoid, mixed)
Finning
Sculling
Child attempts these strokes while being pulled through water. Instructor may stand behind child's head and resist backward propulsion to aid in co-contraction.

Moderate Spastic Quadriplegia and Diplegia
Finning/sculling
Elementary backstroke
Breaststroke

Moderate Athetosis
Finning/sculling
Elementary backstroke

Hemiplegia
Finning/sculling
Child should be encouraged to use only the involved arm initially.
Sidestroke
Involved side should be on top of the water. Child may use inverted scissors kick. (Note that flutter kicks can increase extensor tone, which can result in scissoring gait in the ambulatory child.)

There are a number of contra-indications for aquatic therapy which basically include either issues which may place the child in a dangerous situation in the water such as frequent seizure activity, or issues in which the child may contaminate the water for other swimmers such as having large open infected wounds. There are also a number of situations, which call for extra precautions by the therapist to avoid injury to the patient or the therapist, such as children with severe unpredictable behavior problems.

Each of the different patterns of neurologic involvement require a specific consideration of the swimming strokes the therapist should focus on teaching the child. As an example, the child with hemiplegia and little use of one arm will have little success with a crawling stroke. However, focusing on using the involved arm is an excellent therapy modality and is often stressed during therapeutic sessions. For most of these children the sidestroke will be much more effective as a recreational swimming pattern.

Other Aquatic Treatment Approaches

There are several therapy methods that can be integrated into one practice as the need arises. Watsu, the water-based version of Shiatsu, was developed by a shiatsu master from northern California. The provider always performs Watsu in a hands-on manner. The patient is usually held or cradled in warm water while the provider stabilizes or moves one segment of the body, resulting in a stretch of another segment due to the drag affect. The client remains passive while the provider combines the unique qualities of the water with rhythmic flow. This combination of meridian therapy and massage can calm and relax the patient who is overly excited or experiencing pain.

The Halliwick Method was developed by James McMillan while teaching swimming to handicapped children and is based upon hydrodynamics and body mechanics. It teaches cognitive skills, breath control, and understanding of body movements in the water. The Halliwick Method combines the unique qualities of the water with rotational control patterns.

The Bad Ragaz Ring Method is a form of active or passive aquatic therapy molded after the principles and movement patterns of Knupfer exercises and proprioceptive neuromuscular facilitation (PNF). The patient is verbally, visually, and/or tactilely instructed in a series of movement or relaxation patterns while positioned horizontally and supported by optional floats around the head, neck, hip, wrists, and ankles. The patterns may be performed passively for relaxation/flexibility or actively with assistance or resistance for strengthening.

Berta and Karl Bobath originated the Neurodevelopmental Treatment Approach to treat individuals with pathophysiology of the central nervous system, specifically children with CP and adults with hemiplegia. Treatment involves active participation of the patients and direct handling to optimize function with gradual withdrawal of direct input by the therapist

Pool Design/Accessibility

Ideal pool design requires consideration of multiple factors to accommodate for various disabilities and therapies (Table R6). It is especially important for the pool facility to be accessible to wheelchairs (Figure R3). It is also important to have an accessible changing area, which is not usually available for adult-sized individuals unless there are special adaptations (Figure R4).

Multidisciplinary Approach

Every team member plays a part in addressing patient's needs. Oral hygiene, toilet hygiene, dressing/undressing skills, and showering before or after pool sessions can be incorporated in an aquatics program provided by occupational therapists. Speech therapists can take advantage of water resistance to promote increased voice projection and verbalization while physical therapists are working on functional mobility.

In conclusion, aquatic therapy is an entertaining and efficient way to enhance the quality of life for children with CP. Children are naturally drawn to the aquatic environment, enabling the practitioner to use this pleasant

Table R6. Pool design/accessibility.

Decks
Skid-resistant flooring in the pool area and locker rooms

Depth of water
Zero depth entries to 3 feet is ideal for toddlers and infants. Depending on pool size and therapeutic program, the water depth should meet the needs of the treatment plan. Four and one-half feet of water works well with school age children. Ten feet of water is needed if diving is part of the program.

Air and water temperature
Water temperature for a therapeutic pool should be between 92° and 96°F. Recreation pool water should be between 86° and 88°F. The air temperature should be within 5° of the water to prevent condensation. Too high or low temperatures can affect both the equipment and the participants. Maintaining the ideal water temperature plays an important role in balancing water chemistry.

Pool entries and exits
Zero entry ramps, steps with railing(s), ladders, and hydraulic lifts can benefit patients with different functional levels.

Locker rooms/showers
Wheelchair-accessible locker rooms with mat tables

Safety equipment
All safety equipment required by the state and providing facility to prevent accidents and to meet any medical emergencies

Staffing
Pool lifeguard on duty at all times when program in operation
Qualified licensed therapist to perform aquatic sessions

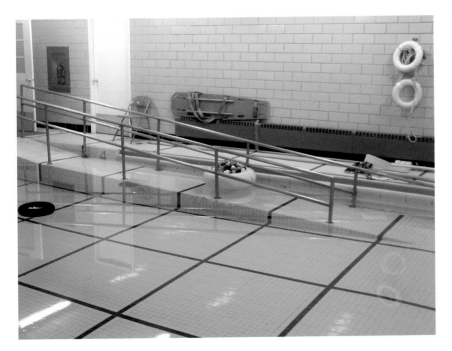

Figure R3. As children grow to adult size, the ability to get a child into and out of the pool for hydrotherapy is an important element of the facility. The wheelchair ramp as is shown here is a very safe, simple, and efficient mechanism to make the pool accessible.

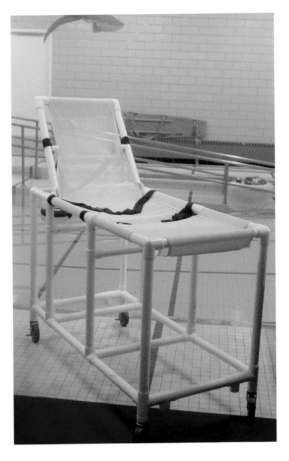

Figure R4. One problem in doing hydrotherapy for large individuals who are totally dependent for dressing and movement is finding changing rooms or tables. Low-cost solutions can easily be developed using construction and plumbing supplies. A volunteer for the school constructed this changing table.

Table R7. Community resources.

American Red Cross
17th and D Streets, NW
Washington, DC 20006
http://www.redcross.org

National Recreation and Park Association
3101 Park Center Drive
Alexandria, VA 22302
http://www.nrpa.org

Boys and Girls Club of America
National Headquarters
1230 W. Peachtree Street, NW
Atlanta, GA 30309
http://www.bgca.org

Table R8. Recommended reading.

Campion MR. Hydrotherapy in Pediatrics, 2nd Ed. Oxford: Butterworth-Heinemann, 1991.

Harris SR, Thompson M. Water as learning environment for facilitating gross motor skills in deaf-blind children. Phys Occup Ther Pediatr 1983;3:1:75–82.

Langendorfer S, Bruya LD. Aquatic Readiness: Developing Water Competence in Young Children. Champion, IL: Human Kinetics. 1995.

Routi RG, Morris DM, Cole AJ. Aquatic rehabilitation. Philadelphia: Lippincott-Raven, 1997.

Martin K. Therapeutic pool activities for young children in a community facility. Phys Occup Ther Pediatr 1983;3:1:59–74.

atmosphere to carry out therapeutic goals along with building confidence and having fun. Aquatic therapy is a great adjunct to traditional land-based therapy, improving such goals as range of motion, coordination, functional mobility, and a lifelong opportunity for fitness. There are many methods to use water for therapy and recreation with many different people developing recommendations and reporting what works and does not work (Tables R7 and R8).

7. Assistive Devices
Mary Bolton, PT

Most children with CP will need assistive devices for standing and walking during their lifetime. There are many assistive device styles, accessories, and options in the durable medical equipment market. Choosing the walker that offers the appropriate support but allows the greatest degree of mobility is of utmost importance. Therefore, it is crucial to have several of these devices available for trial when evaluating a child for the use of assistive equipment.

When a child is being assessed for a walker, the initial evaluation is very extensive. The key factor is the child's ability to weight bear on her lower extremities. When evaluating younger children, hold them upright with their feet in contact with the ground and note their ability to support themselves. Noting the ability to take weight with transfers is key when evaluating older children. Information from the parents, therapists, teachers, and other caregivers will increase your understanding of the child's needs and potential. The ability to dissociate the lower extremities from each other is essential for walking, but is difficult for children with extensor tone. Stepping reactions should occur with the drive to stand and move. A thorough evaluation of the child's range of motion is needed. Contractures of the lower extremity will have a significant effect on the child's ability to stand upright. Evaluate the ability and strength used to hold the body upright with her arms. The arms may function in a variety of positions for weight bearing, such as extended elbows, or flexed with the arms supported on platforms.

The child's functional mobility should also be assessed. Their usage of floor or upright movement enables the therapist to view weightbearing control, weight-shifting ability, cognitive motivation, and problem-solving skills. Observation of transfers from sit to stand, stand to pivot, and floor to stand is of value. The child's use of a wheelchair, the style and maneuvering skills, provides further information about vision, strength, endurance, and cognitive and environmental awareness. Any durable medical equipment that is used to help the child's positioning or ability to stand upright should also be used and evaluated.

With their knowledge of the child's equipment use at home and school, the parents are often able to provide additional background information for the assistive device evaluation. A history of the type of equipment the child has tried and how well she performed with it is helpful. You also will need to know what equipment is currently in use. Parents may have ideas about their child's current needs and desires. In addition, determine if any surgeries or medical interventions (bracing, Botox injections, etc.) are proposed in the future, which may influence the recommendations for walking aids.

Many times the school or home therapists involved with the child's care have important information regarding the assessment of the child's walking needs, but they are limited by equipment availability and options. Access to the Internet often increases information about equipment, although it may not always be available to try with the child. Working with local durable medical equipment vendors and/or contacting the equipment manufacturers directly is always an option.

Standers are helpful for children who need significant postural support, lack ability or understanding of how to support themselves on their arms, and have limited cognitive understanding (by developmental age or actual limited cognitive development) of how to use a walking device. The first step is to determine if a supine, prone, or upright stander is most appropriate for the position desired. Children who need more extension strength including head control, arm weightbearing facilitation, and can actively engage in standing would benefit from a prone stander (Figure R5). Children with increased extension posturing or decreased postural control due to weakness or low tone generally benefit from initiating upright standing at a slower rate. A supine stander allows for a slower progression into the upright posture and ease with blood pressure and circulation problems. The upright stander has many varieties from full trunk support to lower lumbar control. They are often used with children who can move to standing with a stand

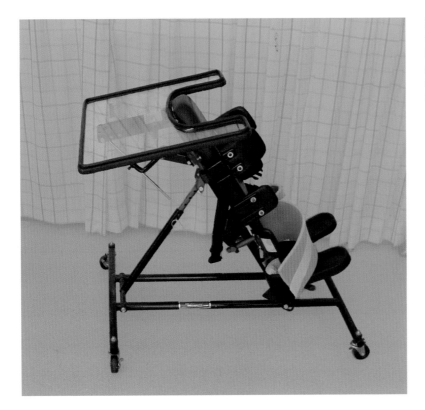

Figure R5. Prone standers such as this are very useful but require measuring to fit the individual child. It is also ideal to have the equipment at the evaluation site so the parent can see how big it is and see how the child responds to the device.

transfer and need to increase their overall standing tolerance, whether it is due to limited range of motion, strength, or overall endurance. This type of stander with additional bracing can be used for lower extremity weakness. All these different stander styles have a variety of options, accessories and special features. There are boundless possibilities limited only by the manufacturer's creativity.

When a child begins to show the ability to bear weight on her legs and attempts to weight shift as she steps, she is usually ready for a walking aid. These walking devices vary from maximum assistance control, as in a gait trainer, to walkers, canes, and crutches.

A gait trainer is usually most appropriate for a child with increased postural tone, limited pelvic and lower extremity dissociation, and the inability to weight shift with caregiver support. Such children have a desire to move and interact with their environment but are limited by their ability to do so independently. Gait trainers align the body's center of gravity over the feet, prevent trunk lateral flexion, and offer weightbearing support through a seat. The gait trainer helps to stabilize the trunk and pelvis so the legs can move independently for stepping. For the child that adducts her legs, stepping straps can assist in abducting the legs. Arm supports are optional. The child is able to propel the device by stepping. The trunk is aligned with trunk/hip guides, straps, or pads. Gait trainers are like ring walkers or baby walkers that offer more support, have variable sizes, and the capability for limited wheel direction. For safety of the older and more mature child, the gait trainer's base of support is much larger, but this is often found to be large and cumbersome in a home setting. Also, the large child needs to be lifted or moved into the trainer making it difficult for a single caretaker to manage safely. Although not functional for the older child, the trainer is ideal for the younger one who needs stabilization and is beginning to demonstrate ambulation skills.

A walker is usually beneficial when a child shows potential for weight bearing, is initiating stepping, but has limited weight shift, balance, muscle endurance, or coordination. There are a variety of walkers to use for assessment. Forward and posterior walkers are available and include many accessories and options. The most important determinant in choosing a walker is how the child actually functions with it. It is valuable, as with all equipment, to have a large selection of walker styles, sizes, and upper extremity support devices to try. Additional items such as wheels, brakes, seats, and pelvic guides can be added or interchanged later. Generally, watching the child's emotional reaction and movement ability will guide the therapist in narrowing down the style of walker that is most appropriate for that child. Some children need multiple sessions or extended periods to adjust to the equipment, especially if it is their first time using it. The younger child may be more accustomed to walking with their arms in a variety of positions including hands held high, leaning on furniture, or pushing walking toys. A child with this experience may accept the posterior walker easier than an older child who has become accustomed to using a front walker. The larger child also has an easier time with maneuvering the forward walker, because the base of support on the large-size posterior walkers becomes too cumbersome. A posterior walker is most suitable for a child who advances the supportive device too far forward or has excessive trunk flexion. A forward walker is appropriate for children who need less upper extremity support for postural alignment and have more fluent weight shift patterns. These walkers generally are lighter and more compact.

Children who need relatively little assistance for balance, fall occasionally, and have difficulty with longer community distances or unleveled surfaces may benefit from the assistance of a cane or crutches. The child is usually 6 years or older, and reports using their walker less often, leans on furniture for assistance, or prefers to be mildly supported by another person. Canes and crutches come in a variety of styles and designs. Canes are beneficial for children who have occasional falls, and are gradually getting slower than their peers and entering their teenage years. The therapist will need an array of sizes, base options, and grip styles to determine the most appropriate equipment for the child's comfort level and need. Some individuals use canes for safety in larger school settings and community outings; however, forearm crutches are by far the most useful assistive devices for individuals with CP.

Determining the best assistive equipment should not be a rushed decision. It will impact on the child's continued development and ability to interact and move in her world. Sometimes more than one device is necessary, perhaps a walker for school distances and a cane for the smaller crowded home. Selecting the best equipment for the child should not be limited by evaluation time. Remember, the goal is walking with the best postural alignment, convenience for usage, efficiency, and walking speed. The parent and child should be satisfied and confident with the recommendation.

8. Seating Systems
Denise Peischl, BSE, Liz Koczur, MPT, and Carrie Strine, OTR/L

No other area of technology for children with CP has shown any greater growth than that in mobility systems and seating components. There is no facility where you will not find consensus among the caregivers that an appropriate prescription for a seating device needs to include the family, the treating therapist, the physician, the equipment vendor, and, for the complex cases, a rehabilitation engineer. Guidelines for seating systems are outlined in Tables R9 through R17. Because wheelchairs are always large devices

---

Table R9. Seating systems.

Laterals (trunk supports mounted on the backrest)
(+) Support patient in an upright posture
(+) Lateral support for safety in transport
(+) Proximal stability to enhance distal mobility
(−) Decreases amount of lateral mobility patient has

Curved laterals
(+) Curve around patient's trunk to help decrease forward flexion of the trunk
(−) May make transfers difficult
(−) Requires swing-away hardware for transfers

Straight laterals
(+) Easier for patient to move in and out
(+) Easier for transfers
(−) Does not block forward flexion of the trunk

Summer/Winter Bracket Hardware (Slide adjustment on back of chair allows caregiver to move lateral in and out for heavier clothing); user is unable to access
(+) Easy to use: no tools required
(+) Allows width adjustability for changes in season (i.e., winter coat)
(+) Allows for growth adjustability without tools
(−) Extra parts to chair that could be removed and lost

Swing-away hardware (Push lever on side of lateral, allows it to open at an angle)
(+) Moves lateral out of the way for ease of transfers
(−) Additional hinge; creates a weak spot for potential break
(−) Not considered heavy duty for aggressive support

Table R10. Seating systems.

Hip guides (Pads usually mounted to frame of chair or underneath cushion cover to keeps hips in alignment. Hip guides mounted to chair can come in any length, usually full, three-quarter length, or just around the pelvis.)
(+) Keep hips centered in middle of chair
(+) Able to maintain hip position with accommodating for growth
(+) Narrows in width for midline alignment
(−) Adds to overall weight of chair
(−) Cumbersome when folding chair
(−) Makes transfers difficult

Table R11. Seating systems.

Knee adductors (Pads usually mounted to footrest hangers that assist in keeping knees from frog-leg position. Point of contact is on lateral femoral epicondyle.)
(+) Assists to maintain neutral alignment of lower extremities
(−) May come out of alignment due to moving parts (multiaxis joints)
(−) Makes transfers difficult
(−) Cumbersome

Knee block (Positioned in front of the knee to prevent sliding out of wheelchair in conjunction with seatbelt)
(+) Prevents sliding out
(−) Cannot be used when knee or hip integrity is in question
(−) Difficult for transfers

Abductor (Also called a pommel – used to abduct knees)
(+) Decreases adduction, maintaining good lower extremity alignment
(+) Can flip down to get out of the way for transfers
(−) If positioned incorrectly can cause groin problems
(−) Cumbersome
(−) Difficult for independent function

Table R12. Seating systems.

Shoulder retractor pads (Aggressive positioning option to retract the shoulders. Mounted off backrest padded brackets to hold shoulders against backrest.)
(+) Retract shoulders
(−) Difficult to position
(−) Cumbersome
(−) Adds weight to wheelchair
(−) Not intended for a user who uses trunk flexion/extension for functional reach

Sub-ASIS bar (aggressive positioning option to immobilize the pelvis)
(+) Controls pelvic thrusting usually caused by high tone
(+) Maintains constant position of individual while seated in wheelchair
(+) Controls pelvic rotation
(−) Could cause skin breakdown in ASIS joint if incorrectly set
(−) Difficult to assess tolerance of patient who is cognitively impaired
(−) Cannot be easily adjusted

Trunk positioners
Chest harness (Nylon or Neoprene vest-like apparatus)
(+) Assists to keep client's trunk upright
(+) Used for safety in transport (along with conventional lock downs)
(−) Does not have a good line of pull to promote shoulder retraction

Chest strap (Velcro strap with or without D-ring positioned across trunk)
(+) Assists client to keep from flexing trunk forward
(+) Safety in transport
(+) Easy to put on/off
(−) Not an aggressive trunk positioner

Shoulder straps (Neoprene or nylon padded straps with line of pull on trunk proximal to the shoulder complex)
(+) Aggressive positioner to promote shoulder retraction
(+) Improves clients trunk stability
(+) Safety in transport
(−) Needs to be snug to work correctly
(−) Does not allow client much freedom of trunk movement

Hemi-harness (Upside-down Y-shaped shoulder harness)
(+) Aggressive positioner to promote unilateral shoulder retraction
(+) Allows client to use unaffected limb and trunk for functional reach
(−) Gives stability to only one side
(−) Client may be able to move out of it

Table R13. Seating systems.

Pelvic Positioners

Pushbutton seatbelt
(+) Simple, easy to operate
(+) Some manufacturers produce varieties that require less pressure to undo
(+) Durable
(−) Sometimes too hard for users without fine motor control

Airplane seatbelt (Flip-up seatbelt)
(+) Simple, easy to operate
(+) Easy to undo with gross hand movement
(+) Durable
(−) Big metal buckle can be cumbersome

Fastex buckle seatbelt
(+) Difficult to unlatch, user attempt to remove may create safety issue
(−) Not durable

Padded seatbelt
(+) Comfort
(+) Allows user/caregiver to make snug without "cutting into" user

Single-pull padded seatbelt (One D-ring on seatbelt makes for a better line of pull for user/caregiver to make snug.)
(+) Easy to get snug fit
(+) Assists to reduce tone
(+) Durable
(−) Bulky

Double-pull padded seatbelt (Two D-rings on seatbelt allows user/caregiver to pull equally on both sides of pelvis to make snug.)
(+) Easy to get a snug fit
(+) Easily adjustable
(+) Good for extensor tone reduction
(+) Assists with decreasing pelvic rotation
(−) Bulky

Reverse seatbelt (Seatbelt attaches behind user so they are unable to remove themselves.)
(+) Safety
(−) Difficult for caregivers to reach
(−) Not good for tone reduction or pelvic positioning

Seatbelt rigidizer (Hard plastic cover over one or both sides of seatbelt)
(+) Puts seatbelt in a good position for user to easily retrieve and buckle
(−) May get in the way for transfers

Pelvis Positioning Strap (Y-type strap coming up between legs for abduction)
(+) Alternative pelvic positioning to hip belt or sub-ASIS bar
(+) May work well with children under 2 years of age
(−) Not effective in reducing tone
(−) Does not control pelvic rotation
(−) Requires constant skin monitoring for irritation and abrasion

compared with the child's size, when determining the functional use of the device one must very carefully consider the patient, the family environment and family goals, and the community environment where the device will be used (Figure R6). Many of the specific indications and contraindications are not well defined or widely agreed upon in the rehabilitation community. As with all interventions, there are pluses and minuses and these are included for consideration (see Tables R9–R17).

After the team evaluation and all the specific components for the wheelchair are agreed upon, excellent documentation qualifying the need for each component must be generated. This thorough documentation can then be formulated into prescription form and a detailed letter of medical necessity to qualify the medical need for the wheelchair. Failure to provide the documentation of medical necessity often leads to the denial of key components of the seating system. An example letter of medical necessity is as follows:

Table R14. Seating systems.

Backrests

Flat backrest
(+) Solid support for pelvis and spine
(+) Easy to mount hardware to it
(+) Compliments other positioning devices (i.e., laterals, headrest, etc.)
(+) Allows use of growth-oriented hardware
(−) No accommodation for spinal deformity
(−) Adds weight to wheelchair
(−) Prevent folding of wheelchair unless removed

I backrest (Flat back made in the shape of the capital letter I)
(+) Allow laterals to be moved in close to trunk without significant offset hardware
(+, −) All positive and negative components of a flat backrest
(−) Need to measure correctly for adequate support
(−) If moving back between posts, posts may interfere with lateral maneuverability

Curved backrest (Slightly concave, made of wood and foam)
(+) Minimal contour for lateral stability
(−) More difficult to mount lateral hardware than to a flat backrest

Premolded contoured backrest (Commercially available contoured back, i.e., Jay)
(+) May come with pressure relief areas along spine
(+) Minimal contour for lateral stability
(−) Sometimes difficult to fit for pediatric population

Custom-molded contoured backrest (Practitioner uses foam to mold backrest for individual patients. Foam in place can be completed at appointment, however, some molds must be sent to manufacturer to be completed.)
(+) Accommodation for spinal deformity
(+) Individual for user
(+) Foam in place may be changed easily
(−) User may have to wait for custom mold
(−) Requires knowledgeable practitioner to measure for or produce an accurate mold of the child's spine

Bi-angular backrest (Flat backrest with hinge in lumbar area to give patient increased spinal extension)
(+) Assists with upright positioning
(−) Difficult to get correct specifications
(−) Not adjustable

Sling backrest (Nylon padded backrest)
(+) Easy to fold
(−) Promotes kyphotic posture
(−) No adjustability

Adjustable tension backrest (Six to eight hook-and-loop straps positioned horizontally on sling back)
(+) Maintains constant tension on backrest
(+) Promotes upright posture
(+) Easy to fold chair
(+) Allows minimal concavity for minimal lateral stability
(−) Unable to mount any hardware on it for laterals or headrest
(−) Maintains minimal amount of sling

Date

To Whom It May Concern:

Kevin Jones is an 11-year-old male with a primary diagnosis of quadriplegic CP. Kevin was seen in the Seating Clinic at the duPont Hospital for Children on August 15, 2003 for evaluation and prescription of a new seating system, which is necessary to meet his seating and mobility needs.

Kevin presents with the following: he is on a bowel and bladder program; his hearing and vision are within normal limits; he has increased tone in his upper extremities, and increased tone in his lower extremities; his head control is fair; his trunk control is poor; his spine is flexible. Kevin has knee flexion

Table R15. Seating systems.

Foot Positioners

Calf strap (Hook-and-loop strap positioned in front or behind calf)
(+) Minimal positioning for knee flexion/extension
(+) Easily removable
(−) Not an aggressive positioner
(−) Usually used with another type of foot positioner

Heel loop (Strap mounted to posterior part of footplate)
(+) Assists in keeping foot from sliding posteriorly off footplate
(−) Not an aggressive positioner
(−) Sometimes in the way to flip up footplate

Ankle strap (Hook-and-loop or D-ring strap mounted to footplate, positioned across ankle)
(+) Assists in keeping foot on footplate
(−) Not aggressive, many users are able to pull feet out

Toe loop (Hook-and-loop or D-ring strap mounted on footplate, positioned across metatarsals)
(+) Assists to keep foot on footplate
(+) Used in conjunction with ankle strap can help to prevent forefoot rotation
(−) Bulky

Ankle hugger (Neoprene strap mounted to footplate, encompasses entire circumference of ankle)
(+) Padded, comfortable
(+) Allows minimal movement
(+) Difficult for user to pull out of it
(−) Bulky
(−) Does not control forefoot movement

Shoe holder (Heavy-duty plastic piece that shoe sits in and is strapped into)
(+) Aggressive positioning
(+) Difficult for user to pull out of it
(+) Controls forefoot and rear foot motion
(−) Bulky
(−) Must get correct size

Table R16. Seating systems.

Cushions

Flat cushion (Minimal cushioning on a firm surface)
(+) Supports client's pelvis and limbs
(+) Easy to transfer into and out of
(+) Inexpensive
(+) Requires minimal maintenance
(−) No positioning for orthopaedic deformities

Pre-molded contour foam cushion
(+) Gives minimal – moderate contour to accommodate for orthopaedic deformities
(+) Supports patient's pelvis and limbs
(+) Requires minimal maintenance
(−) Increased contour may make it difficult to transfer into and out of

Gel cushion (Cushions using foam and a pressure-relieving fluid)
(+) Pressure relieving get positioned under bony prominences
(+) May come with different contours to accommodate for orthopaedic deformities
(+) Firm – good for pelvic stability
(−) Requires caregiver/patient maintenance
(−) Increased contour may make it difficult for patient to move into and out of

Air cushion (Pressure-relieving cushions using air regulation to maintain cushion firmness)
(+) Great for pressure relief under bony prominences
(−) High level of patient/caregiver maintenance
(−) Minimal pelvic stability
(−) Difficult for patient to transfer on/off of

Incontinent cover (One type of removable cover, prevents urine from soaking cushion)
(+) Maintains integrity of cushion
(−) Positions urine under patient

Table R17. Seating systems.

Trays

Full lap tray
(+) Supports individual's upper body
(+) Good for cognitive stimulation and feeding issues
(−) Needs to be removed for transport

Clear tray
(+) Allows client to see lower half of body
(+) Pictures can be placed under the tray
(−) More expensive than wood

Wood tray
(+) Durable
(+) Supports individual's upper body
(−) Individual unable to see through

Half-lap tray (Fits on one armrest; used for patients with hemiplegia)
(+) Supports affected side of patient
(+) Allows patient to freely use unaffected side to propel wheelchair
(+) Firm surface for work, etc.
(+) Patient can independently remove
(−) Difficult for patient to independently put on
(−) Sometimes desk space is too small for patient to work effectively

Easel tray
(+) Supports book/objects in a better line of vision for patient
(−) Takes up a lot of space on tray
(−) Not for a patient with aggressive behavior
(−) Cumbersome

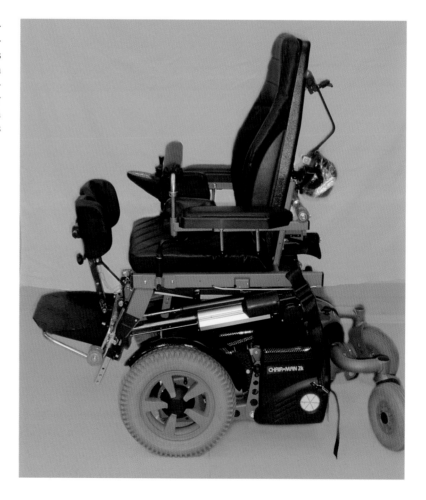

Figure R6. The process of making an assessment and writing the prescription for a wheelchair requires evaluating many elements. This is ideally done in a multidisciplinary team with therapist, rehabilitation engineer, parent, and physician. This process is especially true for very sophisticated power chairs with multiple features, which may cost as much as $30,000.

contractures; he is independent in power wheelchair mobility; he is dependent for transfers; he is verbal in communication; and cognitively he is age appropriate.

His current wheelchair is a Quickie P200 power wheelchair, which is three years old. Due to growth and weight gain, this system no longer accommodates Kevin's seating and mobility needs. His P200 is a 17-inch wheelchair and currently Kevin's hip measurement is 19 inches. It is evident that this wheelchair no longer accommodates his needs.

The seating goals for Kevin are to increase mobility, increase efficiency, enhance function, maintain posture, increase independence, protect skin, provide comfort, and provide safety.

Upon evaluation, the seating team recommends the following be prescribed for Kevin: Action Arrow wheelchair with 4-pole motors and weight-shifting power tilt-in-space; 14-inch wheels with flat free fillers and rubber knobby tires; Q-tronics electronics – joystick with 1/8 inch jacks; swing-away mount on right side; 24 NF gel batteries; low seat-to-floor height; 70 degree hangers with angle-adjustable footplates; height-adjustable desk length on right and full length on left; clear tray with top drop hardware and tray support extension and joystick cutout; Cloud cushion; AEL flat swing-away laterals 5×6; solid curved I-back; small curved OttoBock headrest with hardware; TRCM with mounting bracket; TASH C5 adapter; TASH microlite switch; color: black with twilight.

Specific components and indications:

Basic Motorized Wheelchair	• Unable to ambulate or propel a manual wheelchair • Has functional use of one UE • Low/decreasing endurance
Motorized W/C with adjustable electronics	• Special switch configuration necessary due to upper extremity weakness • Increased sensitivity adjustability to decrease spasms of client and/or allow use of ECU with w/c • Capability to adjust speed, excel; to allow better control and safety in use
TRCM w/TASH switch	• Alternate switch for tilting due to limited strength, especially when in tilt and working against gravity • Maintains constant access to tilt regardless of degree of tilt
High strength	• Strong base of support for tilt • Outdoor terrain
Power tilt	• Independent weight shift for position change • Pressure relief • Reduce/eliminate shear • Reduce spasms • Personal hygiene
Adjustable height arm	• Support to tray at right height • Upper body support and balance • Ease of transfer
Angle-adjustable footplates	• Ankle contractures • Ankle braces • Reduce extensor thrust in LEs • Knee contractures – prevent feet from resting on standard footplate
Solid seat	• Pelvic stability • Avoid sling effect, adduction of knees

Cloud cushion	• Pressure relief for bony prominences
	• Contour for pelvic stability
Jay back	• Pressure relief along spine
	• Min/mod lateral and lumbar support and contour
	• Built-in capability for growth
Solid back	• Upright posture
	• Prevent/minimize kyphosis
	• Trunk stability
Laterals	• Encourage midline trunk position and correct/delay scoliosis
	• Compensate for lack of trunk control
	• Safety
	• Assist with transfer, locks for strength
Headrest	• Poor head control due to low tone
	• Active flexion/hyperextension of head
	• Posterior and/or lateral support
	• ATNR
	• Safety in transport
	• Facilitate breathing
Tray (clear)	• Upper arm and trunk support
	• Functional surface for schoolwork
	• Inability to access desks, tables, etc.
	• Base for augmentative communication device, computer
Seat belt	• Pelvic positioning – prevent sliding out
	• Safety
Anti-tippers	• Safety
Large casters	• Rugged terrain, smoother ride
Flat-free fillers	• Prevent flat tires
	• Reduce maintenance

Should you have any questions regarding these recommendations for Kevin, do not hesitate to call us at (302) 999-9999. We hope that you will be able to accommodate these needs in an expedient manner. Thank you for your co-operation and assistance in this matter.

Sincerely,

Freeman Miller, MD

9. M.O.V.E.™ (Mobility Opportunities Via Education) Curriculum
Kristin Capone, PT, MEd, Diana Hoopes, PT, Deborah Kiser, MS, PT, and Beth Rolph, MPT

The M.O.V.E.™ Curriculum is an activity-based curriculum designed to teach individuals basic functional motor skills needed for adult life. These skills allow them to enjoy a more inclusive lifestyle because movement is an integral part of everyday life. People with physical disabilities often require assistance to participate in these everyday activities, such as moving to the bed or bathroom, to school, or to their place of work. The MOVE curriculum provides a framework for teaching the skills necessary for individuals with disabilities to gain greater physical independence. It combines functional body movements with an instructional process designed to help people acquire increasing amounts of independence in sitting, standing, and walking.

Linda Bidabe, founder and author of the MOVE curriculum, realized the need for a functional mobility curriculum when she observed that 21-year-old students were graduating from her school with fewer skills than they had when they entered school. She believed that the "developmental model" was not meeting the needs of students with severe disabilities because these students learned skills at a very slow rate and would take years to develop some of the early developmental skills such as rolling or prone propping on elbows. Therefore, the students would never accomplish functional mobility skills in sitting, standing, and walking.[35]

This program is for any child or adult who is not independently sitting, standing, or walking. This includes those with both significant motor disabilities and mental retardation. Whether in a special school or a regular classroom setting, MOVE provides the student increased opportunities to participate in life activities with their peers without disabilities. Progress in the program can help reduce the time needed for custodial care, increase the child's self esteem, and promote acceptance by peers.

Contraindications to consider before starting the MOVE curriculum include circulatory disease, respiratory distress, brittle bones, muscle contractures, curvature of the spine, hip dislocation, foot and ankle abnormalities, pain or discomfort, or a head that is too large to be supported by the neck. Medical or physical therapy consultation is recommended for any student with possible contraindications to obtain clearance for the exercise and weight-bearing activities. Exclusion from the program is limited to those individuals whose medical needs contraindicate the need to sit, stand, or walk.

The MOVE program is based upon the teaming of special education instruction with therapeutic methods and includes ecologic inventory, prioritization of goals, chronologically age-appropriate skills, task analysis, prompts for partial participation, prompt reduction, and the four different stages of learning: acquisition, fluency, maintenance, and generalization. It is divided into six steps. In step one, the student participates in the Top-Down Motor Milestone(TM) Test that evaluates his or her ability in 16 basic motor skills that are necessary for functioning in the home and community. The motor skills are age appropriate and based on a top-down model of needs rather than the traditional developmental programs based on sequential motor skills acquisition of infants.

Following the test, the student, parents, and/or caregivers are briefly interviewed in step two, to determine activities important to the family at the present time and in the future. An activity is defined as a specific event such as, " I want to be able to walk across the stage to get my diploma." Step three analyzes the activities to determine the motor skills (from the Top-Down Motor Milestone™ Test) necessary to perform the activity, for example, walking forward or maintaining standing.

In step four, the amount of assistance needed by the student to perform the selected activities at the time of testing is recorded on the Prompt Reduction Plan Sheets provided in the assessment booklet. A plan is then formulated in step five to systematically reduce assistance over the instructional period. In the final step, step six, the skills are taught using the teaching sections of the curriculum to provide suggestions based on individual student needs.

To teach certain skills the MOVE curriculum utilizes equipment such as regular classroom chairs, adapted chairs, mobile standers, and gait trainers that are designed to support the student while they are practicing a skill (Figures R7 and R8). The equipment is not a substitute for teaching but rather a support to make instruction possible. Dependence upon equipment is continually reduced until the individual achieves as much independence as possible.

Figure R7. The development of gait trainers with a high degree of modularity has been driven in part by the philosophy of the MOVE program to have children up weight bearing and moving in the device, which gives the amount of support the child needs. The goal is then to gradually reduce the amount of support as the child develops strength and motor skills.

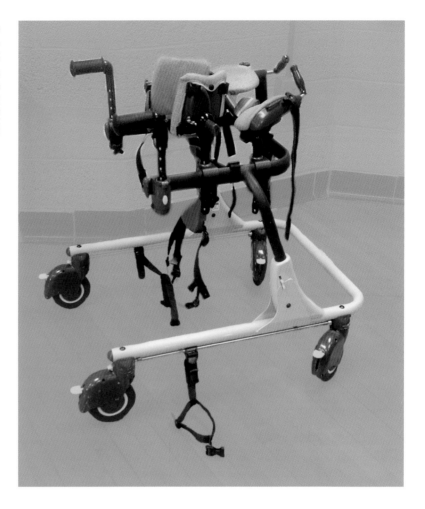

Figure R8. An important aspect of the MOVE program is the ability to get individuals into weightbearing positions, which is difficult for adult-sized adolescents. The development of mechanical lift walkers makes this process much easier for the caregivers.

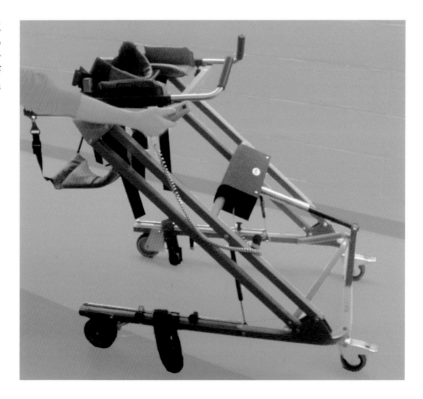

MOVE is designed to embed mobility skill practice into functional everyday routines. As a result, MOVE can occur at school, in a facility, at home, or in the community, thus providing opportunities for multiple repetitions. MOVE is successfully implemented by therapists, educators, paraprofessionals, parents, and anyone who interacts with the individual.

The structured teaching approach used in the MOVE curriculum is validated in the article, Mobility Opportunities Via Education (MOVE): Theoretical Foundations, by Barnes and Whinnery,[36] which describes its use of natural environments, functional activities, scaffolding, partial participation, and use of contemporary motor theories related to teaching functional mobility skills.

The John G. Leach School, the nation's first MOVE model site, completed a pilot study in 1998 to evaluate the effectiveness of the MOVE curriculum. Eleven students (ages 4 to 18 years) with a variety of severe disabilities participated in the six steps of the MOVE program. After a 5-month period of instruction, improvements in sitting, standing, and walking were achieved. Improvements were also noted in the areas of communication, alertness, and overall health. Because of the success of the pilot program the MOVE curriculum was adopted for schoolwide use.

For example, a 5-year-old boy with a diagnosis of Cornelia–DeLang syndrome began the MOVE program at Leach School because he was nonweight bearing and intolerant of positions other than supine, as well as unable to communicate or play with his peers and siblings. Following daily practice in a mobile stander, he increased his tolerance for weight bearing. As support from the equipment was reduced, the student was able to practice standing as part of his classroom routines such as diaper changes and getting in and out of his classroom chair. Over a 3-year period he progressed from walking with full support in a gait trainer to walking with one hand held or pushing a forward rolling walker. This gain has led to increased social interaction and independent exploration of his environment.

10. Occupational Therapy Extremity Evaluation
Marilyn Marnie King, OTR/L

Individuals with CP may present with spasticity that causes dynamic or fixed contractures. Typical orthopaedic deformities include shoulder excessive external rotation, elbow flexion, pronation, ulnar deviation, wrist flexion, thumb adduction, tight finger flexion, and swan neck fingers. Surgery should improve these areas, but some children use their limits for function and may not do better. Examples are children who use augmentative communication aids and need a pronated arm or whose ability to point requires wrist flexion (tight tenodesis).

Brief Description of Surgeries to Treat the Upper Extremity

Surgeries to lengthen tendons or to transfer muscles to balance power and tone are frequently performed on the child with spastic CP, although never on children with dystonia, nor those with undulating fanning of fingers, nor those with rigid extension of the arm and flexion of the wrist. The Green transfer is the transfer of the flexor carpi ulnaris (FCU) to the extensor carpi radialis brevis (ECRB). There are variations that include tying flexors into the finger extensors and the palmaris longus (PL) into the extensor pollicis longus (EPL) thumb extensors. Prognosis is progressively improved with the following skills of the patient: good intelligence and motivation to follow through with splinting and treatment exercises, good sensation and proprioception, patience versus poor attention span, realistic expectations, the ability to isolate wrist flexion from finger extension, and good volitional release.

Goals to achieve through surgery usually include two of the following, which are listed in order of certainty: improved cosmesis, meaning the wrist is placed in neutral, improved ability to keep the hand clean and odor free, improved ease of dressing, improved ability to see where the fingers are grasping, which further improves the potential for eye–hand coordination, and improved function of the hand, which is the least successfully achieved. A realistic order of achievement relative to improved function of the hand includes mass grasp, mass release, helper limb, tip pinch to index to middle fingers, lateral key pinch, grasp and turn object, cylindrical fist lacking 1 inch from palm, mass finger abduction/adduction, and finally, but rarely, individual isolated finger positions (such as sign language alphabet), finger magic tricks, shadow pictures with hands, rotating isospheres in palm, and fast activities such as spinning a top, snapping fingers, clapping, stirring, and shaking.

The surgeon's evaluation includes the effect the patient's body motions have on the increased wrist flexion, the patient's timing in throwing, and the posture of the arm with the use of the body during reaching, grasping, and running. If the child uses synkinesis or mirroring motions from the sounder side, the functional use will not be as good. Families' coping skills and unrealistic anticipated use of the extremity after surgery often present a dichotomy of expectation that the surgery will cure the functional deficit as compared to the more realistic prospect that the appearance of the arm will improve. The surgeon's recommendations to therapists are to keep splints small, compact, and simple (no outriggers) with focus on assisting function over cosmetic splinting. The dorsal wrist cock-up splint is recommended for functional protection. It provides extension support with the palmar arch preserved, as well as providing lateral borders to control the ulnar drift. By being on the dorsum, the splint does not rest against the trunk and is easier for the child to self-apply with the wrist strap being easier to handle. A night resting splint may be indicated if the fingers cannot extend (tight tenodesis) with the wrist, which following surgery is now in greater extension. The appropriate time for surgery is after the child is 6 years old; the ideal time is between 8 and 12 years old because of the child's greater understanding, cooperation, and ability to participate in the decision. There is a common range of problems of the upper extremity observed in children with CP for which a specific treatment is usually defined based on the identified deformity (Table R18).

Splinting

Usually following muscle transfer surgery the patient is casted for 4 to 6 weeks. Upon cast removal, the surgeon recommends that the patient wear a wrist cock-up splint at 20° to 30° extension for protection to prevent forceful wrist flexion (transfers) for 1 month with an hour or two off each day while sitting and bathing. After that period the child wears the splint at nighttime only. By 4 to 6 months the splint is worn only as protection as ambulation balance/roughness requires. The night resting splint is recommended for 6 months to a year, depending on severity of tone.

Upper extremity splinting for children who are not postoperative may pose some challenges. If a child is totally uncooperative and noncompliant about using splints, the family should not fight the child so as to lose sleep or create psychologic barriers. Generally, the following splinting is recommended for children with contractures caused by CP. The child between 1 and 4 years old who is not yet a candidate for surgery may benefit from a soft

Table R18. Typical problems and surgical intervention.

Shoulder
P: Instability, dislocation
D: Joint laxity, athetosis
Tx: Decrease ROM to shoulder, increase strength around shoulder, tie/tether elbow to belt or wheelchair, avoid surgery if possible

Shoulder
P: Axilla hygiene, difficulty with dressing, getting through doors
D: External rotation of "high guard" or "flying bird" deformity
Tx: Release pectorals, tighten internal rotators or do a rotation osteotomy of humerus

Elbow
P: Dress, hygiene, cosmesis
D: Flexion contracture (surgery will weaken biceps strength)
Tx: Elbow extension splint, surgery to lengthen biceps, brachialis, elbow extension splint at night, AROM

Forearm
P: Palm out of sight, unable to see object pinched
D: Pronated arm
Tx: Reroute pronator teres to supinate, cast to above elbow to hold supination

Wrist
P: Poor appearance of flexed wrist, difficulty dressing or being dressed, unable to see what is in pinch, unable to easily touch thumb to index tip
D: Wrist flexed, ulnar deviated, forearm pronated, fingers flexed
Tx: If AROM of finger extension occurs with wrist flexion, then Green transfer (flexi carpi ulnaris to extensor carpi radialis brevis). If AROM is only wrist extension, then flexi carpi ulnaris may be transferred to finger extensors. If there is ulnar drift, plicate extensor carpi radialis longus. Lengthen flexor digitorum sublimis if strength is less than "poor" or 2/5. A wrist cock-up splint (in 20° extension) is needed for 3 months to prevent overstretch of flexor carpi ulnaris if wrist is flexed accidentally. A wrist/resting hand splint in progressive finger and wrist extension to increase the tenodesis excursion is needed if the child cannot open his fingers with the wrist in extension.

Fingers
P: Child cannot grasp, joints lock, swan neck deformity
D: Joint laxity, intrinsics – function
Tx: Tighten tenodesis with flexor digitorum sublimis

Thumb
P: Hygiene
D: Cortical position
Tx: "Rules of Thumb" – Lengthen a short muscle; shorten a long muscle; fuse an unstable thumb; augment a weak muscle (transferring from site of more power)

Thumb
P: Poor grasp, hygiene, cosmesis, web space contraction (House Type 1)
D: Contracted abductor pollicis, active interphalangeal joint extension and abduction of thumb
Tx: Abductor pollicis release (Matev) to increase web space

Thumb
P: Poor grasp, hygiene and cosmesis (House type 2)
D: Flexed metacarpal phalangeal of thumb but some variable function of IP flexion and extension
Tx: Shorten or augment EPL with PL/BR/FDS; augment abductor pollicis with BR/PL or lengthen adductor longus

Thumb
P: Poor grasp, hygiene, cosmesis (House type 3)
D: MCP extension contraction (hyperextension)
Tx: Adductor pollicis release, MCP fusion or plication; augment abductor pollicis longus with BR/FPL; lengthen extensor pollicis longus/EPB

P= Problem, D=Deformity, Tx= Treatment

Benik thumb abductor splint with wrist extension stabilized with integrated thermoplastic (molded by microwaving the splint to fit the thumb) during the day. At night, a dorsal resting splint is required if there is thumb abductor tightness and tight tenodesis. The splint should hold the thumb, fingers, and wrist in extension to stretch the tenodesis (no outriggers). If the resting position of the elbow is approximately 90° and passive range of motion (ROM) of elbow extension is approximately −50°, a long resting splint that incorporates the elbow may be used at night, or an elbow extension splint may be used as well. Air splints may be used for elbow extension for 10 minutes during crawling, keyboard use, and arm-reaching play. Soft neoprene supinator "twister" splints may also be used during activity. These may be constructed with a Benik splint and a long neoprene strip spiraling up the forearm, or may be obtained readymade from an orthotics manufacturer. The child 4 to 9 years old should wear the same night splints as above, but not wear the splints as much during the day and only for function. Unfortunately, the adolescent splinting program is often futile due to dissatisfaction with cosmesis and lack of compliance.

Cerebral Palsy Functional Scoring Levels: Scoring Scales

There are many ways to classify the levels of function of the child with CP. Reasons for a classification system include being able to compare outcomes of similar children, noticing trends in abilities of these similar children to be able to help predict the type of care the child will need, and the effectiveness of hand surgery. Table R25 includes scoring scales that help quantify the use of the hand and upper extremity so that there can be a presurgery and postsurgery comparison with objectivity. Functional limitations are influenced by a variety of issues each child faces. There are many different assessment tools based on the goals of the measurement. Many of these are commercially available (see Table R25).

Green's Scale is a quick progressive description of use of the upper extremity by the child with CP and reflects cognitive, sensory, reflexive, and orthopaedic limits in a concise list that families can understand. This scale permits the child, family, physician, therapist, etc. to rate the following function for both upper extremities and can be used before and after surgery. The expectation of improving one level after surgery is realistic. The Green's Scale categorizes use of the upper extremities as poor, fair, good, and excellent. The term POOR is applied to describe the function of the upper extremity capable of lifting paper weight only, having poor or absent grasp and release, and poor control. FAIR is used to describe the upper extremity having a helping hand without effectual use in dressing, has fair control, and slow, not effective grasp/release. The term GOOD describes the upper extremity with a good helping hand, good grasp/release, and good control. EXCELLENT is used to explain the upper extremity having good use in dressing, eating, and general activities, effective grasp/release, and excellent control.

The A.I. duPont Hospital for Children's (AIDHC) Clinic Scale was designed to classify the upper extremity functional ability of children with CP. This orthopaedist's scale is used in a busy clinic and requires no equipment to administer. By assessing the child's movement both actively and passively and with parent report on use of the limb, the examiner can use the data to assist in treatment planning. Level of function is categorized in a series of types from 0 through V (Table R19). Parents of children with CP are asked to assess the use their child makes of her hands by way of an upper extremity questionnaire (Table R20). A correlation is being studied between the parents' assessments and the functional types as determined by the surgeons, as well as the outcomes after surgery. Generally, after surgical intervention functional type is increased by one level, thereby improving the collective functional activities of most children.

The Quality of Upper Extremity Skills Test (QUEST) is used to measure hand function by evaluating four domains: dissociated movement, grasp, protective extension, and weight bearing. It is designed for use with children

Table R19. Functional report: Upper extremity (UE) functional classification for CP (AIDHC).

_____ R _____L   Type 0 (No function, position interferes)
_____ No contractures
_____ With dynamic contractures
_____ With fixed contractures

_____ R _____L   Type I (Uses hand as paperweight or swipe only, poor or absent grasp and release, poor control)
_____ No contractures
_____ With dynamic contractures
_____ With fixed contractures

_____ R _____L   Type II (Mass grasp, poor active control)
_____ No contractures
_____ With dynamic contractures
_____ With fixed contractures

_____ R _____L   Type III (Can actively grasp/release slow and place object with some accuracy)
_____ No contractures
_____ With dynamic contractures
_____ With fixed contractures

_____ R _____L   Type IV (Shows some fine pinch such as holding pen, some key pinch with thumb)
_____ No contractures
_____ With dynamic contractures
_____ With Fixed contractures

_____ R _____L   Type V (Normal to near-normal function; fine opposition of thumb; can do buttons and tie shoes)
_____ No contractures
_____ With dynamic contractures
_____ With fixed contractures

who have neuromotor dysfunction with spasticity and has been validated for use in children from 18 months to 8 years of age and correlates strongly with the Peabody Developmental Fine Motor Scales. The House Scale describes the thumb position in progressive degrees of contracture.

The Shriner's Hospital (South Carolina) Upper Extremity Test (SHUE) is currently under development and evaluation. It is a series of activities to permit observation of function that the child with hemiplegic CP demonstrates. The therapist observes joint positions for the following contractures while performing a variety of functional activities. Joint position during elbow extension is viewed while the child throws a large therapy ball, bounces a ball, places a sticker on a ball, and ties shoelaces. Having the child place a sticker on a large ball, open a wallet, use a knife and fork with Theraputty, hold a wallet, and throw and bounce a large therapy ball allows joint position during wrist extension to be viewed. Observation of joint position during supination can be observed by having the child place her palm on the opposite-side cheek and during the palm-up hand-slap activity "give me five" and receive five. The joint position of thumb (open web, neutral web, thumb in palm) function can be viewed during activities such as removing paper money from a wallet, removing a sticker from a sheet, holding paper when cutting it with scissors, and opening the top of a large-mouth thermos.

Table R20. Upper extremity questionaire.

Instructions: Please answer questions 1 through 5. When answering yes to a question, please circle any and all comments (a through d) that apply.

My child uses the involved arm very little. Yes_____   No_____
I find it difficult to adequately cleanse the elbow of my child.
I find it difficult to adequately cleanse the wrist of my child.
My child's arm (s) make it difficult to dress because of the positions.

My child can use the involved arm somewhat. Yes_____   No_____
My child can position the arm/hand on his/her own.
My child tends to use the involved hand/arm as a paperweight or post while the opposite extremity performs a task.
My child can use the involved arm to turn switches on and off.

My child has some ability to hold large objects in the affected hand. Yes_____   No_____
My child seems to have difficulty managing small objects (i.e. pick up a pen).
If my child uses a walker, he/she can use the involved arm to hold the walker.
My child has the ability to place objects (i.e. blocks) into my hand or a container when asked.

My child has some ability to dress alone. Yes_____   No_____
My child can use the involved hand to pull up his/her pants
My child can use the involved hand to zip a zipper (holds the tab end).
My child can use the involved hand to do buttons.
My child can use the involved hand to turn doorknobs.

My child can use the involved hand fairly well. Yes_____   No_____
My child can tie his/her own shoes (not velcro straps)
My child can draw with the involved hand (i.e. make stick figures).
My child's thumb tends to get in the way during tasks.

The results of this questionnaire are compared to an answer key. A perfect score adds up to 21 points. Each item is worth one point if the item is not a problem for the child to perform.

Tenodesis effect is assessed by holding the finger straight and measuring the range of passive wrist extension. Spontaneous use of the limb can be determined by observing the child's use of both hands during activities such as ball catch, stabilizing objects, and tying shoelaces. For information about SHUE, contact the Occupational Therapy Department of the Shriner's Hospital of South Carolina in Greenville, SC at (864)240-6277.

Overall Evaluation of CP in Occupational Therapy

For an overall perspective of CP, one may use some general scoring scales for CP from an occupational therapy point of view to evaluate tone, trunk, and neck control as well as fine motor control of the upper extremities.[37] To achieve this perspective one must assess the following: type of CP, therapy issues as indicated, associated problems, sensory integration, cognitive integration, and psychosocial skills. Young children with CP also are having neurologic development , therefore maintaining a developmental perspective of function especially functional development of hand use is important (Figure R9).

The types of CP include those with motor cortex lesions (hemiplegia, quadriplegia, spastic, diplegia), basal ganglia lesions (fluctuating tone, dystonia, diakinesis athetosis), and cerebellar lesions (ataxia).

A   B

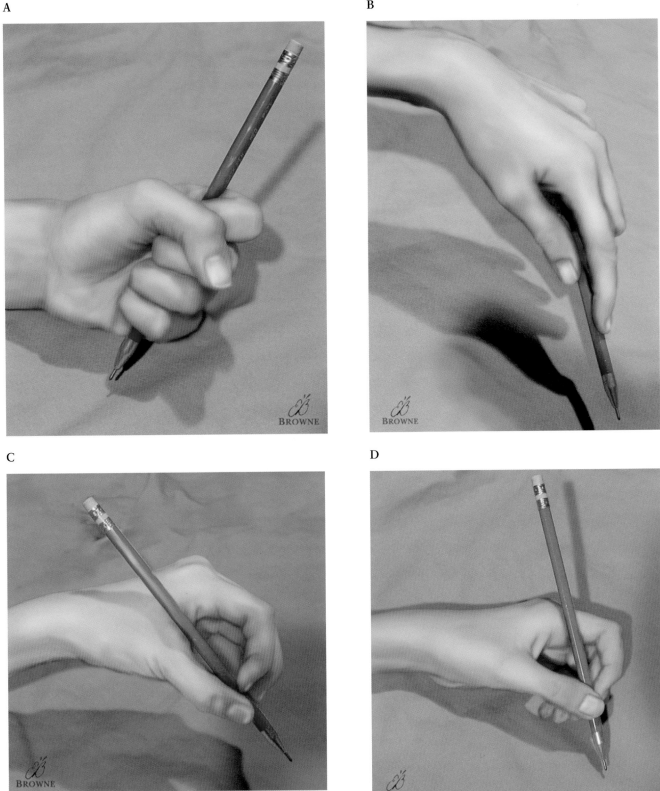

C   D

Figure R9. Hand grasp and position can be classified by developmental stage. Palmar-supinated grasp predominates from age 1 to 2 years (A). When the hand is used it is usually fisted, wrist slightly flexed, and supinated with movement being produced by motion of the whole arm. Between 2 and 3 years of age, digital-pronated grasp predominates with finger grasp, straight pronated ulnar deviated wrist in which movement mainly occurs in the forearm (B). From age 3 to 4 years, static tripod posture predominates in which there is rather crude finger grasp and most motion occurs in the wrist (C). Between 4 and 6 years of age, dynamic tripod postures becomes the norm in which there is better fine grasp with the fingers and motion is occurring in the fingers (D).

Issues to address in therapy as indicated are varied and first include the neuromuscular components and how they affect self-care.[38] In that category, the quality and distribution of tone (spasticity, athetosis, both, athetosis with tonic spasms, choreoathetosis, flaccid, ataxia) is considered using a spasticity scale such as Ashworth's Scale[39] or a general description of the spasticity.[40] Next, range of motion is assessed for patterns that may lead to scoliosis, kyphosis, forearm pronation, wrist flexion, swan neck finger deformities, hip subluxation, contractures of elbow/hip adduction, knee flexion, and ankle plantarflexion, etc. Focus is then directed toward quality of movement and includes evaluation of position and the need for hand/wrist splints, and of posture and the need for equipment for seating, wheelchair, bath and toilet supports, etc. Finally, reflexes and reactions such as symmetric tonic neck reflex (STNR), asymmetric tonic neck reflex (ATNR), positive supporting obligatory, and slow protective balance are considered. There are many additional and detailed upper extremity reflexes[41] (Table R21).

Associated problems include seizures, hearing difficulties, eye musculature imbalance, vision problems, mental retardation, obesity, urinary tract infection, and malnutrition/failure to thrive.

Sensory integration assessment includes the evaluation of sensory awareness and sensorimotor processing components and how they affect occupations of work, leisure, and self-care:[38] tactile, proprioceptive, vestibular, visual, auditory, gustatory, and olfactory. Also, through perceptual components and how they affect occupations of work, leisure and self-care:[38] stereognosis, kinesthesia, body scheme, right–left discrimination, form constancy, position in space, visual closure, figure ground, depth perception, and topographic orientation.

Cognitive integration is determined by assessing arousal, attention, orientation, memory, problem solving, and generalization of learning.

Assessment of psychosocial skills and psychologic components incorporates the evaluation of personality characteristics such as lability, passivity and dependence, resistance to change, and frustration.

Occupational Therapy Evaluation Before Proposed Surgery

Because the surgical procedure(s) produce a biomechanical change, the occupational therapy evaluation encompasses both orthopaedic and functional components. To obtain active/passive ROM (A/PROM) measurement of both upper extremities, a standard goniometry of the upper extremities is performed as well as the passive stretch of the tenodesis and spasticity interference. Evaluation of active ROM includes joint measurement as well as observation of patterns and synergistic motions. If the angle of ulnar deviation is severe, it will make it difficult for the child to see what is being grasped. Severe wrist flexion decreases the ability of the index pad to touch the thumb and mechanical advantage is lost, although it may make opening the fingers easier for pointer use. Swan neck deformities frequently occur with the child's overall finger and wrist extension effort. Synergistic movements that indicate primitive reflexes or spasticity influences are noted. These motions will decrease the ease or ability for large improvements from surgery. Primitive reflexes include Moro or startle reflex, ATNR, STNR, or extensor thrust used to flex the shoulders for arm positioning. Associated reactions may include synkinesis demonstrated by mirroring motions of the stronger extremity, overflow, and oral grimace or tongue use during activities. Basic reflexes that may still persist will decrease the effectiveness of coordinated smooth movement and subsequent function.

Table R21. Upper extremity reflexes.

Hoffmann's sign	A finger flick of the index finger produces clawing of fingers and thumb.
Klippel and Weil thumb sign	Quick extension of fingers causes flexion and adduction of thumb.
Chaddock's wrist sign	Stroking the ulnar side of the forearm near the wrist causes flexion of the wrist with extension fanning of the fingers.
Gordon's finger sign	Pressure exerted over the pisiform bone results in flexion of the fingers or the thumb and index finger.
Tromner's sign	The finger flexion reflex is sharp tap on the palmar surface or the tips of the middle three fingers producing prompt flexion of the fingers.
Babinski's pronation sign	The patient places his hands in approximation with the palms upward and the examiner jars them several times with his own hands from below. The affected hand will fall in pronation, the sound limb remaining horizontal.
Bechterew's sign	The patient flexes and then relaxes both forearms. The paralyzed forearm falls back more slowly and in a jerky manner, even when contractures are mild.
Leri's sign	Upon forceful passive flexion of the wrist and fingers, there is absence of normal flexion of the elbow
Mayer's sign	Absence of normal adduction and opposition of the thumb upon passive forceful flexion of the proximal phalanges (MP joint), especially of the third and fourth fingers of the supinated hand. This procedure may be painful and will decrease cooperation of the patient.
Souque's sign	In attempting to raise the paralyzed arm, the fingers spread out and remain separated.
Sterling's sign	Adduction of a paretic arm occurs upon forceful active adduction, against resistance of the unaffected normal arm.
Strumpell's pronation sign	Upon flexing the forearm, the dorsum of the hand instead of the palm approaches the shoulder.
Forced grasping	Firm radial directed stroking by the examiner's fingers across the subject's palm causes a grasp reaction of the hand.
Kleist's hooking sign	Reactive flexion of the fingers of the affected hand upon pressure exerted by the examiner's hand against the flexor surface of the finger tips
Oral motor	Decreased chest mobility, decreased lip closure, tongue thrust affecting feeding, swallowing, drooling, articulation, dysarthria
Palmo-mental	A vertical stroke along the radial border of the child's thumb will produce a contraction of the chin (mental muscles) if abnormal.

Evaluation of passive ROM is impacted by muscle tone, which can be assessed by Hoffman's sign, finger flick elicits thumb flexion clonus; Klippel–Weil sign, flexed fingers quickly extended elicits thumb flexion/adduction or clonus; and Ashworth's spasticity scale using the elbow extension test.[40] There are many associated reflexes[41] (see Table R21).

How the range interferes with function, such as difficulty dressing when placing flexed wrists into sleeves, or externally rotated arms getting caught when rolling wheelchairs through doors, is also evaluated. Tenodesis tightness will require a resting hand splint with the wrist placed in the best extension/finger extension after surgery because the FCU to ECRB procedure will increase the tenodesis tightness when the wrist is extended. Skin maceration may be due to a deep wrist crease, fisted hand, and/or antecubital fossa.

A significant aspect of upper extremity function is grasp and the functional use of both arms. Many of the children evaluated are functionally and/or cognitively very limited; thus, selecting the best evaluation test is challenging. A simple observation of how the child is able to stabilize objects, such as wrist as a weight on paper, holding a jar to open with the other hand, or perform a grasp–release task will give a pre- and postassessment measure for each child. Unilateral tests will also give more specific details in actual prehension. Doing functional activities of daily living (ADL) such as dressing, buttoning, and toileting will also give a degree of integrated use of the hands. Basic control is observed for extrinsic and intrinsic hand muscle skill: supination and pronation, wrist flexion, extension, ulnar and radial deviation, finger flexion, extension, ability to abduct and adduct fingers, make an opposed pinch, and form the sign language alphabet characters (which tests isolation of fingers). Grasp strength (Dynamometer or bulbs) and pinch strength[41] is tested by how the child can perform as well as noting the angle of the wrist (usually flexion) during the grasp.

Basic grasp–release is required for the next screening. Some abnormal grasp patterns work well (Figure R10) whereas other patterns are not effective (Figure R11); for example, grasping a 1-inch cube and then releasing it into a coffee can, or stacking 1-inch cubes. The wrist angle (flexion and ulnar drift) is measured while the child is picking up and releasing large objects such as a soda bottle/can, medium-sized objects such as a 1-inch block or checker, and small-sized objects such as a pencil or Cheerio. These dexterity tests require good control of the hand and are frequently not possible with children having involved CP.

The Jebsen Hand Test is composed of seven short timed subtests that assess writing, turning cards, picking up small objects, simulated feeding, stacking checkers, lifting empty 3-inch cans, and lifting 1-pound, 3-inch cans (weight) and is normed for individuals age 6 and up.[43] Each subtest is normalized so one subtest may be useful. Thumb abduction is particularly examined with the can pick-up test. The Physical Capacities Evaluation (PCE) includes both unilateral and bilateral subtests but are normed for ages 18 through 68. The Purdue Pegboard, Crawford Small Parts, and Minnesota Rate of Manipulation (MMRT) Tests are more prevocational with endurance being one of the parameters tested.

For children with more advanced physical and cognitive skills, it is helpful to use a bilateral functional test. Observe how the child is able to stabilize objects such as paper against the wrist, holding a jar to open with the other hand, opening a wallet (take money out), unscrewing 3-inch and smaller jars, buttoning, putting on socks, taking off a sticker from a sheet, and taking a cap off a pen or marker. Doing functional ADLs such as dressing, buttoning, and toileting will also give a degree of integrated use of the hands, but will not give a numerical score or norm. Standardized tests may be too long for the attention or cognitive level of the child, too advanced, or have a prevocational focus. Therapists should consider the Peabody Developmental Scales of Fine Motor Skills for children age 4 to 14, or the Bruininks–Oseretski Test of Motor Proficiency for ages 4 to 14, and the Pennsylvania Bi-Manual for children age 17 and up. Clinical observations must be made as to the altered grasp patterns and other postural compensations, etc. Commenting about the child's ability to follow directions and the use of arms and whether the limb interferes with being dressed all give measures to compare after surgery.

After surgery, the child will need a protective wrist cock-up splint with the wrist in about 20° extension to wear continuously with brief breaks during

A

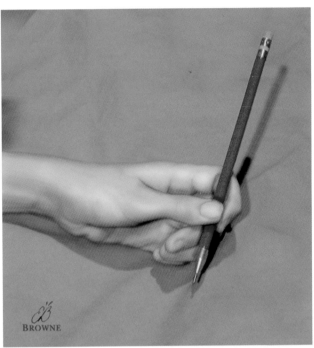

Figure R10. Some individuals develop abnormal but relatively efficient grasps with the tripod grasp being common (A). Also, the quadruped grasp (B) and the adapted tripod grasp are relatively efficient. Stabilizing the pencil between the index and long fingers may look clumsy, but it is an efficient grasp for individuals (C).

B

C

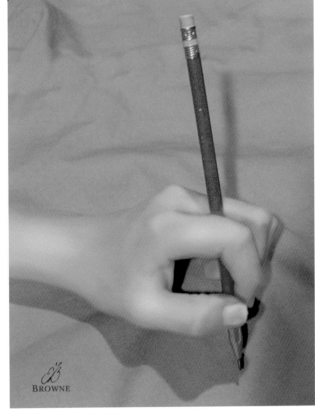

A

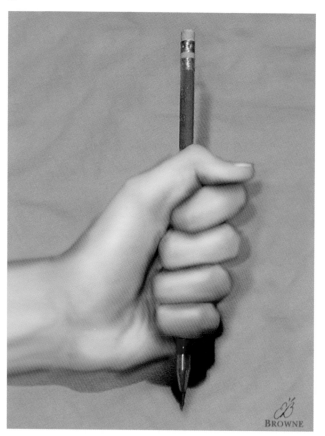

Figure R11. Inefficient grasps that develop in children with cerebral palsy include the transpalmar grasp, which is similar to the very immature grasp (A). Other more abnormal inefficient patterns include the supinated grasp (B), interdigital brace grasp (C), thumb tuck grasp (D), index curl grasp (E,F,G,), and the thumb wrap grasp (H).

B

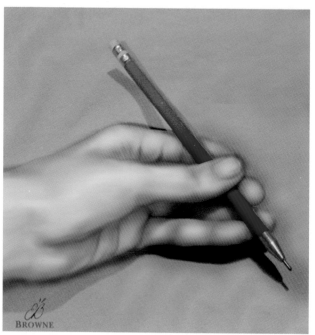

C

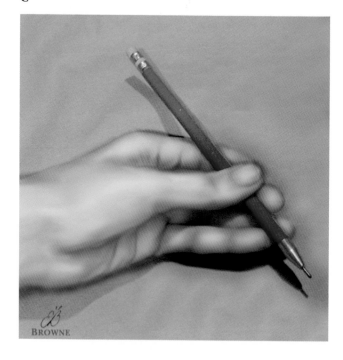

D

E

F

G

Figure R11 (continued).

Figure R11 (continued).

H

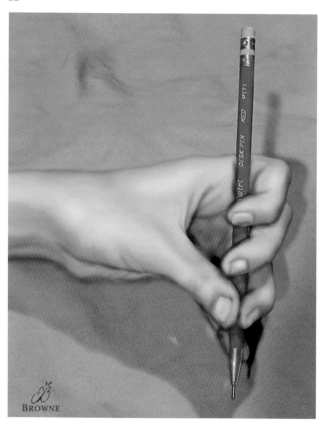

bathing and at meal times for 2 to 3 months, and for 4 to 6 months during ambulation to prevent sudden wrist flexion that may strain or injure the muscle transfers. A night resting splint with the wrist in progressively more extension to stretch the tenodesis may be indicated. Synergy or Aquaplast is used due to the strength and ease of moldability. A dorsal wrist cock-up splint is used because it is easier for the child to put on herself, controls simultaneously the wrist extension and the ulnar drift, places less splint material in the palm, and does not rely on the straps to keep the wrist stable.

Sensory testing is done to help determine if the hand has enough sensation to encourage spontaneous use of the limb. A quick screen is testing the stereognosis differentiation of a 1-inch foam block or wood block. Texture discrimination is tested in the 2- to 3-year-old, object identification in the 4- to 5-year-old, graphesthesia in the 6- to 9-year-old, and two-point discrimination in the older child. Sharp/dull sensation is tested with a paper clip and is done on all the children. The collected clinical data are recorded on a standardized worksheet (Table R22). These published evaluation instruments are available from a number of resources (see Table R25).

Treatment Precautions Following Surgery

If a FCU to ECRB transfer was performed, one should avoid forceful passive wrist flexion and resistive wrist flexion or extension during the first 2 months after cast removal. This precaution is recommended to assure that the muscle transfers are not ruptured.

Table R22. AIDHC occupational therapy clinic evaluation worksheet.

CP Hand/Pre- and Post-surgery

NAME: _____

ID#: _____   DOB: _____

DATE: _____

Referred by: _____   OTR Initials: _____

Dx: CP (Circle type)   SPASTIC   FLACCID   ATHETOID   QUAD   HEMIPLEGIC – R ____ L ____

Proposed procedure & which extremity: _____

Purpose for surgery: (Circle)   Increase wrist extension, supination, thumb abduction, elbow extension, other: _____

Pre-op ____ / ____ / ____   Surgery ____ / ____ / ____   Post-op ____   Post-op (4–6 wks.) ____   Post-op (6 mos.) ____

Dominance: R ____ L ____   Ambulation: (Circle)   W/C   W/Aids   Walks

Resting position of limb:

	SITTING R / L	STAND R / L	WALK R / L	RUN R / L	(Circle)
SHOULDER	/	/	/	/	PROTRACTED/RETRACTED/ABDUC
ELBOW	/	/	/	/	FLEXED/EXTENDED
FOREARM	/	/	/	/	SUPINATED/PRONATED
WRIST	/	/	/	/	FLEXED/EXTENDED
Wrist Deviation	/	/	/	/	RADIAL/ULNAR
HAND	/	/	/	/	FISTED/OPEN
THUMB	/	/	/	/	CORTICAL/ADDucted/ABDucted

Deformities: (List digits/joints)   Swan-neck Y ____ N ____   Boutonniere's Y ____ N ____

Strength/ROM	R A/PROM	L A/PROM	MMT 0-5 R/L
SHOULDER			
SHOULDER /			
SHOULDER ABD			
SHOULDER ADD			
SHOULDER INT ROT			
SHOULDER EXT ROT			
ELBOW V			
ELBOW/			
SUPINATION			
PRONATION			
WRIST V			
WRIST/			
ULNAR DEVIATION			
FINGERS (GROSS)			

(continued)

Table R22. Continued

PROM: TENODESIS ON STRETCH: WITH FINGERS HELD IN EXTENSION,
WHAT IS PASSIVE EXTENSION OF WRIST? R _____ L _____

ABILITY TO FOLLOW DIRECTIONS: (Circle) GOOD FAIR UNABLE

COMMUNICATION EFFECTIVENESS: (Circle)

CLEAR MILDLY UNCLEAR SPECIAL SYSTEM: _____

Comments _____

STRENGTH OF GRASP and WRIST ANGLE: R _____ # _____
L _____ # _____

TIP PINCH: R _____ # _____
L _____ # _____

LATERAL PINCH: R _____ # _____
L _____ # _____

OPPOSITION: R: THUMB to Index Y/N, to 3 Y/N, to 4 Y/N, to 5 Y/N
L: THUMB to Index Y/N, to 3 Y/N, to 4 Y/N, to 5 Y/N

GRASP/RELEASE AND TENODESIS INFLUENCE (Indicate R or L):

TIP PINCH: R _____ # _____
L _____ # _____

LATERAL PINCH: R _____ # _____
L _____ # _____

OPPOSITION: R: THUMB to Index Y/N, to 3 Y/N, to 4 Y/N, to 5 Y/N
L: THUMB to Index Y/N, to 3 Y/N, to 4 Y/N, to 5 Y/N

GRASP/RELEASE AND TENODESIS INFLUENCE (Indicate R or L):

0   1   2   3   0 = UNABLE, NO RELEASE

CUBE _____ 1 = RELEASE C WRIST FLEXED >40 DEG

PENCIL _____ 2 = RELEASE C WRIST NEUTRAL

SPOON/FORK _____ 3 = RELEASE C WRIST EXT. >20 DEG

CUP_____

CHEERIO PICK UP _____ Uses mirroring of other hand (Synkinesis)
Yes = Abnormal   No = Normal

CHEERIO TO MOUTH _____ Y/N

UNSCREW A 3″ LID _____ Y/N

JEBSEN HAND TEST (If possible): (Seconds) R _____ L _____ Standard Deviation _____

Comments _____

Write 30 letter sentence _____

Turn over 5 cards _____

Pick up 6 small objects _____

Use spoon—5 beans _____

Stack 4 checkers_____

Pick up 5 empty cans _____

Pick up 5 1# cans_____

(continued)

Table R22. Continued

REFLEX OVERFLOW: (Circle)

    STARTLE - Y/N

    HOFFMAN'S (finger claw with index flick) - Y/N

    KLIPPEL+WEIL (quick flexed fingers are extended, thumb flexes and adducts) - Y/N

SENSATION SCREEN:

    STEREOGNOSIS (Distinguish 1″ cube of foam from 1″ block of wood) - R=Y/N   L=Y/N

    SHARP/DULL - R=Y/N   L=Y/N

    2PT DISCRIMIN (Thumb and index tips 1/4″) - R=Y/N   L=Y/N

FUNCTIONAL REPORT: (AIDHC) UE Functional Classification for CP (Circle)

R/L   Type 0 (No function)
        No contractures _____   With dynamic contractures _____   With fixed contractures _____

R/L   Type I (Uses hand as paperweight or swipe only, poor or absent grasp and release, poor control)
        No contractures _____   With dynamic contractures _____   With fixed contractures _____

R/L   Type II (Mass grasp, poor active control)
        No contractures _____   With dynamic contractures _____   With fixed contractures _____

R/L   Type III (Can actively grasp/release slow and place object with some accuracy)
        No contractures _____   With dynamic contractures _____   With fixed contractures _____

R/L   Type IV (Shows some fine pinch such as holding pen, some key pinch with thumb)
        No contractures _____   With dynamic contractures _____   With fixed contractures _____

R/L   Type V (Normal to near normal function; fine opposition of thumb; can do buttons and tie shoes)
        No contractures _____   With dynamic contractures _____   With fixed contractures _____

PARENTAL REPORT: Limb interferes with dressing self (Circle)   R=Y/N   L=Y/N

SPLINTS:

PRIOR to surgery _____

AFTER surgery _____

NIGHT RESTING with hand at maximum tenodesis stretch _____

WRIST COCK-UP (For protection during ambulation)_____

SUPINATION _____

OTHER _____

VIDEO/PHOTO OF HAND GRASPING OBJECT: (Circle)

Start position   Grasp block   Pick up Cheerio   Other_____

TREATMENT RECOMMENDATIONS: _____

SURGERY EXPECTATIONS: (Review post-surgery home program and show types of splints)

                                                         _____

                                                         Therapist

Occupational Therapy Treatment Goals Following Surgery

Occupational therapy goals are to improve scar formation, avoid swelling, maintain normal position of the wrist, and prevent muscle transfers from being avulsed. Gentle restoration of grasp is also a goal, but does not include resistive strengthening or passive stretching of wrist flexion for several months. Therapy goals are progressive and begin with improving the coordination of grasp (mass grasp, and then refined grasp if feasible). Next is coordination of grasp–release accuracy and grasp with supination/pronation. Focus is then directed at improving the tripod pinch accuracy. Finally, isolated finger control (if feasible) is improved, using many in-hand manipulation activities. Examples are sign language or hand gestures, rotation of two isospheres in the palm, performing peg activities with progressively finer pegs and using resistive tools to strengthen grasp while working with the pegs, and bilateral/bimanual hobbies such as hand sewing, leather lacing, cooking, working with dough/clay, and erector set assembly.

Generally, use of the new arm and hand positions shows favorable results of improving appearance (cosmesis) and advances one functional type (AIDCH orthopaedic score) or progresses one level of the Green's scale in about 2 months; results are best at 6 months, and grip strength recovers in about 6 months.

Photography: Position with Grasp/Release Effort

Photographs obtained before and after surgery will assist documentation to help quantify the outcome. Typically the following activities are photographed if the child can perform them: resting position of the limb (elbow, wrist, and fingers), also called the "attitude" of the limb, best opening of the hand (finger extension and thumb abduction) in combination with the wrist (flexion, ulnar deviation), supination/pronation, elbow flexion/extension, shoulder position (internal or external rotation), and functional grasp and release (thumb/wrist position), which includes the child's attempts at grasping a pen on table, releasing a 1-inch cube into a coffee can, and lifting and placing a 3-inch can (from the Jebsen test). Some grasp or pen-holding patterns have a high risk for developing fatigue or writer's cramp if these postures are used over long periods of time (Figure R12).

Informational/Instructional Handouts for Families and Home Therapist

Families require written instructions and instructional handouts can be standardized. Examples include information pertaining to splint care (completed for the family when the splints are made), and postsurgery guidelines for the family and home therapist (Tables R23 and R24).

Prediction of Functional Outcomes

The more abnormal the reflexes and sensory awareness, the less function even after surgery. A combination of more than one of these systems will decrease use of the limb. Surgery will improve the position of the limb but not improve the sensory control of the limb. If influence of grasp–release skill is present before surgery, it should be better following surgery performed to improve wrist extension because the fingers and thumb will be in a better

A

B

C

D

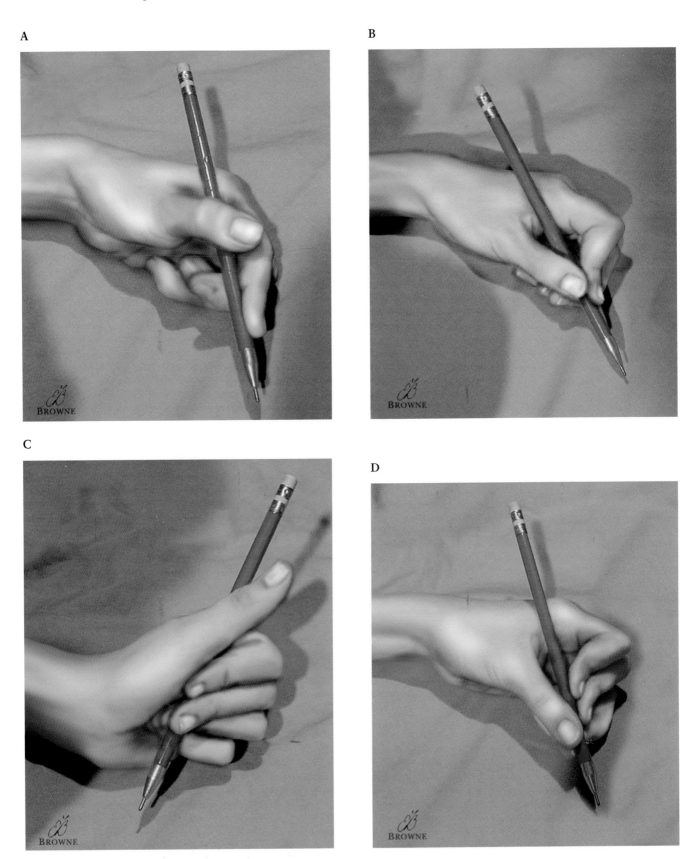

Figure R12. Some grasp patterns that develop have a high risk of leading the writers cramp if the individual does a significant amount of writing. The adducted thumb posture (A) and combinations of digit hyperextension grasps (B–D) are at-risk positions.

Table R23. Therapy services: splint care.

Purpose of Splint: This splint was prescribed by your doctor for:

_____ preventing deformity

_____ proper positioning to correct deformity

_____ increasing range of motion (gentle stretching)

_____ permitting exercise of specific muscles

_____ stabilizing for better use of involved limb

_____ protecting weak muscles, bones and/or joints

_____ permitting complete rest or healing of the limb, joints, or muscle transfers

_____ preventing the child from removing tubes, bandages, or interfering with healing

Wearing Instructions:

First, build up the length of time using the splint by wearing it about an hour and then remove it, and examine the skin for red marks. If these marks disappear within one-half hour, then wear the splint for _____ hours.

Usage:

_____ Night use Build up the length of time wearing the splint by 1 hour until reaching 5 hours; then wear all night.

_____ Day use   Wear _____ hour(s) on, and _____ hour(s) off

Instructions:

If there is pain or redness that does not resolve in one hour, contact the therapist. If sweating occurs, try sprinkling powder (without talc), cornstarch, or placing thin absorbent cotton such as a sock or stockinette between the skin and splint. Dampening the splint, shaking baking soda on the splint and rising it off can eliminate odor from body perspiration.

Be sure the splint straps are not so tight that circulation is cut off. One way to test this is to pinch the nails of the limb in the splint. The toe or finger should turn white, and then pink. If the toe or finger does NOT become pink again or develops a darker color, Recheck the fit of the splint and loosen the strap slightly.

Care of Splint:

The materials in the splint are affected by heat, so take care that it is not left near heat producing areas such as the television and radiator, or left in an enclosed car, or on a sunlit windowsill. Store the splint in a safe area away from pets and where dogs cannot get them; dogs will chew them! The splint should be washed in lukewarm water and mild soap or alcohol. Acetone (fingernail polish remover) and other chemicals should not be used near the splint.

Follow-Up:

Therapists prefer to periodically examine the splint to ensure proper fit if it is used to progressively correct deformity. Please obtain your insurance referral and then call for an appointment if you are not regularly in therapy.

Material Used: _____

_____   _____
     Therapist Constructing Splint   Phone Number

_____
          Date Constructed

Splint Care Home Program
AIDHC/MK, 1989
AIDHC 2001 Home Therapy Program

biomechanical position to grasp items on a table. If skill with influence of sensation is diminished, the use of the limb in dynamic, quick situations will be diminished. Automatic or spontaneous use of the limb will also be reduced. Influence of primitive reflexes will hinder good control or speed of control. These changes may cause a child to avoid the use of the limb.

Table R24. CP surgery: FCU to ECRB and other surgeries.

Guidelines for Family & Occupational Therapist

The main goals of surgery for the arm of a child with cerebral palsy or spasticity of the flexors are: (Check applicable)

____ less skin maceration from tight position (thumb, wrist, elbow creases, even axilla)

____ easier cleaning of these creases

____ a better appearance of the limb at rest

____ a better position of the wrist to permit easier dressing, for care-giver or individual improved ability to see what is in the hand or pinch

____ to improve a cylindrical helping-grasp

____ to improve the grasp-release but not with the expectation of a faster, normal fine

____ pincer grasp or controlled release combined with supination (enhanced dexterity)

The most common surgery is the FCU>ECRL/B which is to transfer the muscle that causes the wrist to flex and ulnarly deviate (the flexor carpi ulnaris or FCU) and transfer it to the insertion of the wrist extensor tendon (the extensor carpi radialis longus and brevis also called ECRL+B or extensor digitorum communis EDC). Associated surgeries usually performed at the same time include biceps release or lengthening, thumb abductor augmentation or thumb adductor release, pronator teres release or rerouting. Following the surgery, the arm is casted for 1 month in a position that stretches the muscles out of the deforming posture. This cast position is typically with the elbow held at 60 degrees of flexion, forearm supinated (palm toward face), and wrist extended (hand away from palm) to about 50 degrees. ROM during cast wear should occur to the shoulder and fingers several times daily to prevent stiffness.

About 1 month after surgery, the surgical dressing/cast is removed and a wrist cock-up splint for protection during ambulation or at school is made the same day as the cast removal. This splint permits grasp but prevents wrist flexion, protecting the transfer while it heals and is to be worn continuously for a period of one to two months. A night resting splint with the wrist, fingers and thumb in full extension is frequently ordered to stretch the tenodesis so that grasp-release is more effective during the day. A supination splint or elbow extension splint may also be ordered.

Home exercises include stretching the joints that were released. Elbow extension, wrist extension and thumb abduction should be done. There should be no active or passive wrist flexion for two months.

Early therapy includes gentle scar massage after the scabs are gone, monitoring swelling, monitoring scar maturation (absorbable sutures), and general wound management. Stretching should be done for the thumb into abduction and extension, the wrist into extension only, the forearm into supination and the elbow into extension. These should be done two to three times per day. The wrist splint should be worn continuously and only removed during the day for therapy or for bathing once the patient is transferred into the tub. The splint is worn all night for the next six weeks, and possibly up to six months. If the child is walking, the splint must be worn to protect the wrist from forceful flexion, which could tear the FCU transfer to the ECRB during the two to three month healing period.

For the therapist at home or school: There is a need to clarify confusion between typical hand therapy for peripheral injuries versus therapy following hand surgery for CNS involvement and spasticity such as CP. These outcome expectations differ greatly. For children with CP who have muscle transfers to balance the power of wrist flexors, the wrist cock-up splint is not intended to create a thumb post, which could cause rubbing due to spasticity, would not permit passive stretching out of the thumb-in-palm tendencies, would limit the thumb to only a pincer thumb post and would interfere with healing of palmar incisions. Instead the use of the wrist cock-up splint is to afford protection for the tendon transfers during healing by preventing fast forceful wrist flexion. The surgery together with the cock-up splint allows some mass cylindrical grasp and pinch early. If the child has a pincer grasp, it is encouraged. A pincer grasp can be assisted with a soft stretchy neoprene strap attached to the wrist cock-up splint to hold the thumb in the necessary abduction and extension and may be removed when walking, holding crutches, doing thumb stretches, etc. A firm functional thumb-post splint is only provided later if there is functional ability to pinch and use the pinch, and if the child has the ability to follow directions for that pinch. If there is some grasp and release, the family can gather a bowl of 1-inch to 3-inch sized items to pick up and move as part of games (hard, soft, fuzzy, rough, i.e., dice, cans, cubes/blocks, Legos, bristle blocks, etc.). Start with picking up and putting down of items. If successful and not frustrating, have the child pick up and put the items into slots, stack, or place on a target like a checkerboard, Tic-Tac-Toe, etc. If the child has better grasp control, try picking up coins, paperclips, buttons, playing cards, etc. Combining grasp with turning the wrist can be tried next, for example buttoning clothes, wind-up toys etc., but these are not usually possible for children with CP.

If there are further questions, please call your therapist at _____ .

11. Intrathecal Baclofen Pumps
Maura McManus, MD, FAAPMR, FAAP

Neurosurgical interventions have been brought into wide use during the past 10 to 15 years. The first is that of dorsal root rhizotomies, which has met with mixed reviews. Recent meta-analysis of affected patients demonstrates that if there is any benefit it is only in a few points of improvement and not dramatic functional improvements. Use of intrathecal baclofen in the pediatric patient having CP has yielded as good a reduction in tone as dorsal rhizotomy and does not represent an ablative procedure. This is important because, unlike rhizotomies, it is entirely reversible.

Table R25. Evaluation sources.

Crawford Small Parts from Psychological Corp, 1-800-872-1726

DeMatteo C, Law M, Russell D, Pollock N, Rosenbaum P, Walter S. The reliability and validity of the Quality of Upper Extremity Skills Test (QUEST). Phys Occup Ther Pediatr 1993;13(2):1–18.

Bruinink RH. "Bruinink-Oseretsky Test of Motor Proficiency." Circle Pines MN: American Guidance Service, 1978.

Jebsen RH. An objective and standardized test of hand function. Arch Phys Med Rehab 1969; 50:311, 1969. (Unilateral hand dexterity test made from household objects)

Mathiowitz V, Rogers SL, Dowe-Keval M, Donohoe L, Rennells C. The Purdue Pegboard: norms for 14- to 19-year olds. Am J Occup Ther 1986;40(3):174–179.

Minnesota Rate of Manipulation Test. Published by American Guidance Service, Inc., Publishers Building, Circle Pines, MN 55014

Peabody Developmental Motor Scales (PDMS-2) by M. Rhonda Folio, Rebecca R. Fewell, Austin, TX: Pro-ed. Order Number 9281 from Pro-ed, 8700 Shoal Creek Boulevard, Austin TX, 78757-6897, 1-800-897-3202

Physical Capacities Evaluation of Hand Skill (PCE). In: Bell E, Jurek K, Wilson T. Hand skill: a gauge for treatment. Am J Occup Ther 1976;30(2):80–86.

Schmidt R, Toews J. Grip strength as a measured by Jaymar dynamometer. Arch Phys Med Rehab 1970; 51:321.

Shriners Hospital, Greenville, SC. "SHUE" Evaluation. Contact the Occupational Therapy Dept. at 864-240-6277.

Taylor N, Sand PL, Jebsen RH. Evaluation of hand function in children. Arch Phys Med Rehab Mar 1973;54:129–135 (Jebsen Hand Test: Pediatric Norms).

Tiffin J, Asher E. Purdue Pegboard: norms and studies of reliability and validity. J Appl Psychol 1948;32:234. (Purdue Pegboard is available from Lafayette Instrument, 1-800-428-7545.)

Spasticity is the most common motor disorder in CP and is seen in approximately two thirds of the population.[45,56,84] It is a component of the upper motor neuron syndrome and is described as a velocity-dependent increase in resistance to passive stretch associated with increased deep tendon reflexes (DTR). Spasticity is probably due to an imbalance between inhibitory and excitatory impulses that terminate on or near the alpha motor neurons in the spinal cord.[56,63,64] In CP, there is believed to be a deficiency of descending impulses that typically stimulate the release of the inhibitory neurotransmitter gamma-aminobutyric acid (GABA). GABA acts presynaptically to inhibit the release of excitatory neurotransmitters such as glutamate and aspartate, resulting in relative excess of excitatory impulses and resultant hypertonia.[45,59,64]

Although some spasticity may be necessary for function in children with neurologic impairment, it is often a problem that can be difficult to treat. Spasticity may cause pain, limit sleep, lead to joint deformity, and interfere with function. It may also interfere with care including transfers, toileting, bathing, and dressing.[59,68,71]

Multiple approaches are available for treatment of spasticity in patients with CP. These include physical and occupational therapy for stretching, positioning, and bracing. Oral medications have been used as well as local treatments such as Botox injections and phenol motor point block injections.[56,59,68] Orthopaedic surgery may be necessary, and this may include soft-tissue releases and/or osteotomies.[84] Neurosurgical procedures such as selective dorsal rhizotomy are also available.[44,79] The goals for treatment should be realistic and individualized and they need to be agreed upon by patient, family/caregiver, and medical team. Ideally, a multidisciplinary team should be involved in the decision making. Such a team may include physical and occupational therapists, nurse, physiatrist, neurologist, orthopaedist, neurosurgeon, patient, and family.

Several oral medications have been used to reduce tone, including diazepam, baclofen, dantrolene, tizanidine, and clonidine. Although they can decrease spasticity, their sedating side effects are not well tolerated in children.[59,68,90]

Baclofen has been noted to be moderately helpful when taken orally for spasticity of spinal origin in adults. It has been relatively unhelpful in treating spasticity of cerebral origin, especially in children with CP. It is lipophilic and crosses the blood–brain barrier poorly. Intrathecal baclofen has been shown to reduce spasticity with fewer side effects.[68]

Pharmacology of Baclofen

Baclofen (lioresal) is an analogue of GABA, which is the main inhibitory neurotransmitter in the central nervous system (CNS). Intrathecal baclofen diffuses into the superficial layers of the dorsal gray matter of the spinal cord (layers II–III) where $GABA_B$ receptors are believed to be located.[70,82] These receptors have been noted in the brainstem as well. Muller et al. noted the concentration of baclofen in the cerebrospinal fluid (CSF) is 10 times higher then levels achieved by oral administration.[76] Also, there is a concentration gradient from the lumbar to cervical region of 4 to 1.[70]

History

In 1984 Penn and Kroin pioneered the use of intrathecal baclofen for spasticity in patients with multiple sclerosis and spinal cord injury.[70] Albright et al. did their first study in 1991 and a follow-up study in 1993 noting successful decrease in spasticity in patients with spasticity of cerebral origin.[45,46] In 1992 the Federal Drug Administration (FDA) approved the use of intrathecal baclofen in the form of the Medtronic SyncroMed implantable infusion system for treatment of spasticity of spinal origin. This same treatment was approved by the FDA for treatment of spasticity of cerebral origin in adults in 1992, but it was not approved for use in children until 1997.[46]

Criteria

For the success of intrathecal baclofen, careful patient selection is critical. Patients with moderately severe spasticity of spinal and cerebral origin (i.e., CP, traumatic or anoxic brain injury) have been successfully treated with intrathecal baclofen.[46,73,88] Patients with dystonia have also responded to this treatment, often at higher doses.[47] Patients with athetosis, ataxia, and myoclonus have not noted improvement. Spasticity is considered severe with Ashworth scores of greater than 3.[51] Spasticity and dystonia are believed to be problematic when they are generalized and significantly interfere with movement, positioning, or care. Patients may also experience spasticity-related pain during the day and at night, and this sometimes limits sleep. Many patients are at risk of severe joint deformity.[84] Other important issues to consider include the following[62]: the patient must have significant body mass to maintain the pump, the patient and family need to understand and accept the cosmesis of the pump, the entire team must agree upon appropriate goals, and the patient and family must be motivated to achieve these goals and be committed to the follow-up required to maintain the pump's function. Ideally, the previous assessments should be made with a multidisciplinary team in a spasticity management clinic where families can have access to adequate information. Gait analysis should be part of the evaluation in ambulatory patients.[74]

The following are additional clinical considerations, not contraindications, for intrathecal baclofen pump implantation.[62] A trial of oral baclofen is not a prerequisite for patients with spasticity of cerebral origin. Patients who have had a spinal fusion cannot undergo a trial, but this not a contraindication for pump implantation. A history of seizures is not a contraindication to intrathecal baclofen therapy. The presence of a ventriculoperitoneal (VP) shunt is not a contraindication. Patients with VP shunts may require less baclofen. Prior soft-tissue lengthenings, tendon releases, and selective dorsal rhizotomy are not contraindications. For patients with cervical or trunk weakness, the benefits of baclofen in reducing extremity spasticity must be weighed against the potential for loss of the patient's function if trunk and cervical tone is reduced. Some patients and families may be reluctant to undergo the destructive invasive procedure. The reversible nature of intrathecal baclofen may be especially important.

Screening Trial and Pump Implantation

Once a patient is felt to be a potential candidate, a screening trial is scheduled. Because of the risk of respiratory depression during the trial, it is probably most appropriately performed in a hospital on a general nursing floor.[83] Early on the day of the trial, a baseline physical exam is completed, and a lumbar puncture is performed. The test dose of either 50, 75, or 100 μg is injected into the intrathecal space. If conscious sedation is used, a short-acting sedative such as midazolam may be used in conjunction.[65] After the lumbar puncture is performed and intrathecal baclofen is injected, patients should remain flat for at least 1 hour to avoid spinal headache. Spasticity scores/Ashworth or modified Ashworth scores are recorded preinjection and at 2-hour intervals postinjection as patients are followed for 6 to 8 hours. It takes 1 to 2 hours for the baclofen to penetrate the spinal cord to produce clinical effect. Peak effect is believed to be at 4 hours.[75] Aside from noting Ashworth scores, it is important to assess patients out of bed in their seating/wheelchair system.[52] It is often difficult to obtain a functional assessment during the screening trial. Evaluation of mobility in an ambulator may be challenging as underlying weakness may limit function during the trial. Such a patient may still be a candidate for the pump because a lower dose of intrathecal baclofen can be programmed through the pump than can be achieved during the trial.[58] Although bolus injections are preferred for screening trial, continuous infusion trials using an externally placed catheter can be performed; this is important in patients in whom dystonia is being evaluated.[47,53] If the patient had a clinically significant response to intrathecal baclofen (i.e., Ashworth or modified Ashworth scores decreasing by 1 or more), the pump implantation is scheduled.

The intrathecal baclofen delivery system consists of a programmable subcutaneously implanted pump with a reservoir attached to an intraspinal catheter (Medtronics, Inc., Minnapolis, MN). The adult-sized pump with an 18-ml reservoir is 7.5 cm by 2.8 cm (similar to the size of a hockey puck). A pediatric-sized pump with a 10-ml reservoir is available. It is one third thinner, but has the same diameter as the adult-sized pump.[62] Because they are close in size, it might be difficult to justify using the pediatric-sized pump, which will need to be refilled much more frequently.

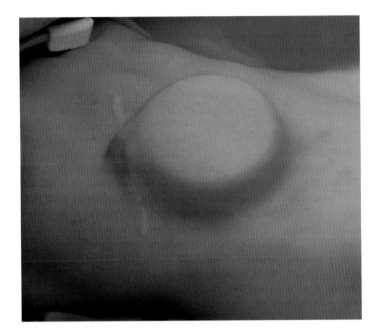

Figure R13. Baclofen pumps may be very prominent in thin children. Implanting the pump under the fascia makes it less prominent, and it is very important to implant the pump so the scar is not overlying the implant, as this has a higher risk of breaking down than normal skin

The pump is inserted under general anesthesia into a lateral abdominal subcutaneous location or under the external oblique and rectus fascia (Figure R13). A catheter is tunneled subcutaneously and connected to an intrathecal catheter. The catheter enters the subarachnoid space of the spinal canal at the lumbar spinal level.[46,62] The catheter can be placed at various heights depending on whether upper extremity relaxation is also a goal. To increase the effect of intrathecal baclofen on the upper extremities, the catheter can be placed at midthoracic level (T6–T7) rather than T11–T12.[60] The mean dosing may also be lower. The pump is programmed to deliver a continuous infusion, which assists with diffusion of baclofen into the spinal cord.

Postoperatively the patient remains supine for 48 hours to limit spinal leak and headache. For nonambulators, postoperative dose adjustments can be made daily even during bed rest. For ambulators, it may be necessary to wait until they are cleared to be out of bed to ambulate before adjusting the dose.[60,65] Adjustments should be made once daily while in the hospital postoperatively. The first follow-up visit should be at 7 to 10 days and then monthly for the first 6 months. It may take 6 to 9 months to gradually titrate the dose to the desired clinical response. In some cases, the dose may need adjustment for the first 2 years after implantation.[46,73] Typically, the dose of intrathecal baclofen is not related to age or weight. As noted above, patients with VP shunt may require a lower dose.

The pump reservoir is refilled by percutaneous puncture through a septum in the pump at intervals of 1 to 3 months. Dosage adjustments are made via an external computer/programmer and transmitted to the pump by a handheld radiofrequency wand. The pump can be programmed to deliver the baclofen in several modes including simple continuous infusion, complex continuous infusion (i.e., rate changes at set times during the day), and bolus infusion mode.[62]

Complications

Complications seen with the intrathecal baclofen infusion system may be related to the medication, the pump, the catheter, or the surgical procedure.

Complications related to the medication may be seen during the trial, immediately postoperatively, or during maintenance therapy especially at the time of dose adjustments. Common adverse affects of the medication include somnolence, headache, nausea, vomiting, hypotonia, dizziness, and increased constipation. Transient urinary retention/hesitation has been noted after dose adjustment, and this appears to respond to decreasing the dose.[66,77] The most serious side effects of medication overdose include respiratory depression and loss of consciousness progressing to coma. There is no specific antidote for treating overdose, but reports suggest that intravenous (IV) physostigmine may reverse the central effects, most notably drowsiness and respiratory depression.[76] Pediatric dosage of physostigmine is 0.02 mg/kg IV, with no more than 0.5 mg/min. This dose may be repeated at 5- to 10-minute intervals if necessary, with a maximum dose of 2 mg.[62]

Complications of intrathecal baclofen withdrawal have been well documented in the literature; they include rapid increase in spasticity, irritability, hallucinations, seizures, and pruritus without rash. Muscle rigidity, rhabdomyolysis, multiorgan system failure, and death have been reported but are quite rare.[87]

Other complications are more easily divided into immediate postoperative and late complications. Immediate postoperative complications include infection at pump or catheter site, meningitis, wound dehiscence, seroma, or cerebrospinal fluid (CSF) leak.[46,72,73] Infections have lead to pump removal, but the overall number of postoperative infections has decreased with use of prophylactic antibiotics. CSF leak may be suspected if postoperative spinal headache persists. Fluid collection and/or leakage at the catheter site in the lumbar region may also present as a CSF leak. Such a leak usually seals off within 1 to 2 days but may take as long as 2 to 3 weeks. If the spinal leak persists, a blood patch may be considered.[65]

Late complications can involve pump and catheter problems and skin breakdown, as well as human error. Skin breakdown over the pump site has been seen under braces or seatbelts. Close monitoring of pump site and adjustments to wheelchairs and braces can limit this problem. Human error can lead to programming errors, improper filling of the reservoir, and errors in dosing concentration. The highest probability of seeing these problems is within 48 hours after refill.[83]

Pump problems may include positional and mechanical problems. Pumps have been reported to flip over, especially in obese patients, and more secure suturing may limit this. Mechanical problems include battery failure and rotor lock problems. Low battery level can be detected by interrogating the pump. Current batteries, placed since 1999, have a longer lifespan of 7 years, rather than 4 years as observed in the original pumps. With a low reservoir volume, less than 2 ml, the pump will slow the rate automatically, and this can lead to an underinfusion of programmed dose. If a rotor lock problem develops, this may also present with the patient receiving less medication than was programmed. This can be evaluated by obtaining an X-ray of the pump to identify the roller and repeat X-ray in 24 hours should reveal roller-changing position.[62]

Catheter problems can include a kink, fracture, blockage, migration, and disconnection. Patients can present with signs of limited clinical response or even clinical withdrawal. After interrogating the pump, a radiologic examination with anteroposterior and lateral views of the pump and catheter system should be obtained. If an X-ray provides minimal information, a check of the catheter patency to the site of delivery with either contrast media or radiolabeled indium is indicated.[62] Follow-up X-rays are reviewed after radiopaque solution is injected. After radiolabeled indium is used, serial nuclear medicine scans over 12 to 24 hours are reviewed.[85] After the cause of intrathecal baclofen interruption is determined, either surgical repair, revision, or replacement of system components is carried out. Catheter problems overall have been reduced since catheters have been made more flexible and since the one-catheter system has replaced the two-catheter system.

Outcomes

The benefits of intrathecal baclofen have been published in the spinal cord injury literature and more recently in the CP literature.[46,49,50,81] Functional improvements and improved quality of life have been reported in the treatment of both spasticity and dystonia. These benefits include increased comfort and ease of positioning, with increased seating tolerance and decreased caregiver burden; this has been reported in areas of bathing, toileting, and dressing. Decreased pain and improved sleep have also been noted.[46,50,52] Many families have reported increased smiling, engaging, and socializing at home and at school. Functional improvement has been noted in upper extremities as well as lower extremities.[48]

Although the benefits of intrathecal baclofen in the spastic quadriplegic population are well documented, the role of intrathecal baclofen in ambulatory patients is not as clear.[50,72,73] One study by Albright et al. investigated functional improvement in ambulators, marginal ambulators, and nonambulators. Of 24 patients, clinicians noted functional improvement in 9, no change in 12, and worsening function in 3. Subjectively, 20 of 24 of these families felt gait had improved.[58] This is a promising study even without formal gait analysis. Pre- and postintrathecal baclofen gait analysis will likely add significant information.[74] Intrathecal baclofen treatment in CP may reduce the need for subsequent orthopaedic surgery related to spasticity and may decrease the need for multiple orthopaedic procedures.[57]

Some challenges to outcome include the fact that there is more effect from intrathecal baclofen on lower extremities then upper extremities. If patients and families feel strongly about optimizing upper extremity function, they need to be aware that standing, transfers, and ambulation may be lost.

One great advantage of intrathecal baclofen compared to selective dorsal rhizotomy is that the dose of intrathecal baclofen can be titrated to carefully reduce tone while not completely eliminating it.[48] This has been demonstrated to be very helpful in children who have significant spasticity with lower extremity weakness who inherently use some of the spasticity in their lower extremities to ambulate. Another advantage is if patients and families are not completely satisfied with the intrathecal baclofen therapy, the system may be removed.

Summary

Intrathecal baclofen treatment has been shown to successfully decrease generalized spasticity in patients with CP. The benefits in spastic quadraplegic patients have been demonstrated. While there does seem to be a functional benefit in ambulatory patients, the role of intrathecal baclofen in this group is not as clear. This continues to need further study, particularly with gait analysis.

Success of the intrathecal baclofen therapy does seem to be related to appropriate patient selection, setting of achievable goals, patient and family motivation and compliance, and dedicated multidisciplinary team.

References

1. DeGangi, GA, Royeen C. Current practice among neurodevelopmental treatment association members. Am J Occup Ther 1994;48(9)803–9.
2. Bly L. A historical and current view of the basis of NDT. Pediatr Phys Ther 1991; 131–5.
3. Slominski AH. Winthrop Phelps and the Children's Rehabilitation Institute. Management of motor disorders of children with cerebral palsy. In: Scrutton D, ed. Management of the Motor Disorders of Children with Cerebral Palsy. London: Spastics International Medical Publications, 1984:59–74.
4. Damiano DL, Vaughan CL, Abel MF. Muscle response to heavy resistance exercise in children with spastic cerebral palsy. Dev Med Child Neurol 1995;37:731–9.
5. Wiley ME, Damiano DL. Lower-extremity strength profiles in spastic cerebral palsy. Dev Med Child Neurol 1998;40:100–7.
6. Faigenbaum AD, Westcott WL, Loud RL, Long C. The effects of different resistance training protocols on muscular strength and endurance development in children. Pediatrics 1999;104:e5.
7. Lockwood RJ, Keyes AM. Conditioning with Physical Disabilities. Champaign, IL: Human Kinetics, 1994.
8. American Academy of Pediatrics. 1990. Strength training, weight and power lifting by children and adolescents (RE9196). Committee on Sports Medicine 1989–1990. http://www.aap.org/policy/03327
9. MacPhail HEA, Kramer JF. Effect of isokinetic strength training on functional ability and walking efficiency in adolescents with cerebral palsy. Dev Med Child Neurol 1995;37:763–75.
10. Darrah J, Wessel J, Nearingburg P, O'Connor M. Evaluation of a community fitness program for adolescents with cerebral palsy. Pediatr Phys Ther 1999;11: 18–23.
11. Darrah J, Fan JSW, Chen LC, Nunweiler J, Watkins B. Review of the effects of progressive resisted muscle strengthening in children with cerebral palsy: a clinical consensus exercise. Pediatr Phys Ther 1997;9:12–7.
12. Horvat M. Effects of a progressive resistance-training program on an individual with spastic cerebral palsy. Am Correct Ther J 1987;41:7–11.
13. McCubbin JA, Shasby GB. Effects of isokinetic exercise on adolescents with cerebral palsy. Adapted Physical Activity Quarterly 1985;2:56–64.
14. Johnson LM, Nelson MJ, McCormack CM, Mulligan HF. The effect of plantarflexor muscle strengthening on the gait and range of motion at the ankle in ambulant children with cerebral palsy: a pilot study. N Z J Physiother 1998;26: 8–14.
15. Damiano DL, Kelly LE, Vaughan CL. Effects of a quadriceps femoris strengthening program on crouch gait in children with cerebral palsy. Phys Ther 1995; 75:658–67.
16. Damiano DL, Abel MF. Functional outcomes of strength training in spastic cerebral palsy. Arch Phys Med Rehabil 1998;79:119–125.
17. Carr JH, Shepherd R. Neurological rehabilitation: optimizing motor performance. Theoretical consideration in balance assessment. Aust J Physiother 2001; 47:89–100.
18. Long C. Handbook of Pediatric Physical Therapy. Baltimore: Williams & Wilkins, 1995:198–200.
19. Woolacott, MH, Shumway-Cook A. Development of posture and gait across the lifespan. In: Long C. Handbook of Pediatric Physical Therapy. Baltimore: Williams & Wilkins, 1995:198–200.
20. Nasher LM, Shuymway-Cook A, Marin O. Stance posture control in select groups of children with cerebral palsy: deficits in sensory organization and muscular coordination. Exp Brain Res 1983;49:393–409.
21. Gentile AM. Skill acquisition. Aust J Physiotherapy 2001;47:89–100.
22. Michaud LJ. Electrical stimulation in children. In: Pediatric Rehabiltation State of the Art Reviews. Physical Medical Rehabilitation, Vol. 14, No. 2. Philadelphia: Hanley and Belfus, year:347–362.

23. Reed B. The physiology of neuromuscular electrical stimulation. Pediatr Phys Ther 1997;9:100. As adapted from Baker LL, McNeal DR, Benton LA. Neuromuscular Electrical Stimulation: A Practical Guide, 3rd ed. Downey, CA: Los Amigos Research and Education Institute, 1993.

24. Bertoti DB. Effect of therapeutic horseback riding on posture in children with cerebral palsy. Phys Ther 1988;68:1505–1512.

25. Heine B, Benjamin J. Introduction to hippotherapy. Adv Phys Ther PT Assist 2000;June:11–13.

26. Haehl V, C Giulinai, C Lewis. Influence of hippotherapy on the kinematics and functional performance of two children with cerebral palsy. Pediatr Phys Ther 1999;11:89–101.

27. MacKinnon JR, Therapeutic horseback riding: a review of the literature. Phys Occup Ther Pediatr 1995;15:1–15.

28. MacKinnon JRA study of therapeutic effects of horseback riding for children with cerebral palsy. Phys Occup Ther Pediatr 1995;15:17–30.

29. MacPhail HEA, J Edwards, J Golding, et al. Trunk postural reactions in children with and without cerebral palsy during therapeutic horseback riding. Pediatr Phys Ther 1998;10:143–7.

30. McCloskey S. The effects of hippotherapy on gait in children with neuromuscular disorders. AHA News Summer 2000;10–14.

31. McGibbon NH Andrade CK, Widener G, Cintas H, et al. Effect of an equine-movement program on gait, energy expenditure, and motor function in children with spastic cerebral palsy: a pilot study. Dev Med Child Neurol 1998;40:754–62.

32. Quest Therapeutic Services, Inc. Hippotherapy volunteer information packet. 461 Cann Rd., West Chester, PA 19382. (610) 692-0350. e-mail:SandraMcCloskey @msn.com

33. North American Riding for the Handicapped Association (www.narha.org/PDFFiles/tr_cp.pdf).

34. Thorpe DE, Reilly MA. The effects of aquatic resistive exercise on lower extremity strength, energy expenditure, function mobility, balance and self-perception in an adult with cerebral palsy: a retrospective case report. Aquat Phys Ther 2000;8(2):18–24.

35. Bidabe L. M.O.V.E.: (Mobility Opportunities Via Education) Curriculum. Bakersfield, CA: Kern County Superintendent of Schools, 1990.

36. Barnes SB, Whinnery KW. Mobility opportunities via education (MOVE): theoretical foundations. Phys Disab 1997;16(1):33–46.

37. Case-Smith J, Allen A, Pratt PN. Occupational Therapy for Children, Vol. 3. St. Louis: Mosby, 1996.

38. Dunn W, ed. Pediatric Occupational Therapy. Thorofare, NJ: Slack, 1991.

39. Damiano DL, Quinlivan JM, Owen BF, Payne P, Nelson KC, Abel MF. What does the Ashworth scale really measure and are instrumented measures more valid and precise? Dev Med Child Psychol 2002;44(2):112–118.

40. Pedretti L. Occupational Therapy, Practice Skills for Physical Dysfunction. St. Louis: Mosby, 1985:89.

41. Chusid JG, McDonald JJ. Correlative Neuroanatomy and Functional Neurology. Los Altos, CA: Lange, 1964:212 (persistent reflexes in the UE and hand).

42. Mathiowitz V. Grip and pinch strength: norms for 6-19 year olds. Am J Occup Ther 1986; 40:705–711.

43. Jebsen RH. An objective and standardized test of hand function. Arch Phys Med Rehabil 1969;50:311.

44. Abbott R. Selective rhizotomy for treatment of childhood spasticity. J Child Neurol 1996;11:S36–42.

45. Albright AL, Cervi A, Singletary J. Intrathecal baclofen for spasticity in cerebral palsy. JAMA 1991;265:1418–22.

46. Albright AL, Barron WB, Fasick MP, Polinko P, Janosky J. Continuous intrathecal baclofen infusion for spasticity of cerebral origin. JAMA 1993; 270:2475–7.

47. Albright AL, Barry MJ, Fasick P, Barron W, Schultz B. Continuous intrathecal baclofen for symptomatic generalized dystonia. Neurosurgery 1996;38:934–9.

48. Albright AL, Barry MJ, Fasick MP, Janosky J. Effects of continuous intrathecal baclofen infusion and selective dorsal rhizotomy on upper extremity spasticity. Pediatr Neurosurg 1995;23:82–85.

49. Armstrong RW. Intrathecal baclofen and spasticity: what do we know and what do we need to know? Dev Med Child Neurol 1992;34:739–745.

50. Armstrong RW, Steinbok P, Cochrane DD, Kube S, Fife SE, Farrell K. Intrathecally administered baclofen for the treatment of children with spasticity of cerebral palsy. J Neurosurg 1997;87:409–14.

51. Ashworth B. Preliminary trial of carisoprodol in multiple sclerosis. Practitioner 1964;192:540–2.

52. Barry MJ, Albright AL, Shultz BL. Intrathecal baclofen therapy and the role of the physical therapist. Pediatr Phys Ther 2000;12:77–86.

53. Butler C, Cambell S. Evidence of the effects of intrathecal baclofen for spastic and dystonic cerebral palsy. AACPDM Treatment Outcomes Committee Review Panel. Dev Med Child Neurol 2000;42:634–45.

54. Campbell SK, Almeida GL, Penn RD, Corcos DM. The effects of intrathecally administered baclofen on function in patients with spasticity. Phys Therapy 1995; 75:352–62.

55. Frost F, Nanninga J, Penn R. Intrathecal baclofen infusion: effects on bladder management programs in patients with myelopathy. Am J Phys Med Rehabil 1989;68:112–5.

56. Gans B, Glenn M. In Glenn M, Whyte J, eds. The Practical Management of Spasticity in Children and Adults. Philadelphia: Lea & Febiger, 1990:1–7.

57. Geszten PC, Albright AL, Johnstone GF. Intrathecal baclofen infusion and subsequent orthopedic surgery in patients with cerebral palsy. J Neurosurg 1998; 88:1009–13.

58. Gerszten PC, Albright AL, Barry MJ. Effect on ambulation of continuous intrathecal baclofen infusion. Pediatr Neurosurg 1997;27:40–4.

59. Gormley ME Jr. Management of spasticity in children. Part 2: Oral and intrathecal baclofen. J Head Trauma Rehabil 1999;2:207–9.

60. Grabb PA, Guin-Renfroe S, Meythaler JM. Midthoracic catheter placement for intrathecal baclofen administration in children with quadriplegic spasticity. Neurosurgery 1999;45:833–7.

61. ITB technical note. The effects of magnetic resonance imaging (MRI) on Medtronic drug infusion systems. Minneapolis: Medtronic Inc., 2000.

62. ITB product monograph. Minneapolis: Medtronic Inc., 1998.

63. Katz R. Management of spasticity. Am J Phys Med Rehabil 1988; 67:108–116.

64. Katz RT, Campagnolo DI. Pharmacologic management of spasticity. Phys Med Rehabil State Art Rev 1994;8:473–80.

65. Keenan C, Alexander M, Sung I, Miller F, Dabney K. Intrathecal baclofen for treatment of spasticity in children. Phys Med Rehabil State Art Rev 2000;12: 275–83.

66. Keisswetter H, Schober W. Lioresal in the treatment of neurogenic bladder dysfunction. Urol Int 1975;30:63–71.

67. Kofler M, Kronenberg MF, Rifici C, Saltuari L, Bauer G. Epileptic seizures associated with intrathecal baclofen application. Neurology 1994; 44:25–7.

68. Krach LE. Pharmacotherapy of spasticity: Oral medications and intrathecal baclofen. J Child Neurol 2001;16:31–36.

69. Kroin JS. Intrathecal drug administration, present use and future trends. Clin Pharmacokinet 1992;22:319–26.

70. Kroin JS, Ali A, York M, Penn RD. The distribution of medication along the spinal cord after chronic intrathecal administration. Neurosurgery 1993;33:226–30.

71. Massagli TL. Spasticity and its management in children. Phys Med Rehabil Clin N Am 1991;2:867–89.

72. Meythaler JM, Guin-Renfroe S, Law C, Grabb P, Hadley MN. Continuously infused intrathecal baclofen over 12 months for spastic hypertonia in adolescents and adults with cerebral palsy. Arch Phys Med Rehabil 2001;82:155–61.

73. Meythaler JM, Guin-Renfroe S, Grabb P, Hadley MN. Long-term continuously infused intrathecal baclofen for spastic-dystonic hypertonia in traumatic brain injury: 1-year experience. Arch Phys Med Rehabil 1999;80:13–9.

74. Miller F. Gait analysis in cerebral palsy. In: Dormans JP, Pellegrino L, eds. Caring for the Child with Cerebral Palsy. Need publisher information, 1998:169–191.

75. Muller H, Zierski J, Dralle D. Pharmacokinetics of intrathecal baclofen in spasticity. In: Muller X, Zierski J, Penn RD, eds. Local-Spinal Therapy of Spasticity. Berlin: Springer, 1988:223–6.

76. Muller-Schwefe G, Penn RD. Physostigmine in the treatment of intrathecal baclofen overdose. Report of three cases. J Neurosurg 1989;71:273–5.

77. Nanninga JB, Frost F, Penn R. Effect of intrathecal baclofen on bladder and sphincter control. J Urol 1989;142:101–5.

78. Parise M, Garcia-Larrea L, Sindou M, Mauguiere F. Clinical use of polysynaptic flexion reflexes in the management of spasticity with intrathecal baclofen. Electroencephalogr Clin Neurophysiol 1997;105:141–8.

79. Peacock W, Straudt L. Functional outcomes following selective posterior rhizotomy in children with cerebral palsy. J Neurosurg 1991;74:380–5.

80. Penn R , Savoy SM, Corcos D, et al. Intrathecal baclofen for severe spinal spasticity. N Engl J Med 1989;320:1517–21.

81. Penn RD, Kroin JS. Intrathecal baclofen alleviates spinal cord spasticity. Lancet 1984;1:1078.

82. Price GW, Wilkins GP, Turnbull MJ, Bowery NG. Are baclofen-sensitive GABAb receptors present on primary afferent terminals of the spinal cord? Nature 1984; 307:71–4.

83. Rawlins P. Patient management of cerebral origin spasticity with intrathecal baclofen. J Neurosci Nurs 1998;30:32–46.

84. Ried S, Pellegrino L, Albinson-Scull S, Dormans JP. The management of spasticity. In: Dormans JP, Pellegrino L, eds. Caring for the Child with Cerebral Palsy. Baltimore: Brookes, 1998:99–123.

85. Rosenson AS, Ali A, Fordham EW, Penn RD. Indium-111 DTPA flow study to evaluate surgically implanted drug pump delivery system. Clin Nucl Med 1990; 15:154–6.

86. Rymer WZ, Katz RT. Mechanisms of spastic hypertonia. Phys Med Rehabil State Art Rev 1994;8:441–54.

87. Sampathkumar P, Scanlon PD, Plevak DJ. Baclofen withdrawal presenting as multi-organ system failure. J Neurosurg 1998;88:562–3.

88. Tilton A, Nadell J, Massirer B, Miller M. Intrathecal baclofen therapy for treating severe spasticity in pediatric patient with anoxic brain injury. Clinical Case Study. Medtronic Inc., Minneapolis, 1999.

89. Young RR, Delwaide PJ. Drug therapy spasticity (first of two parts). N Engl J Med 1981;304(1):28–33.

90. Young RR, Delwaide PJ. Drug therapy spasticity (second of two parts). New Engl J Med 1981;304(2):96–9.

Index

Springer

Printed in Singapore